To my parents and beautiful wife and children

Pacing
Individual Strategies for Optimal Performance

Kevin G. Thompson, PhD

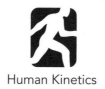

Human Kinetics

Thompson, Kevin G., 1966-
  Pacing : individual strategies for optimal performance / Kevin G. Thompson, PhD.
    pages cm
  Includes bibliographical references and index.
  1. Sports--Physiological aspects. 2. Sports--Psychological aspects. 3. Cardiac pacing. I. Title.
  RC1235.T57 2014
  613.7'1--dc23
                                    2014013036

ISBN (print): 978-1-4504-2123-2

The web addresses cited in this text were current as of April 2014, unless otherwise noted.

Acquisitions Editor: Tom Heine; **Developmental Editor:** Carla Zych; **Managing Editor:** Tyler M. Wolpert; **Copyeditor:** Patsy Fortney; **Indexer:** Alisha Jeddeloh; **Permissions Manager:** Martha Gullo; **Graphic Designer:** Nancy Rasmus; **Graphic Artist:** Tara Welsch; **Cover Designer:** Keith Blomberg; **Photograph (cover):** Swimmer: Christophe Schmid/Fotolia; Speed Skater and Rower: Photodisc; Bicyclists: © Human Kinetics; **Photo Asset Manager:** Laura Fitch; **Photo Production Manager:** Jason Allen; **Art Manager:** Kelly Hendren; **Associate Art Manager:** Alan L. Wilborn; **Illustrations:** © Human Kinetics, unless otherwise noted; **Printer:** Sheridan Books

Human Kinetics books are available at special discounts for bulk purchase. Special editions or book excerpts can also be created to specification. For details, contact the Special Sales Manager at Human Kinetics.

Printed in the United States of America   10 9 8 7 6 5 4 3 2 1

The paper in this book is certified under a sustainable forestry program.

Human Kinetics
Website: www.HumanKinetics.com

United States: Human Kinetics
P.O. Box 5076
Champaign, IL 61825-5076
800-747-4457
e-mail: humank@hkusa.com

Canada: Human Kinetics
475 Devonshire Road Unit 100
Windsor, ON N8Y 2L5
800-465-7301 (in Canada only)
e-mail: info@hkcanada.com

Europe: Human Kinetics
107 Bradford Road
Stanningley
Leeds LS28 6AT, United Kingdom
+44 (0) 113 255 5665
e-mail: hk@hkeurope.com

Australia: Human Kinetics
57A Price Avenue
Lower Mitcham, South Australia 5062
08 8372 0999
e-mail: info@hkaustralia.com

New Zealand: Human Kinetics
P.O. Box 80
Torrens Park, South Australia 5062
0800 222 062
e-mail: info@hknewzealand.com

E5602

contents

Modern day coaches and sports scientists combine their collective expertise to plan training, monitor responses, analyse technique, and optimize arousal for best competitive performance. On the other hand, less of this kind of collective expertise is applied to the specific tactics that their charges employ on race day. This book may well change that trend, because Kevin Thompson and a specially selected group of practically minded scholars demonstrate how scientists and coaches may develop closer relationships at the business end of performance; and share practical and scientific knowledge to enhance tactical awareness and planning.

Most of us have witnessed athletes, and unfortunately sometimes our own, making a mess of their competition performance because of poor tactics. This book focusses on methods of judging effort or pace throughout the performance to achieve the desired outcome and it does so in a most comprehensive and effective manner, combining case studies and experiences of internationally successful athletes with scientific studies

The authors tackle many questions that coaches deliberate, even agonize over, leading up to important competitions. Uncertainty prevails even in the elite echelons of sport, and even in the best coaches. On the other hand, coaches themselves have made great inroads into methods of improving human athletic performance; these inroads are usually derived from personal experience, from their own trial and error in the big arenas. Scientists too have made their contributions to improved human athletic performance, explaining why certain athletes achieve greatness and why novel coaching methods work. This type of contribution is important, because discovering why things work provides the framework for the refinements of methods that further enhance performance.

Understanding the mechanisms of improving athletic performance also allows coaches to work from first principles. This obviates the need to simply copy successful coaches' ideas, risky in itself because these ideas may not apply to other athletes. Pacing is a clear case in point. Athletes have always known that holding back on initial pace in all but the short sprints is likely to improve overall competition performance, but with a solid understanding of pacing, coaches and scientists can plan racing and game strategies to match individual physical and psychological profiles, their training and the environmental conditions. We are all aware that races are sometimes won and lost by milliseconds, so very small refinements in race tactics and pacing can have very large consequences. Similarly, to win games team-sport players have to carefully judge when to attack decisively and when to defend patiently.

Kevin Thompson and the other contributors to this book are scientists who have dedicated much of their scientific careers to understanding the nuances of pacing. Chances are you will be surprised by the breadth of knowledge in this area these men have compiled, much of it having emerged over the last two decades. Consider how you would answer a few of the questions tackled by our expert contributors:

What is the best way to distribute energy during a race…is it *always* best to hold back in the early stages?

If this is not always the case, when is it not the case?

Are there general rules that apply to all athletes or is pacing very much an individual thing? How do we know what sort of athlete is best suited to a particular strategy?

Can we change this characteristic in an athlete?

What is the underlying cause of fatigue that determines the optimal pacing strategy, and how does this vary in events of different durations?

Can the perception of fatigue and the impairment of muscle function be controlled or modified?

Does the practice of drafting used so regularly in cycling provide any benefit when used in other sports?

How do the wind, temperature and humidity affect pacing strategies?

Not all that straightforward, is it? For coaches whose pre-race comments are confined to standard reminders to "Be careful to sit at the back of the pack running into the wind" or "Don't go too hard in the first lap," this book will be an eye-opener, providing a new perspective on pacing. A new coaching perspective can lead to new breakthrough in an athlete's performance, reward and satisfaction for all, and isn't that what competitive sport is all about?

Professor Richard D. Telford, AM, PhD, FACSM, FSMA

Pacing in sport is critical for reaching an end point, the finish, in the shortest possible time or ahead of the competition. In many sports, the objective is to outscore the competition; in those sports pacing is often used tactically to score at the right time, when chances of success are most likely. Therefore, in virtually every type of athletic endeavour, pacing is a prerequisite for success. Athletes must maintain enough metabolic capacity to avoid fatiguing before the end of the event, and so a pacing strategy is required.

The pacing strategy for any event depends on the sport, the environment, the equipment and the athlete's psychological and physiological characteristics. The brain plays a key role as it processes complex internal and external information and establishes, maintains and adapts the pacing strategy during training practices and competition. The brain calculates the distance remaining against the current rate of energy production and usage, the energy reserves left and developing fatigue. It then decides the level of force production possible to reach the finish and activates the muscles accordingly. But is it fallible? The answer is clearly a resounding yes! Marathon runners and Ironman participants are acutely aware of the consequences of a pacing strategy that goes wrong, because it can lead to a catastrophic deterioration in race speed and even collapse. Such a collapse can be due to a medical condition that manifests only under an extreme exercise challenge or because of insufficient energy levels, overheating or dehydration. However, we must also acknowledge the strong psychological drive that pushes some competitors beyond their optimal pacing strategy (St Clair Gibson et al. 2013). Why this happens, even in well-trained and experienced athletes, is a complex question, but the fact that it does demonstrates that pacing is a critical skill with the potential to make or break sport performance.

This book describes the history, nature, role and use of pacing in athletic events. This book is written for coaches, athletes and readers with a general interest in sport, as well as those studying sport-related subjects or who might be starting to research the science of pacing in sport. Part I explores the history, nature and role of pacing and explains what is known about the mechanisms that control pacing, from both a physiological and a psychological perspective. These chapters draw on the evidence base developed from scientific studies to describe and explain how athletes set, regulate and execute their pacing strategies during competition. The final chapter of part I builds on the understanding of the mechanisms that regulate exercise and underpin the athlete's selected pacing strategy, by discussing pacing strategies that might optimise athletic performance.

Part II addresses pacing in relation to a wide variety of sports. Included are chapters on the time-dependent sports of swimming, cycling, speed skating, running, triathlon and rowing, in which the application and importance of pacing is most obvious. However, also included are chapters on racket sports (tennis and squash) and several team-based sports (Association football, Australian Rules football, rugby, and basketball), in which the application and importance of pacing may be less apparent. Interviews with world-class athletes and coaches accompany many of the sport chapters. These anecdotal reports give real-life views of and insights into how pacing affects athletes' preparations. The athlete and coach accounts help to marry current sport practice with the sport science research on pacing. These chapters demonstrate that an understanding of pacing is critical in most, if not all, sports.

Athletes need to be able to recognise when the pacing strategy is not working during a competition and to adjust it accordingly. Especially when the stakes are high and the distractions are plentiful, they may be so excited that they forget or fail to execute the pacing strategy they have planned and practised in training. It takes a special athlete to execute an optimal pacing strategy during the very highest levels of competition, such as the Olympic Games or a major championship final, when emotions are hard to control.

A famous, and perhaps unexpected, example of an athlete reading the situation and implementing a deliberate pacing strategy in a crucial contest can be found in one of the most celebrated fights in boxing history—the 1974 Rumble in the Jungle between George Foreman and Muhammad Ali for the world heavyweight boxing championship. Insiders later said that Foreman and his handlers had actually prayed in the dressing room before the fight for Foreman not to kill Ali, so high was the expectation that Foreman was too strong for him. From the beginning of the bout, Foreman was highly motivated and aggressive, hurting Ali and pinning him against the ropes in the early rounds. It was then that Ali made a fight-winning, pacing-based decision.

'I didn't really plan what happened that night', Ali said. 'But when a fighter gets in the ring, he has to adjust according to the conditions he faces. Against George, the ring was slow. Dancing all night, my legs would have got tired. And George was following me too close, cutting off the ring. In the first round, I used more energy staying away from him than he used chasing me. So between rounds, I decided to do what I did in training when I got tired.' Ali covered up and stayed on the ropes for long periods, much to the dismay of his trainer, who feared he would be hurt. But Ali managed to survive the tirade of punches, and by round 7, Foreman was visibly fatiguing. In round 8, Ali was able to land a final combination of punches to knock out the exhausted Foreman.

The importance of pacing has been acknowledged for thousands of years, as Aesop's fable of the tortoise and the hare illustrates. The hare's victory was captured in the phrase 'Don't brag about your lightning pace, for slow and steady won the race!' The need to pace physical activity has been evident throughout human history. Early humans made critical decisions about how long and how far to persist with a hunt and whether to target a fast animal or a tired and weak one who might be less able to escape. The phrase that armies 'walk on their stomachs' conveys a clear recognition that managing energy resources is a proven historical prerequisite for success. Generals who paced the march to battle appropriately and managed their food and water supplies well brought strong, energetic troops into battle, where they often triumphed over their weary, underfed opponents.

In more modern times, the need for pacing permeates most facets of our lives. Parents and teachers teach children how to regulate their academic and extracurricular activities with appropriate pacing strategies. An aspiration of many young and middle-aged adults is to achieve the prized work–life balance, which relates in part to pacing their activities both inside and outside the workplace. Even an elderly person's weekly shopping trip can be an object lesson in pacing—energy levels, current health and fitness, the load of the shopping bags, the availability of rest stops, the transportation options and weather conditions must be calculated when deciding whether to venture out.

Perhaps surprisingly, given the historic significance of pacing and the common application of pacing strategies in sport coaching, widespread scientific interest in pacing did not develop until the early 1990s, although pacing-related studies had been sporadically conducted well before then. As described in chapter 3, as far back as 1898, Dr Norman Triplett of Indiana University wrote an enlightening manuscript discussing aspects of pacing during cycling races from a scientific perspective. However, many of the ideas and theories he put forward have been challenged and investigated in earnest only over the past 25 years.

It is fitting that chapter 1, which describes the fundamental need for pacing during exercise from a historical and contemporary perspective, was written by Professor Carl Foster and Dr Jos de Koning (with assistance from colleagues at the University of Wisconsin at La Crosse, USA; VU University, Amsterdam, Netherlands; and the University of Applied Sciences, Bochum, Germany), as these two scientists and their co-workers have blazed the trail that many of us are now following. Indeed, the research papers published in 1993 and 1994 by Professor Foster and his colleagues have galvanised a generation of sport scientists to undertake research in this area. Chapter 2 defines and examines the pacing strategies that are commonly observed in sport, including the all-out pacing strategy in 100 m sprinting in track and field, positive pacing evident in 1 km cycling and 100 m swimming events, and parabolic pacing often observed in the sport of rowing. Chapters 3 and 4 follow with an overview of the physiology of pacing and the psychology of pacing, respectively, laying out what we now know about the mechanisms that control pacing as well as the limitations of our current understanding. Chapter 5 brings this information together to outline how pacing strategies might be manipulated through various training and other interventions and what factors coaches and athletes should consider when planning pacing strategies

Possessing a clear understanding of pacing strategies that optimise performance seems fundamental if coaches are to train athletes appropriately for their particular athletic events. Focusing only on the overall performance outcome when improvement is noted does not inform the coach or athlete as to which aspect of the performance improved or how to ensure that it is sustained. Relevant questions abound: Did the athlete improve the start, midportion and end portion of the race or just one of these elements? How and why did the improvement occur? Was it due to technical improvements, fitness improvements or a combination of the two? Was the athlete psychologically better able to compete?

Research into the psychological aspects of pacing is yielding a number of surprising and useful findings that are explored in this book. Interestingly, when you ask elite athletes to complete a maximal time trial or a graded step test to exhaustion and then to report their perceived exertion, they typically do not describe the effort at the end of the trial as maximal. Why? Well, it might be that they want to believe that they have something left in reserve at the end, to feel more confident. Alternatively, perhaps the brain has actually ensured that they do have something left in reserve—and perhaps they are consciously aware of it. A cleverly designed 2012 study by Stone and colleagues, described in detail in chapter 5, examined whether athletes maintain an energy reserve to draw from only under extreme circumstances and whether their impressions of how much energy they have left are accurate.

Clearly, there is a psychological component to pacing. It's possible that humans do keep something in reserve, even when attempting to exercise maximally. This mechanism might be subconscious, operating without the athlete's being aware of it. Can elite athletes, through repeatedly exercising at a high intensity during training, learn how to delve into this reserve, if it exists? Similarly, should the coach, having determined how best to pace a particular race distance, devise a pacing profile that gives the athlete a greater chance of dipping into this reserve? Perhaps it is true that the more we learn about pacing, the better armed we are to push the boundaries of human performance. It is also true that the physical and psychological underpinnings of pacing are complex.

A significant debate among exercise physiologists in the last 10 years or so has been whether the brain dictates the pacing strategy to avoid a catastrophic failure in a physiological system that would be detrimental to exercise performance or health. This is thought to be related to the body's drive to maintain a constant internal environment known as homeostasis through the regulation of a number of fundamental physiological processes. Sport science researchers are investigating whether the brain might limit how much the athlete's physiology can be perturbed during exercise by adjusting muscle activation to maintain a safe level of performance. There is supporting evidence for this theory in short- to long-term endurance events; however, evidence is less compelling for short events lasting only a few seconds to a few minutes. This book examines the evidence that is unfolding in these areas and others as well as the questions that arise from the evidence.

During exercise, the brain, through the sensory nervous system, processes massive amounts of complex information about what is happening inside the body and external to it (e.g., competitors' pace, wind conditions, air temperature, changing landscape, crowd support). How this information is interpreted to inform the athlete and determine the athlete's pace is not well understood at present; however, sport scientists are looking into this and attempting to shed light on how to develop optimal race pacing strategies and match play tactics.

A related aspect that researchers are exploring is the effect of physical training itself. When you are naive about the race distance, the brain will make a best guess, which might be conservative; if you are highly motivated, it might be overly ambitious! Simply by training, the athlete continually exposes the body's sensory nervous system to stimuli that relay feedback to the brain. By practising racing pace in training, is it possible that athletes not only adapt in terms of changes to their muscle structure and metabolism, but also train the brain to calculate a more successful pacing template? This concept, first described by Ulmer (1996) and known as *teleoanticipation*, is the fundamental tenet of pacing theory. Related questions include how this process might work and how coaches and athletes can take advantage of it.

Part II of this book describes pacing templates and strategies that have been observed across a number of sports. Recent technological advances allow the measurement and recording of an athlete's profile in terms of speed, accelerations, distance travelled, power output and physiological response in actual competitive situations—often in real time. These advances are transforming our understanding of sport performance and sport tactics. By combining these descriptive models of pacing from sporting events with research findings about the physical mechanisms that control pacing, sport scientists are beginning to understand how to optimise pacing to maximise sport performance. This understanding is informing the training practices, competition tactics and pacing strategies of coaches and their athletes. *Pacing: Individual Strategies for Optimal Performance* offers a current, comprehensive review of the science of pacing and its potential applications in various athletic pursuits.

acknowledgments

In writing this book I have been privileged to be able to collaborate with leading sports science researchers, world class coaches and athletes, and talented PhD candidates. I would like to acknowledge the support and wisdom of Professor Carl Foster, Dr Jos J. de Koning, Dr Richard Keegan and Professor Richard "Dick" Telford AM and thank them for writing such well-crafted sections for this book. I need to especially thank Dr Louise Turner for her support in the production of a number of the figures for this book. I also need to thank a number of researchers who contributed ideas and informed my understanding of pacing and were a source of inspiration for this book. These scholars of sport science and exercise regulation (pacing) are: Professor Alan St Clair Gibson, Professor Andrew M. Jones, Professor John S. (Jack) Raglin, Dr Dominic Micklewright, Dr Les Ansley and Dr Duncan French. Can I also thank Dr Richard Akenhead, Dr Thomas Gee, Jocelyn Mara, Graham Mytton, Dr Mark Stone and Dr Kevin Thomas whose PhD work related to pacing greatly informed this book, it has been a pleasure being part of your PhD supervisory committees.

So far, during my career in high performance sport and higher education, I have been fortunate to work alongside many truly inspirational world-class coaches and athletes and long may that continue! Although time and circumstance (moving from the UK to Australia!) did not allow me to interview as many of these amazing people as I would have liked for this book, I am so pleased that a good number were able to give up some of their precious time to provide their fascinating thoughts about pacing. I believe their insight adds significant depth and validity to the chapters. Many, many thanks to: Ben Bright (triathlon), Chris Cook (swimming), Peter Elliott (athletics), Carrie Graf (basketball), Nick Matthew and Chris Robertson (squash), Paul Manning and Shane Sutton (cycling), Paul Thompson (rowing) and Joe Roff and Jake White (rugby union).

Finally I want to thank the Human Kinetics editorial team for their passion and support for *Pacing: Individual Strategies for Optimal Performance*. I am very grateful to Karalynn Thomson, Tom Heine, Carla Zych, Martha Gullo and Tyler Wolpert—your help has been invaluable in producing this book. Many thanks to you all!

part I

Pacing Science and Philosophy

chapter 1

What Is Pacing?

Carl Foster and Jos de Koning with Arjan Bakkum, Sil Kloppenburg, John P. Porcari, Annabelle Splinter, Christian Thiel and Joyce van Tunen

Pacing is the distribution of energy use during exercise. The goal of pacing, which is almost certainly a fundamental quality of exercise, is to achieve the desired outcome without fatigue interfering with the completion of the task or with the person's basic health. The roots of pacing go back to early human history, to our days as hunter-gatherers. In our niche as persistence hunters, we had to make decisions about whether the energetic cost of running a game animal until it died of heat exhaustion was worth the effort expended (Cordain et al. 1998; Eaton, Konner & Shostak 1988; Studdel-Numbers & Wall-Schieffler 2009). This sense of pacing followed humans as our species spread over the world: Migrant groups had to ensure that they didn't deplete their resources on a migration, and armies had to avoid exhausting themselves before getting to the battle.

Although there was some early scientific interest in pacing (Adams & Bernauer 1968; Leger & Ferguson 1974; Robinson et al. 1958), contemporary interest in pacing began in the 1990s (de Koning et al. 1999; Foster et al. 1993, 1994; Ulmer 1996; van Ingen Schenau, de Koning & de Groot 1992). When these lines of research converged with research exploring the central regulation of exercise performance (Ansley, Robson & St Clair Gibson 2004; Lambert, St Clair Gibson & Noakes 2005; Noakes, St Clair Gibson & Lambert 2004, St Clair Gibson & Noakes 2004), the contemporary study of pacing began. For more interested readers, excellent contemporary reviews are available (Abbis & Laursen 2008; Foster, de Koning et al. 2012; Roelands et al. 2013; St Clair Gibson & Foster 2007; St Clair Gibson et al. 2006, 2013; Tucker & Noakes 2009).

In athletics, pacing means controlling the intensity of effort early in a competition so you don't develop such profound fatigue that the overall performance is destroyed, or fall so far behind your competitors (or your pre-race goal) that success can't be attained with an end spurt. The most obvious example to anyone who has ever tried to run a marathon is the process of 'hitting the wall', in which the muscle glycogen or blood glucose level (or both) become critically low before the finish, resulting in an enormous decrease in pace. Indeed, winning or losing a marathon, or achieving a target time, is as much about avoiding hitting the wall as it is about maximal aerobic speed (Foster, Porcari et al. 2012; Karlsson & Saltin 1971). Other clear examples are athletes who are literally staggering during the finishing portion of the race, which is indicative of the massive changes of metabolite concentrations in the muscle during heavy exercise (Jones et al. 2008; Karlsson & Saltin 1970; Skibba et al. 2012; St Clair Gibson et al. 2013), and teams that perform poorly in the closing part of a season because they run out of gas or go stale. Conversely, pacing mistakes can happen in the other direction, when athletes leave too much in reserve at the end of a race that even with a big kick they cannot get to the front of the race by the finish. These athletes cross the line with too much energy left in the tank as a result of a misjudgement of pace during the race.

Pacing is usually thought of in the context of a single competitive event, as in the case of a competitor who works too hard too early and collapses near the finish line, or one who launches an effort too late and finishes very strongly, albeit behind the winner. However, long-term pacing plays a role in many athletic endeavours. Evidence of pacing can be seen in the process of multiday competitions, such as the Grand Tours of cycling, in which competitors pick days in which to increase their effort, but must reduce their efforts on other days to make it through the event (Foster et al. 2005). There is also the concept of seasonal pacing, in which athletes with long competitive seasons seek to achieve a critical balance among competition, training and recovery so they have the physical and emotional reserves to produce their best performances at the critical portion of the season. Athletes who compete or train too hard too early in a season (or tournament) and don't use recovery days to really recover are often exhausted during the championship portion of the season.

When pacing is done right, it is virtually invisible, both to the athlete using it and to those watching the athlete. It represents the natural extension of how the race should be run or how the season should be managed. This simplicity of gauging effort was brilliantly expressed in the concept of teleoanticipation (Ulmer 1996), which suggests that athletes must know where the finish line is and regulate their effort over the course of the entire race from the perspective of the finish line. There is wide experimental support for this concept (Amann et al. 2006, 2008; de Koning et al. 2011a, 2011b; Joseph et al. 2008; Tucker & Noakes 2009), which has been expressed in the concept of exercising with reserve (Swart et al. 2009a, 2009b). Further, although external motivators such as money (Hulleman et al. 2007) and other competitors (Bath et al. 2011) can influence the overall performance level, only rarely (Thiel et al. 2012) does the basic pacing strategy change. Indeed, evidence suggests that the overall pacing strategy is robust enough to remain intact despite deliberate manipulation of the distance completed (Mauger, Jones & Williams 2011).

A reasonable body of evidence indicates that pacing is a learned process, and that a variety of elements, including conscious decisions, prior competitive experience and race simulations performed as part of training, contribute to developing a sense of pace that is appropriate to optimise performance (Corbett, Barwood & Parkhouse 2009; Foster et al. 2009; Micklewright et al. 2010). When pacing becomes obvious, it usually means that there were pacing mistakes, which provide the dramatic examples that we all think of when we think of the term *pacing*. Pacing can also be a powerful competitive tool, allowing athletes to disrupt the performance of their competitors and achieve victory (Thiel et al. 2012). Although the term *pacing* is most specifically used to describe the energy expenditure during an event or season, the difference between using pacing to achieve an optimal performance and using it to disrupt the pacing strategy of competitors is very small. Indeed, the concept of an athlete purposely making a pacing 'mistake' in the middle of an event by deliberately going at a pace that the athlete knows is not sustainable, merely to disrupt the race plan of other competitors, is one of the most interesting aspects of sport. Lastly, to improve performance, at least in events in which success is time based (versus determined by merely finishing in front of other competitors), the athlete must take a calculated risk. If the pace is too much faster than the athlete has achieved before (i.e., the calculated risk is too large), then the failure could be just as obvious and abject as the success could be glorious.

Pacing, even perfectly executed pacing, will not make a champion out of an ordinary athlete. Pacing is clearly much less important than talent, and less important than careful and adequate training, but it is crucial in optimising performance. Correct pacing is the secret to feeling that you are 'on top of the race' or 'getting the best out of yourself' versus having a 'competitive disaster'. Every athlete, from the elite competitor chasing a world record or Olympic victory all the way down to the club runner trying to collect one more T-shirt by completing the event, knows this feeling. There is good evidence that pacing can be learned (Foster et al. 2009), can be practised and can have a profound impact on performance.

In the remainder of this chapter, we examine some examples in which pacing has had a profound impact on the history of sport. Then we talk about how pacing is practised in various events. Lastly, we present some experimental examples of responses to manipulations of pacing and peer into the unexplored aspects of pacing. Because it is every coach's dream to be ahead of the competition, we offer a glimpse of the direction in which the science of pacing will develop in the coming years.

Pacing in the History of Sport

One of the best early examples of the importance of pacing in sport occurred during the 1908 Olympics in London. Italian runner Dorando Pietri took the lead early in the marathon race and was first into the stadium with a time of 2:54:46. However, he was clearly in trouble as he entered the stadium; he turned the wrong way onto the track, collapsed several times and ultimately had to be assisted across the finish line by British officials. For understandable reasons, the British officials did not want American Johnny Hayes (who was running comfortably in second place) to win the Olympic championship. Ultimately, Pietri was disqualified for 'official assistance', an outcome that, even today, makes race officials (particularly medical personnel) reluctant to assist runners who collapse. However, his collapse makes clear the concept that a competition, like an opera, is never over until the fat lady sings. Remarkably, in the absence of overt pacing mistakes, various events have clearly evident pacing profiles (see figure 1.1).

The profile for a given event seems to depend on both the distance (duration) of an event and the medium on which the event is contested (which affects the likelihood of slowing if propulsive power output is lost). In shorter events, and particularly in air-resisted events such as speed skating and track cycling, there is evidence of a more all-out strategy (high early speed with progressive deceleration; de Koning et al. 2011b; Foster et al. 2004), whereas events in more viscous media (swimming, rowing) tend to have a comparatively uniform pace (de Koning et al. 2011b). However, there is such a tactical advantage to 'being ahead of the wake' in rowing that the early pace is often the fastest of the event. Overlapping these effects is a clear tendency to produce a U-shaped pattern

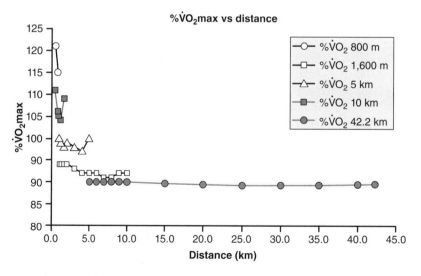

Figure 1.1   Schematic of pacing strategy in high-level athletes in running events of various durations (presented as mean $\dot{V}O_2$max percentages over distance or duration).

(faster, slower, faster) in many middle- and long-distance events (Foster, de Koning et al. 2012; Noakes, Lambert & Hauman 2009; Robertson et al. 2009; Tucker, Lambert & Noakes 2006). Normally, it is thought that power output is reduced during paced races in response to feedback-driven down-regulation of central motor output (the athlete begins to tire, and the brain reduces muscle activation to a more appropriate level to avoid prematurely fatiguing). However, in high-intensity events, true peripheral fatigue may result in a loss of power output despite a preserved or increased motor drive from the brain (Amann et al. 2008; Hettinga et al. 2006).

One candidate for the greatest distance runner of all time was Czech Emil Zatopek. He won gold (10 km) and silver (5 km) medals in 1948 in London. In 1952, in Helsinki, he won gold medals in both the 5 km and 10 km. As the Helsinki Olympic Games concluded, he entered his first marathon. For the first 15 km, he ran with Englishman Jim Peters, who was the leading marathon runner of the era and the pre-race favourite. After 15 km, Zatopek reputedly asked Peters how he thought the race was going. Apparently in an attempt to confuse Zatopek, Peters told him that the pace was too slow, even though the first 15 km had been run at a very good pace. Zatopek promptly accelerated, leaving Peters behind to ultimately fail to finish the race. Zatopek was arguably so much superior to his competitors that pacing (or lack of knowledge about pacing) simply didn't matter to him. Perhaps Zatopek had done so much running under so many circumstances (he was famous for doing intervals in his army boots and for running in place while he stood guard duty in the Czech army) and knew his body so well that pacing, even in an unfamiliar event, was simply second nature to him.

Jim Peters has another contribution to the story of pacing. He set his first marathon world record in 1952 (2:20:42), became the first person to run under 2:20 and ultimately had a lifetime best performance of 2:17:39. In 1954, he competed as a heavy favourite in the Empire Games in Vancouver. Atypical of the usually mild weather in British Columbia and the mild preparation weather experienced by Peters in the UK, the temperature at the start of the race was 28 °C (82.4 °F). Ignoring the hot conditions, which suggested a relatively easy early pace, Peters attacked the race at a near world-record pace. Late in the race he was 15 to 20 minutes ahead of his nearest competitor! However, just as he entered the stadium, he collapsed. With officials failing to intervene, lest they commit a 'Pietri offence', Peters managed to get up, but fell repeatedly and managed to cover only an additional 200 m in a span of 15 minutes before collapsing again, still short of the finish line. At this point he was taken from the track to the medical tent. Reportedly, his rectal temperature after being led to the medical tent was still 39.5 °C (103.1 °F), despite virtually not having run during the preceding 15 minutes. The race was ultimately won in 2:39, a time well within Peters' capability if only he had chosen a pacing strategy appropriate for the conditions. However, as we will see later, Peters essentially had only one pacing strategy to use in competition (full-on attack at the fastest possible speed). Perhaps he would have been better served by practising additional pacing strategies. Peters retired after this race, claiming that the brutal conditions encountered in Vancouver had 'destroyed his killer instinct'.

Two examples in which choosing the appropriate pacing strategy led to good competitive results are provided by Basil Heatley from the UK in the 1964 Olympic marathon in Tokyo and Deena Kastor from the USA in the 2004 Olympic marathon in Athens. In 1964, the undisputed best marathon runner in the world was Abebe Bikila from Ethiopia, who successfully defended his Olympic title with a world record of 2:12:11. Bikila was also the first East African to demonstrate the incredible talent and competitive ability that has led to the dominance of contemporary distance running by East Africans. Recognizing that Bikila was unassailable, Heatley chose to run conservatively during the early portion of the race, and was in eighth place at 30 km. By 40 km he had worked his way up to third place, but was 1 minute and 15 seconds behind Kokichi Tsuburaya of Japan. In the final 2 km, he closed the distance on Tsuburaya, entered the stadium in third place by 10 m and sprinted around the tiring Tsuburaya for the silver medal.

Similarly, in Athens in 2004, the undisputed best marathon runner in the world was Paula Radcliffe of the UK. Despite very hot weather (35 °C; 95 °F), and with the ability to have won a 'kickers race', Radcliffe chose to lead the first half of the race at a very strong pace (just as countryman Jim Peters had done in Vancouver in 1954), before fading from the lead and ultimately failing to finish. Given that she had injuries that had interfered with her preparation, her choice of leading the race in such hot conditions was poorly considered. Kastor, on the other hand, was not favoured for a podium finish based on her pre-Olympic performance. Respecting the heat, she barely warmed up before the race, wore a cooling vest during the warm-up and ran conservatively during the early portion of the race; she then began picking off runners who had gone out aggressively. Ultimately, she won the bronze medal in a performance better than would have been forecast for her, because she chose the right pacing strategy for the event.

Arguably the best single example of choosing, and executing, the right pacing strategy occurred at the 1968 Olympics in Mexico City, in the men's 1500 m event. American Jim Ryun was the best middle-distance runner in the world, with few defeats during the preceding four years and with world records in the 800 m, 1500 m and 1 mile. He had a remarkable last lap. Given that most of the experts were forecasting that the altitude in Mexico City would ensure that most races were likely to be 'wait and kick' strategies, everyone thought that Ryun was likely to become the Olympic champion. Although it was known that the East Africans had lived at altitude, Ryun, like most American and European athletes, had trained extensively at high altitude and was well adapted, at least in terms of the physiological adaptations that occur with altitude training. What Ryun had not done was practise his finishing kick after the challenge of a fast start at altitude. Kenya's Kipchoge Keino anticipated that the only way to challenge Ryun's finishing kick was to set a very aggressive early pace. Keino's first lap in Mexico City was 57 seconds. (Ryun's first lap in the U.S. Olympic trials had been 67 seconds!) Keino never slowed and had a 40 m lead over Ryun as the last lap began. Despite running a very strong last lap, Ryun never challenged Keino's lead.

Ryun ran the race he had prepared for; indeed, he ran better than he ever had at altitude. In conventional terms, he was faultless. However, Keino had the vision and the courage to plan and execute a race that Ryun had neither anticipated nor prepared for. Keino's time of 3:34.9 was only slightly slower than the world record (3:33.1) that Ryun had set while beating Keino the previous year and was equivalent to a 3:50.4 mile (faster than Ryun's existing world record, *despite the altitude*). Keino's effort was perhaps possible in part because of the great range that he had as a runner. In Mexico City, in addition to his performance in the 1500 m, he won the silver medal in the 5000 m and participated in the 10,000 m; and in Munich in 1972, he won a gold medal in the 3000 m steeplechase and a silver in the 1500 m. However, his most important advantage over Ryun was that he was competitively acclimatized to going out fast at high altitude, which Ryun just didn't believe was possible (Daniels & Oldridge 1970). Had Ryun had more experience with fast-start strategies at high altitude, he almost certainly would have made a close race of it. Instead, Keino used a pacing strategy that Ryun had not anticipated to earn a well-deserved victory.

There are many other examples of the right pacing strategy leading to victory. One is the come-from-behind victory in the men's 800 m at the 1972 Munich Olympics. David Wottle from the USA had the best time in the world that year, but had struggled with injuries that reduced his confidence coming into the 800 m final. Immediately after the start, he went to the back of the field, trailing the leaders by more than 10 m after only 200 m of running. At the end of the first lap, he was in last place and looked to be in no position to be competitive. With 300 m to go, he began to move through the field and was in fifth place entering the final 100 m. As the other runners began to slow, he was able to maintain his pace and won in the final steps to the finish. Atypical of the usual pattern in the 800 m (Thiel et al. 2012; Tucker, Lambert & Noakes 2006), Wottle's 400 m splits were exactly equal, demonstrating that sometimes a winning kick is in the failure to slow down, as much as in the ability to accelerate near the finish.

In winter sports, one of the best examples of how a pacing strategy *could* have led to an Olympic gold medal was provided by American speed skater Joey Cheek, in the 1500 m event in the 2002 Olympics in Salt Lake City. Cheek had already won the bronze medal in the 1000 m event and was a true sprinter (he ultimately won the 2005 World Sprint Championships and the gold medal in the 500 m event in 2006 in Torino). In Salt Lake City, the high-altitude venue favoured a fast early pace in speed skating events, because low air resistance minimises speed (power output) losses due to fatigue (de Koning et al. 2005, 2011b; Foster et al. 1994). Earlier in the competition, Jochem Uytdehaage (gold medallist in the 5000 m and 10,000 m) from the Netherlands had broken the world record. His time (1:44.57) was bettered (1:43.95) by American Derek Parra (5000 m silver medallist). Cheek was matched in the next-to-last pairing with defending Olympic champion Adne Sondral from Norway.

Cheek started very quickly; at 700 m he was 0.7 seconds ahead (~11 m) of the pace set by Parra and 1.37 seconds (~21 m) ahead of Sondral. In the third lap Cheek slowed slightly, but was still 0.44 seconds (~7 m) ahead of Parra and 1.75 seconds (~26 m) ahead of Sondral. As Cheek entered the back straight, with 300 m to go, he could be seen to be struggling, the fluidity of his technique gone. Around the last corner and into the final straight, Sondral rapidly closed the distance, passing Cheek for the bronze medal (by 0.08 second) within the last 50 m of the race. Cheek had slowed so profoundly that he lost 1.83 seconds (~27 m) to Parra during the last lap alone, despite the friendly conditions provided by the high-altitude oval in Salt Lake City. Clearly, Cheek had made a calculated risk with a pacing strategy true to his sprinter's roots, believing that he had a reasonable chance of sustaining his early speed. His strategy illustrates an essential aspect of pacing strategy: trying something that might be successful or might end in failure.

Practising Pacing

Pacing is about managing energy resources, about waging what is ultimately a losing battle against distance and fatigue and about having such an exquisite feel for the development of fatigue that you can adjust the rate of energy expenditure repeatedly during an event to allow critical levels of fatigue to occur only at the very end. With the exception of some heroic pacing failures (Dornado Pietri's or Jim Peters' disasters in London and Vancouver or Joey Cheek's effort to unseat two athletes who had beaten the world record in earlier pairs) and some brilliant applications of just the right pace for the conditions and competition (Basil Heatley, Dena Kastor, Kipchoge Keino, David Wottle), pacing is normally completely invisible. A regulatory process so exquisitely successful in so many circumstances, which allows adjustments to account for so many (often changing) variables—competition (Thiel et al. 2012), environment (Abbis et al. 2009; Crewe, Tucker & Noakes 2008; Johnson et al. 2009; Tucker et al. 2007), course (de Koning et al. 2005; Falkner, Parfitt & Eston 2008; Foster et al. 2004; Joseph et al. 2008; Padilla et al. 2000), past training and competition (Eston et al. 2007; Rauch et al 2005) and even the prospect for future competitions (Foster et al. 2005)—cannot operate at the level of a reflex. It must be learned and practised.

There are at least two ways to practise pacing. The first is in preliminary competitions or practice races. With the exception of pure sprints, almost every competitor knows that experience is critical. One of the most striking moments of our experience in the study of pacing came during the 1990-1991 speed skating season. In the middle of that year, we collected several American skaters at the Olympic Oval in Calgary, Canada, to conduct our first real test of our emerging ideas about the importance of pacing. We convinced the skaters to allow us to direct how they skated several 1500 m races, the race that is sort of the common denominator among both sprinters and all-around skaters. In some races, we asked them to skate using their normal pacing pattern: Go out fast and decelerate progressively throughout the event. In others, we asked them to go out more slowly than normal and try to prevent their normal late-race deceleration. In still others, we asked them to go out much faster than normal, almost as if they were skating 1000 m, and to try to hold on. They did what we asked, although they weren't happy about it.

The results of our tests (which today seem obvious) indicated that at high-altitude racing ovals such as the one in Calgary, skaters should go out as fast as possible (Foster et al. 1994). Although Joey Cheek was just a beginning in-line skater in North Carolina then, he essentially defined the wisdom of what became known as the Cheek strategy. However, what was more striking, and much less expected, was a comment by American skater Pat Seltsam. Pat came to us at the end of the skating season and said this:

> You know, I never really understood the 1500 m until you made me skate it in all those really stupid ways. After that, I understood the small things about how I was supposed to feel at different parts of the race. I skated several personal best performances in the last part of the season, not because I was fitter, but because I finally understood the 1500 m.

The point of Seltsam's comment is that you can't make a best performance every time you run a race. Moreover, if you run the race the same way every time, it becomes the only way you can ever run the race. However, we have noticed that most athletes tend to use the same overall strategy for every race. Granting that there are some theoretically optimal strategies (de Koning, Bobbert & Foster 1999; de Koning et al. 2005, 2011b; Noakes, Lambert & Hauman 2009; Tucker, Lambert & Noakes 2006), there may be also a reason to intentionally use suboptimal strategies under certain circumstances, such as to inform the feedback system of how it feels to use such strategies at certain parts of the race.

We suggest that losing (or performing badly) in an unimportant competition is valuable if the athlete learns something about the feel of a different way to run a race. This suggestion is implicit in the concept of the hazard score, which is the relationship between the product of the momentary rate of perceived exertion (RPE) and the percentage of a race left to complete, and the likelihood that the pace will increase or decrease (de Koning et al. 2011a). It is also implicit in the concept of the pacing landscape, which is a three-dimensional representation of the likely relative power output in relation to the length of an event and where in the event the athlete is at any given moment (de Koning, Foster & Hettinga 2011). To properly inform the underlying motor template, or plan, for each event, the athlete must understand what Pat Seltsam called the small things about how you are supposed to feel at different points in the race.

The point about having only one way to run a race is demonstrated in the experience of American runner Mary Decker Slaney in the 3000 m event at the 1984 Olympics. Prior to the Olympics, Slaney had usually run from the front because she was so dominant among American runners that the only way to run at world-class pace was to run from the front. She had succeeded in the 1983 World Championships, winning both the 1500 m and 3000 m events with very good finishing efforts. However, in the Olympics, in which the competition was tougher, she found herself running in the middle of the pack where there was lots of physical interaction among the runners. When South Africa–born Zola Budd, running for Great Britain, moved in front of Slaney after passing her near the 1600 m point, Slaney stepped on Budd's heel, went down and was out of the race. Her shock and outrage at the unfairness of being taken out of a major race by a simple accident rather than by being outrun by a superior athlete is one of the enduring images in the minds of those who follow running. However, the problem that caused her fall was predictable and could have been prevented. With the benefit of hindsight, it's simple to suggest that she and her coach should have recognized that in the Olympic final Slaney would be obligated to run in the middle of the pack, and that both practices and unimportant races should have included frequent practice of the skill of running in the middle of a pack. Even if the pace was slower than Slaney could have maintained, it would have given her experience with the congestion and potential for physical contact that she would experience in the middle of an Olympic final.

The other way to practise pacing strategies is to organise practices around pace variations, either as formal intervals or as a modern variant of the Swedish concept from the 1930s known as fartlek. Thiel and colleagues (2012) observed that during the 2008 Olympic final, the pacing pattern in most middle- and long-distance races was very stochastic, with large changes in pace from lap to lap and even within laps (see figure 1.2). Compared to the relatively even pace during world-record performances, the pacing patterns in most of the distance races in Beijing were chaotic. Wilber and Pitsiladis (2012) noted that Kenyan runners who had recently become quite dominant in distance running would occasionally do training sessions along the lines of three sets of five repetitions of 400 m, in less than 60 seconds per 400 m, with only 110 m of jogging recovery between repetitions. When originally conceived, these very fast, very short recovery intervals were not well understood in terms of the physiological training adaptations they could provoke. However, on reflection, and in light of the observations by Thiel and colleagues (2012) about the pacing at the Beijing Olympics, the so-called secret Kenyan training may just be an example of preparing for the kind of stochastic pace variations necessary in high-level competitions (Martin et al. 2012).

The concept of Kenyan intervals has been around at least since the mid-1970s, when it was recognised that both in training and in races the Kenyans ran with clear and frequent, if subtle, variations in pace. Although it is easy to focus on the physiology of Kenyan runners (which isn't remarkably different from the physiology of top European runners, according to Wilber and Pitsiladis 2012), or the early life experience with altitude (what top athlete doesn't use altitude training these days), perhaps the secret behind the success of the Kenyans and other East Africans is that they are always experimenting with pace variations, always increasing their understanding of the feeling and the consequences of the small things about how they are supposed to feel at any point in a race. The fact that most of these East Africans had run relatively long distances from early childhood, just as means of transportation to school and for family visits, offered them more opportunities to experiment with and gain insight into the world of pacing.

Based on the number of studies that have been performed, it could be concluded that scientists already know how pacing should be done and can simply tell athletes how to pace themselves in their events. However, this is not the case. Although we have more than 20 years of experience in pacing research, we are still learning about the mechanisms that regulate pacing.

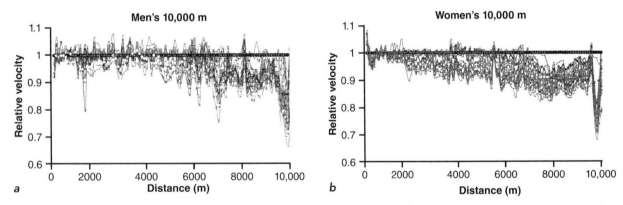

Figure 1.2 Relative pacing patterns in the Beijing Olympic 10,000 m events for (a) men and (b) women, normalized to the pace of the winning runner. The data, based on speed measurements taken every 100 m, reveal a large variability in pace throughout the event as well as a progressively slower relative pace of the non-winning runners.

Data from C. Thiel, C. Foster, W. Banzer, and J.J. de Koning, 2012, "Pacing in Olympic track races: Competitive tactics versus best performance strategy," *Journal of Sports Sciences* 30(11): 1107-1115.

Two examples of the effect of experimental manipulations of pacing strategy (probably originally performed in simplified fashion on the plains of East Africa long ago) provide a good measure of our current understanding of pacing. In the first experimental scenario, we (chapter authors) had good recreational runners run 10 km simulated races on the treadmill. In one race, they ran with a self-paced pattern, trying to improve their best practice time (studies like this always include several preliminary trials before the trial that counts to allow for the control of learning effects on how to run a race). In the other race, runners started at a velocity 5 per cent greater than in their best practice trial—a really fast start, similar to the velocity many of the runners at the Beijing Olympics were obligated to use. In addition to improving their best times, runners were competing with the goal of staying with the pace on a kilometre-by-kilometre basis. The velocity profile in the fast-start race was similar to that seen in Olympic competition (Thiel et al. 2012), with a fast start, a dramatic mid-race deceleration, establishment of a slower, 'tolerable pace' and an end spurt (see figure 1.3). The lap-to-lap variability in running pace during the fast-start race (measured by a statistical technique called the coefficient of variation, or CV) was much greater (7 per cent) than that of the self-paced race (2 per cent). In a few cases, runners improved their times, supporting the concept that pacing is a calculated risk taken with no guarantee as to the outcome. Physiological (HR and blood lactate) and perceived exertion (RPE) responses were markedly elevated early during the fast-paced run, but modulated after the mid-race pace deceleration, and they were similar to the self-paced trial over the last part of the run. These data suggest that runners know the maximal amount of internal 'disturbance' they can tolerate and regulate their pacing, and their physiology, to arrive at the finish just as they reach intolerable levels of disturbance. This supports the concept of running with reserve proposed by Swart and colleagues (2009a, 2009b).

In the second scenario, we organized 3000 m races for similar subjects on the track and recommended that the runners stay with the pack as long as possible. The pacing pattern matched that observed by Thiel and colleagues (2012). When the velocity pattern was normalized to runners who were with the pace entering the last 400 m (versus those who had let go, or dropped back earlier in the race), the velocity pattern was similar to those seen in competition. During the race, the runners who could stay with the pace demonstrated a normal growth of RPE, whereas those who had to let go during the mid-race period demonstrated an accelerated RPE during the first part of the race, which normalized after they reduced their pace. This led to an increased hazard score early in the race in the runners who had to let go (figure 1.4). It also led to a faster and larger value for the summated hazard score, which we thought might better represent the overall effect of running a fast pace early. The accumulated hazard score seemed to predict a smaller end spurt. Despite the strong effect of the hazard score on the behaviour of pace in groups of runners, the individual behaviour of the hazard score was much better at predicting the end spurt occurring late in the race than it was at predicting the mid-race decrease in pace. On the basis of these data, there does not seem to be a unique value of hazard score that predicts the tendency to let go in a race particularly well.

Put simply, The summated hazard score grew more rapidly in the group that was required to drop off the pace, suggesting that the accumulation of fatigue, perhaps more than the momentary hazard score, contributed to the need for runners to drop off. Thus, it appears that although the hazard score remains a theoretically viable concept, it works better for explaining group data than for explaining individual behaviour. Further work is necessary to determine whether the distance scaling of the hazard score should be different (e.g. non-linear). Everyday wisdom in the running community (e.g., that a marathon is half done at the 20-mile mark, or at 75 per cent of the distance completed) suggests that non-linear distance scaling is conceptually valid. However, to date we do not have data indicating what the dimensions of the scaling might be.

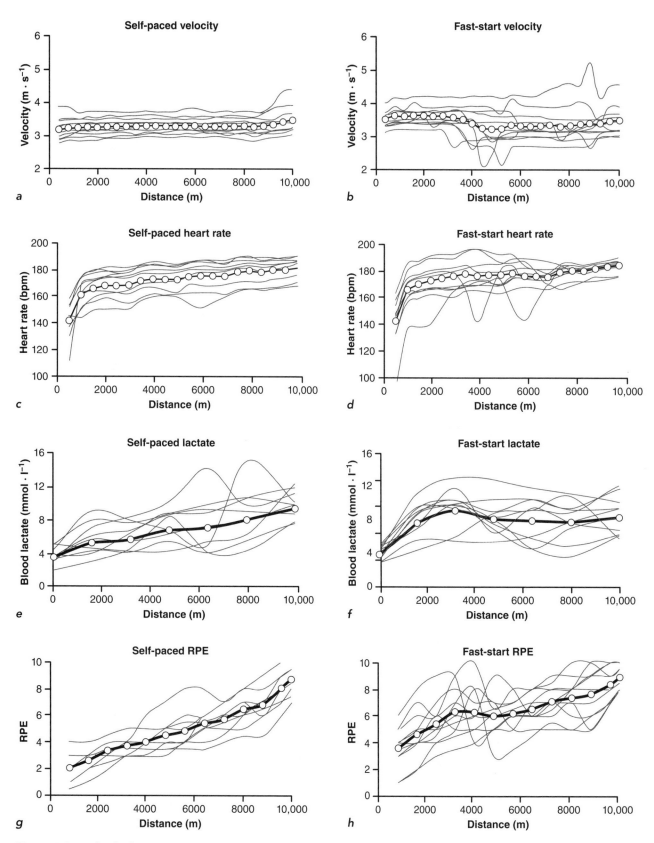

Figure 1.3 Individual responses (heavy line) and mean responses during a self-paced 10 km simulated race on the treadmill (left column) versus results from a race with a faster starting pace (right column). Remarkably, the terminal responses were very similar in both trials, suggesting that the subjects were regulating the degree of homeostatic disturbance to a common level.

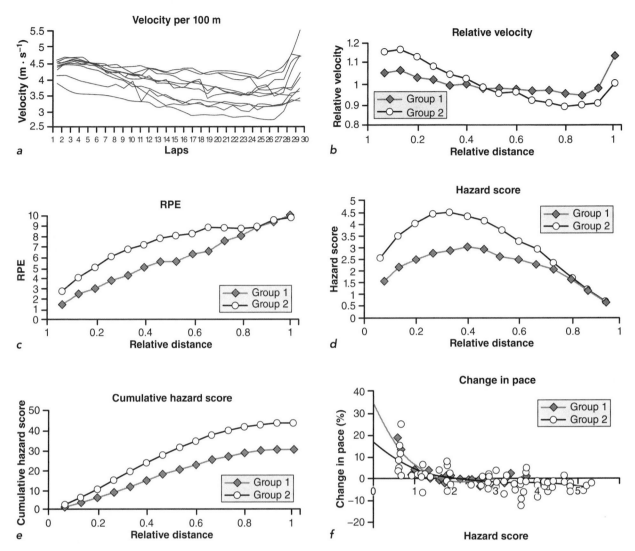

Figure 1.4 Changes in individual pace in each lap of a 3000 m race in which the subjects were instructed to stay with the pacemaker as long as possible, as in high-level competition. Despite the progressive drop off of runners from the front of the pack as the race progressed, all runners demonstrated an end spurt during the last part of the race. Runners who dropped off the pace started relatively faster, but had a progressive deceleration through the body of the race and a relatively smaller end spurt.

Conclusion

Pacing is about the distribution of energy within an event, about how you balance the available energetic resources from aerobic and anaerobic metabolism against time, distance, fatigue and the strategy and tactics of your opponent. Among relatively equally matched competitors, pacing strategy can be the difference in competitive results. For individuals, pacing is about taking reasonable calculated risks of performing better than previously. The importance of pacing is amply illustrated in the rich history of sport. There is good evidence that pacing is learned, either through the creative use of practice races or unimportant competitions, or through the structuring of practice to account for elements of pacing strategy. Ultimately, pacing can be thought of as the feel of competition, a quality that separates the feeling of being on top of the race or having the race under control, from the feeling of being forced to run your opponent's race.

chapter 2

Understanding Pacing Strategies

This chapter introduces the pacing strategies that have been observed across many sports. More detailed and specific descriptions of real-world pacing strategies in selected sports are provided in the sport-specific chapters in part II of this book. The aim of this chapter is to provide a brief overview of the types of pacing strategies and the terms used to refer to them. These general terms can be used to describe pacing strategies across sports from 100 m track sprinting to a soccer match, although for the sake of simplicity the focus of this chapter is on individual rather than team performance.

A key aim of any pacing strategy is to maximise the use of the body's energy stores, whether using energy at a maximal rate, such as when sprinting, or at a submaximal rate, such as when competing in an endurance event. The challenge for the athlete is to develop a pacing strategy that marshals the body's limited energy resources so that the competitive performance is as close to maximal as possible.

Let's look at the example of a competitive cyclist. At the start of a race, the cyclist uses chemical energy derived from the energy stores in the muscles to power the muscle contractions that accelerate the bike towards racing speed. In this scenario, the chemical energy has been converted to what is known as kinetic energy, or the energy an object possesses when it is moving. If the rider manages to ride at an even pace over the remaining race distance, the kinetic energy will be maintained. However, if the rider applies the brakes and loses speed, kinetic energy is lost; alternatively, if the rider accelerates, kinetic energy is gained. On a level racing surface, the rider can maintain a constant speed with proportionately little extra work. Movement is never completely efficient, however, and the rider loses energy through metabolic heat energy production, air resistance, mechanical friction and rolling resistance. Furthermore, the rider inevitably loses kinetic energy and slows down unless additional muscle contractions occur. Of course, these additional contractions require the conversion of more chemical energy, and the continuing conversion eventually depletes the muscles' energy stores. Therefore, the speed that is possible during a race is limited by the rate at which chemical energy can be produced, which in turn depends on which energy pathways (anaerobic or aerobic) are used and also on how much chemical energy can be produced from the body's energy stores and from food taken in during the exercise. This will be addressed in more detail later. Other limiting factors are the side effects of these chemical reactions, such as the creation of waste products and the development of associated heat production, which can also lead to fatigue. In hot environments the production of large amounts of internal heat over a prolonged period can lead to a need to slow down to avoid developing a dangerously high internal temperature or to alleviate considerable discomfort. To conclude, many processes interact during the course of a race and affect the pacing strategy. The sections that follow describe the basic pacing strategies commonly observed in races and explain some of the physiological and biomechanical processes behind them.

Basic Pacing Strategies

Pacing strategies are important because they determine how athletes expend their energy reserves to maximise their performance while minimising the kinetic energy remaining at the finish line. It has been suggested that energy reserves, particularly the anaerobic energy reserve (or capacity), should be fully expended by the end of a race. However, the pacing strategy used to get to that point is critical because expending too much energy too far from the finish line results in a poor performance (Foster et al. 2012). Table 2.1 outlines the six main pacing strategies used in sport.

All-Out Pacing

The all-out pacing strategy is observed in short events in which athletes work at their maximal rate from the start of the event and rapidly fatigue as a result. Once at their peak speed, athletes attempt to maintain that speed and subsequently their kinetic energy by exercising maximally until the end of the event. All-out pacing often results in a negative-split outcome because the majority of the event is spent accelerating from rest to the peak speed; as a result, the second half of the event is typically completed in less time than the first. For example, in the 100 m event in running, the acceleration phase can actually take up to 55 per cent of the race distance. As a result, the race appears to be negatively split because speed is built up over the first half of the race and then largely maintained during the second half of the race. As an interesting aside, the men's 200 m sprint is often run at a slightly higher average speed than the 100 m event because the acceleration phase of the 200 m is proportionately less than that of the 100 m event!

Races that demonstrate an all-out pacing strategy might last for 20 to 30 seconds in some sports and up to 60 seconds in others. This depends on whether the sport is water resisted or air resisted and the type of locomotion involved. The short duration of all-out

Table 2.1 Pacing Strategies Commonly Used in Sport

Pacing strategy	Description
All-out pacing	The athlete works maximally throughout the event.
Positive pacing	The athlete undertakes a fast start, which is not maximal but is at a high enough intensity that the athlete slows down as a result of developing fatigue over the course of the event.
Even pacing	The athlete evenly distributes work across the event. In reality, of course, there must be an initial acceleration phase to get up to racing speed; but thereafter the speed remains relatively constant until the end of the event.
Negative pacing	The athlete starts slowly but then speeds up over the course of the event.
Parabolic pacing	The athlete starts fast, slows down for a period in the middle portion of the event and increases speed towards the end of the event.
Variable pacing	The athlete increases and decreases the pace several times throughout the event. Changes in pace are related to external factors such as the topography of the course and the tactics of other competitors.

pacing events means that the initial start and acceleration phase also have a significant effect on the outcome of the race. Simply developing the body's kinetic energy from rest constitutes a significant part of the overall work (25 to 30 per cent), and the period of acceleration can also take up a significant proportion of the race. The theory is that because the initial acceleration period is proportionately greater in short-distance events than it is in middle- or long-distance events, performance is probably maximised in short-distance races by reaching a terminal speed well before the end of the race and then attempting to maintain it (usually unsuccessfully because fatigue inexorably develops). By doing so, it is thought that the sprint athlete ensures that little kinetic energy remains at the finish of the race and so is not wasted. In general, successful sprinters reach their peak speed as soon as possible and then attempt to maintain it for as long as possible.

In short-duration cycling and speed skating events, an all-out strategy is particularly important because, having achieved their terminal speed, the athletes can maintain a speed close to their peak despite their power output decreasing (see figure 2.1). In 1000 m track cycling, which takes approximately 60 seconds to complete, the riders' mechanical power output can fall off dramatically while their speed falls only by a small amount (Abbiss & Laursen 2008). This is because relatively little mechanical power output is required to maintain the terminal speed compared to when accelerating towards it. Therefore, in an event like this, it is critical to achieve the maximal speed in the shortest possible time because a large proportion of that speed can be maintained even with a reduced power output thereafter. Somewhat analogous to this is a car accelerating to cruising speed: It uses more fuel when accelerating from rest than when at the cruising speed; and of course, the greater the mass and initial acceleration of the car, the greater the rate of fuel use.

However, in sports such as swimming and running, an all-out strategy lasting beyond 30 seconds would be less effective, because the deterioration in speed would become too great and result in a suboptimal overall performance. In swimming, the properties

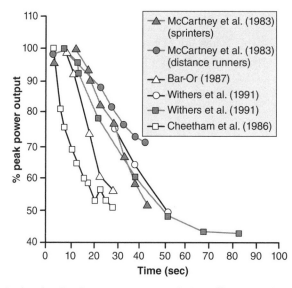

Figure 2.1 A typical reduction in power output during all-out running and cycling exercise. McCartney and colleagues' (1983), Bar-Or's (1987) and Withers and colleagues' (1991) data points relate to cycling exercise. Cheetham and colleagues' (1986) data points relate to sprinting.

With kind permission of Springer Science + Business Media: *Sports Medicine*, "Pacing strategy and athletic performance," 17(2), 1994, pp. 77-85, C. Foster, M. Schrager, A.C. Snyder, and N.N. Thompson, fig. 4, © Adis International Limited. All rights reserved. Data points for cycling exercise relate to O. Bar-Or, 1987, "The Wingate anaerobic test: An update on methodology, reliability and validity," *Sports Medicine* 4: 381-394; N. McCartney, G.J.F. Heigenhauser, A.J. Sargeant, and N.L. Jones, 1983, "A constant velocity cycle ergometer for the study of dynamic muscle function," *Journal of Applied Physiology* 55: 212-217; and R.T. Withers, W.M. Sherman, D.G. Clark, et al., 1991, "Muscle metabolism during 30, 60, and 90s of maximal cycling on an air-braked ergometer," *European Journal of Applied Physiology and Occupational Physiology* 63: 354-362. Data points for sprint running from M.E. Cheetham, L.H. Boobis, S. Brooks, and C. Williams, 1986, "Human muscle metabolism during sprint running," *Journal of Applied Physiology* 61: 54-60.

of water result in increased drag resistance with speed; drag resistance is much less in air-resisted sports. Momentum is therefore easily lost in swimming, and the energy cost is much greater for a given speed, which leads to a faster development of fatigue. Subsequently, only in the 50 m swimming events, which last approximately 21 to 30 seconds, do swimmers attempt an all-out pacing strategy.

Positive Pacing

Positive pacing involves starting the competition at a relatively fast pace, but not maximally. However, the initial exercise intensity is such that the athlete is compelled to slow down over the course of the event, reducing the work being done in the later stages. The sections that follow provide examples of positive pacing in short races (lasting 40 seconds to a few minutes) and in long-distance races lasting 2 hours or more. Positive pacing is also evident in team sports such as association football, in which players are required to sprint on multiple occasions during matches, which has a cumulative physiological effect. The physiological and psychological considerations at play in each of these scenarios are detailed here and in later chapters.

Events Lasting 40 Seconds to a Few Minutes

A positive pacing strategy is often observed in athletes running the 400 m race, which takes more than 40 seconds to complete. In this event, the starting speed is near maximal, and the speed of the athlete diminishes over the course of the race (see figure 2.2).

This strategy is apparent in many sports with races lasting up to a few minutes, although its use depends in part on whether the race is tactical. For example, in the 800 m event, when runners compete at close to world-record pace, most competitors typically run faster over the first half of the race than over the second half; however, in major championship finals, runners may employ the opposite strategy.

A positive pace strategy is more appropriate than an all-out strategy as the race extends beyond 40 seconds or so for several reasons. First, accelerating to the highest possible speed at the start of the event is less important and the starting phase of the race is less significant as a performance indicator. Second it is important to begin sub-maximally to regulate the use of the energy stores so they can be marshalled over the duration of the event. Finally, the length of time that aerodynamic or hydrodynamic resistance is experienced becomes a limiting factor in terms of the energy requirements of the event.

The anaerobic energy pathway is used predominantly during short races to provide the energy for powerful high-frequency muscle contractions. As an event duration lengthens, the energy contribution from the aerobic energy pathway increases. For example, in an event lasting 60 seconds or so, the ratio of anaerobic to aerobic energy contribution

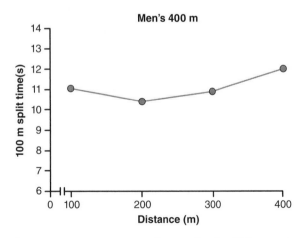

Figure 2.2 A typical positive pacing strategy observed in the 400 m track and field event.

might be approximately 60:40, whereas in an event lasting 3 to 4 minutes, the reverse might be true. The additional aerobic energy contribution in longer events reflects the fact that slow-twitch, or Type I, muscle fibres, which are more fatigue resistant than the fast-twitch, or Type II, muscle fibres, are increasingly recruited in greater proportions. As a result, a greater proportion of the peak speed can be maintained in a positively paced event because a greater proportion of fatigue-resistant slow-twitch muscle fibres are being used. Conversely, in an all-out event, fatigue begins to develop earlier as a result of a more aggressive initial acceleration phase that uses more of the non-fatigue-resistant fast-twitch muscle fibres.

Long-Distance Events (2 Hours and Longer)

Positive pacing has also been observed in events of considerable duration. These races begin with a group of athletes racing together, but at some point competitors select their own exercise intensities and in effect race against themselves, particularly once they have spread out. It has been reported that power output, speed and physiological measures such as heart rate often decline over the course of cycling and triathlon races lasting from 4 to 24 hours (Abbiss & Laursen 2008). This is supported by Esteve-Lanao and colleagues (2008), who discovered that the percentage of the maximum heart rate that competitors in 5 km to 100 km running races sustained decreased systematically with the duration of the event. Proportionally, a long time was spent in the severe exercise domain in the 5 and 10 km events (i.e., heart rate greater than 90 per cent of maximum for 80 to 85 per cent of the total race time). However, this exercise intensity was virtually absent in the ultra-marathon distances. The heavy exercise domain (above lactate threshold) was the predominant exercise intensity in race distances close to or beyond the half-marathon distance (about 40 to 60 per cent of the total running time), whereas time spent in moderate-intensity exercise (below lactate threshold) was negligible in marathon races but predominant in 100 km races (40 per cent of total running time).

A case study of a competitor in the Race Across America demonstrated an almost even pacing strategy. However, this is probably because the exercise domain was moderate throughout (the average stage heart rate range was 109 to 131 beats per minute), suggesting that the race was more a challenge of exercise duration (i.e., exercise capacity) than of the ability to maintain a high exercise intensity (i.e., exercise performance). Interestingly, other factors such as sleep deprivation are a major threat to performance in this type of event, because most participants sleep only 2 to 3 hours per day and cycle 20 hours per day (Schumacher et al. 2011).

In events lasting 2 to 4 hours or longer, the exercise intensity varies depending on the fitness levels of the competitors. For example, highly trained marathon runners can exercise in the heavy-intensity domain (around 80 per cent of $\dot{V}O_2$max, or approximately 85 to 90 per cent of maximum heart rate) during the race, whereas moderately trained runners might compete at lower exercise intensities (less than 70 per cent of $\dot{V}O_2$max, or 75 to 80 per cent of maximum heart rate), while even less well-trained athletes exercise at intensities lower than that (50 per cent of $\dot{V}O_2$max, or 60 per cent of maximum heart rate). In each case energy production is from the aerobic energy pathway, using either glycogen (carbohydrate) stores in the muscles and the liver or fat stores as the substrates for producing energy. Glycogen stores diminish after 1 to 4 hours, depending on the exercise intensity, and so are a limiting factor in maintaining race pace in long-distance events. If you consider that only 250 to 500 grams (8.8 to 17.6 oz) and 100 to 150 grams (3.5 to 5.3 oz) of carbohydrate are stored as glycogen in the muscles and the liver, respectively, with an additional 15 to 20 grams (0.5 to 0.7 oz) present as glucose in body fluids, you can see that carbohydrate sources are limited. Given that carbohydrates might be oxidised at a rate of between 1 to 3 grams (0.03 to 0.1 oz) per minute during endurance exercise, it is clear that these stores will not last long. Therefore, in long-distance events the conversion of fat to energy becomes increasingly important. In fact, long-distance athletes complete long-duration, moderate-intensity (below lactate threshold—60 per cent of $\dot{V}O_2$ max, or approximately 70 per cent of maximal heart rate) training sessions to prompt their fat metabolism to become more efficient so they can use their fat stores to a greater extent when competing at racing speeds and so spare their glycogen stores.

Energy production from fat oxidation is much slower (0.2 to 0.5 grams, or 0.007 to 0.17 oz, per minute) than from glycogen, but the energy content of fat is almost double that of carbohydrate, and so fat is the major source of energy production in ultra-distance events in which the pace of the exercise is relatively slow. However, in long-distance races conducted over only a couple of hours, the pace is faster, requiring athletes to exercise at a heavy exercise intensity. As a result, after about 1.5 to 2 hours, the glycogen content of the exercising muscles becomes depleted. At this time, the take-up of glucose from the blood (blood sugar) into the muscle to support the maintenance of muscle contractions is only modest. This is because the rate of release and the supply of glucose from the breakdown of liver glycogen and from food taken in during the exercise (such as a banana, carbohydrate gel or sport drink) is limited (1 gram, or 0.03 oz, per minute). As a result, the rate of aerobic energy contribution decreases, forcing the athlete to slow down (observed as a positive pacing strategy).

Rauch and colleagues (2005) suggested that a 'glycostat' may exist at the level of the brain that recognises low muscle glycogen content and might directly reduce muscle activation to protect against damage to the body. When marathon runners 'hit the wall', often at 32 km (~75 per cent of the race distance), glycogen stores have become depleted and thus energy for skeletal muscle contraction comes mainly from fat (oxidation) breakdown. This leads to decreased power output from the muscles and a shortage of blood glucose in the brain, affecting limb (motor) control and decision making. In this situation runners might suffer symptoms such as a lack of physical coordination, instability, nausea, muscle spasms, dizziness and extreme physical weakness (Esteve-Lanao et al. 2008; Stevinson & Biddle 1998).

A number of other factors can also cause athletes to slow down during long-distance races and produce a positive pacing profile. In hot conditions, athletes may develop a significantly elevated core body temperature, causing them to slow down to avoid hyperthermia. Muscle damage and a loss of motivation have also been implicated in forcing a reduction in pace, particularly in events lasting beyond 4 hours (Burnley & Jones 2007).

Even Pacing

During prolonged events of greater than 2.5 minutes and up to 60 minutes (i.e., middle- to long-distance events), it has been observed in experimental studies and competitive races that participants and athletes often demonstrate a preference for even pacing (Abbiss & Laursen 2008). It is also apparent that the initial acceleration phase becomes relatively less important to the race outcome as the duration of a race increases (see figure 2.3). Instead, the key consideration becomes speed maintenance, at least in time trial races and races completed at close to world-record pace. Wilberg and Pratt (1988) found that elite Canadian track sprinters used more even-paced profiles than did non-elite riders over 3 to 4 km (1.9 to 2.5 miles), perhaps demonstrating that this is a learned strategy associated with successful performance. In events of this duration, even-paced race strategies relate well to mathematical models which suggest that the race velocity is dictated by the maximal constant force an athlete can exert along with the resistive forces experienced (Abbiss & Laursen 2008).

A key tenet of even pacing is that, by avoiding unnecessary accelerations and decelerations, the athlete is in effect avoiding fluctuations in kinetic energy and is therefore using energy stores most efficiently. There is some evidence that elite rowers adopt a more even pacing strategy than non-elite rowers when repeating 2 km rowing trials (Schabort et al. 1999). Interestingly, a number of recent studies have reported a progressively slower (less aggressive) start to repeated time trials in cyclists and rowers (Corbett, Barwood & Parkhouse 2009; Foster et al. 1993; Thomas et al. 2012a) which suggests that a more even-paced profile develops with practice in well-trained athletes (see figure 2.4). A progressive blunting of the start would minimise physiological fatigue

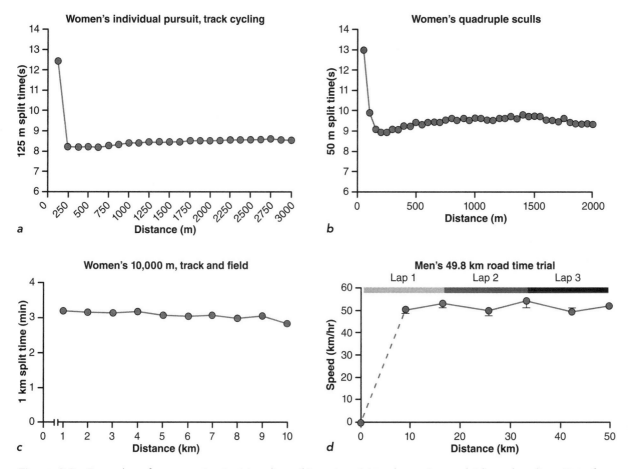

Figure 2.3 Examples of even pacing in (a) cycling, (b) rowing, (c) track running and (d) road cycling. Data from middle- and long-distance world championship events from 2009 to 2011.

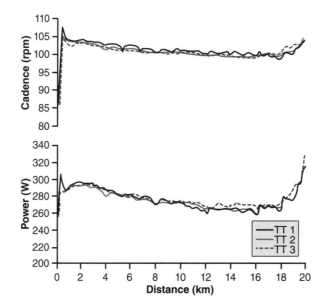

Figure 2.4 Reproducibility of a pacing strategy during simulated 20 km cycling time trials in well-trained cyclists. The first (TT 1) and second (TT 2) time trials show a more aggressive start, which becomes blunted in the third time trial (TT 3) as the cyclists learn to pace more efficiently to allow for a greater sprint finish.

With kind permission from Springer Science + Business Media: *European Journal of Applied Physiology*, "Reproducibility of pacing strategy during simulated 20-km cycling time trials in well-trained cyclists," 112(1), 2012, p. 225, K. Thomas, M.R. Stone, K.G. Thompson, A. Saint Clair Gibson, and L. Ansley, fig. 1, © Springer-Verlag 2011.

early in the event and allow for a better distribution of energy stores across the exercise bout. It also demonstrates that setting an initial pace is difficult to get right and takes practice even for well-trained athletes! As an aside, it is worth mentioning that, if left to self-pace (as in an individual time trial), well-trained athletes can demonstrate remarkable consistency in the ability to reproduce a time trial performance. Stone and colleagues (2011) and Thomas and colleagues (2012a) reported that riders completing 4 km and 20 km time trials on three occasions were able to finish with a time that varied by less than 3 per cent!

Negative Pacing

In contrast with the consequential, rather than deliberate, negative splits seen in all-out pacing discussed earlier in this chapter, true negative pacing is typically observed in middle- and long-distance events. Negative pacing involves an increase in speed over the course of the race and may help decrease aerobic and anaerobic energy use and the associated fatigue-related metabolites early in the exercise bout. Experimental evidence that this is an effective strategy, however, is limited. Thompson and colleagues (2003) reported a reduced heart rate response in a negative-paced 175 m breaststroke swimming time trial compared to even- and positive-paced time trials, but no differences were observed in oxygen uptake measured at the end of the trial, and overall performance was not improved. However, Mattern and colleagues (2001) did note improved performance in a 20 km cycling time trial in a study in which the power output was reduced by 15 per cent below the self-selected pace at the start of the exercise. A reduction in blood lactate concentration (an indirect measure of anaerobic energy metabolism) was also observed during the initial stages of the trial, perhaps indicating a reduced anaerobic energy requirement at the start of the exercise. Fukuba and Whipp (1999) argued that performance is compromised during endurance events if the athlete begins too slowly because metabolic limitations restrict the ability to make up for lost time, even if athletes attempt to do so. The implication is that a negative pacing strategy might lead to underperformance in 30- to 45-minute events which are completed at a severe-exercise intensity.

Parabolic Pacing

An increase in exercise intensity commonly occurs in the last 10 to 20 per cent of middle- and long-distance events (see figure 2.5). In some instances (e.g., 3000 m track cycling), the initial 80 to 90 per cent of a race has been observed to be fairly evenly paced, whereas the final portion has a notable increase in power output and speed (Foster et al. 2004). This practice could be argued to waste kinetic energy because energy that could perhaps have been used earlier is still being expended at the end of the race to accelerate. However, because the consequence of pushing too hard in the middle of a race will be premature fatigue and a large reduction in speed before the final portion, athletes in middle- and long-distance events seem to choose to pace conservatively in the middle portion of races. An end spurt or sprint finish is often in evidence at the end of these races and is a strategy well known to coaches and athletes alike. Surprisingly this strategy has not been well described in scientific studies until recently. This is largely because the analysis of races has been rather crude historically, incorporating only a few measurements (e.g., 2-4 split times) over the course of a race. This has meant that subtle changes in speed could not be detected during race analyses.

Recent advances in technology permit the measurement of power output and speed at high-frequency intervals (e.g., second by second), providing greater resolution to the analysis of sport events. Consequently, researchers and sport performance analysts are increasingly reporting that races are parabolic, demonstrating a distinct downward curve in the power output profile across the race. The additional resolution afforded by more sophisticated measurement tools provides the scientist and coach with much

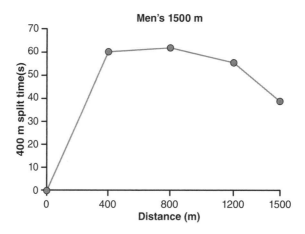

Figure 2.5 A typical men's middle-distance track profile, illustrating a parabolic pacing strategy.

greater insight into the pacing strategies used in sporting events. For example, middle- and long-distance runners often start with an initial high power output to gain forward momentum or an advantageous position in a field of competitors, but the pace decreases during the middle portion of the race before an end spurt in the latter stages. Figure 2.5 shows lap times for the men's 1500 m at the 2009 IAAF Athletics World Championships in Berlin; a parabolic profile is evident. Figure 2.6 also demonstrates a parabolic profile, this time in terms of the percentage of the average speed for a race; this pacing profile is often observed in cycling and running races. It is apparent that an almost even-paced profile occurs in the early stages, but a significant increase in speed takes place towards the end of the event to create a J-shaped profile. The reverse of this, or a reverse J shape, has been observed in 2000 m on-water rowing (Garland 2005). An equal percentage of a reduction and then a gain in speed during a race would be represented by a U-shaped profile in the figure.

When parabolic pacing occurs, the increase in power output at the start and end of the race requires competitors to access their anaerobic capacity. However, the anaerobic

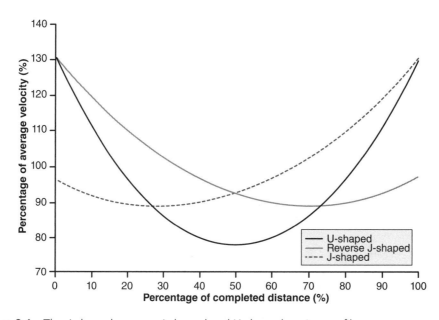

Figure 2.6 The J-shaped, reverse J-shaped and U-shaped pacing profiles.

energy system is limited and produces metabolites associated with fatigue processes. If too much anaerobic capacity is used early in the race, the end spurt will be compromised because too little anaerobic energy production will remain and too much fatigue will have developed. Conventional wisdom states that the body cannot regenerate the anaerobic exercise capacity during middle-distance events, although regeneration might be possible in long-distance events where the race is largely conducted in the heavy-intensity exercise domain. This suggests that judging the start and finish speeds is more critical in middle-distance events.

Hettinga and colleagues (2006) showed that during 4000 m cycling, the anaerobic energy metabolism follows the pacing profile, whereas the aerobic energy contribution increases similarly in even-, positive- and negative-paced trials, irrespective of the pacing strategy. The importance of the anaerobic capacity in achieving a successful parabolic pacing profile was also demonstrated during a study involving 4000 m self-paced cycling trials by Stone and colleagues (2012). They reported that the improvement in performance observed in one of the trials was due to the cyclists' using more of their anaerobic capacity, which allowed them to produce a faster finish (end spurt).

Variable Pacing

For many reasons, athletes sometimes vary their pace throughout an event. Pacing strategies are affected by many external factors including the race type and duration, competitors' paces, environmental conditions (temperature, humidity, altitude, wind) and the topography of the course (flat, uphill, downhill, fast-water, wave formation, depth of a pool, ice conditions). In multistage events, such as the Grand Tours in road cycling, in which athletes compete over many days across varying terrain, evidence suggests that athletes may limit their efforts on a given day and push hard on others (Foster et al. 2012). For example, exercise intensity (as measured by the percentage of maximum heart rate and power output) and the duration of effort have been observed to be greater in high mountain stages than in semi-mountainous stages and flat stages (Padilla et al. 2001; Vogt et al. 2007). A variable, or fluctuating, pacing strategy seems to have been developed by athletes to counter changing outdoor conditions during races. However, only a few studies to date have investigated variable pacing strategies and their effect on athlete performance.

In laboratory-based studies, when the exercise time and total work for a bout of cycling exercise have been matched, physiological responses during even-paced and variable-paced exercise have been shown to be similar, as long as the power output fluctuates within a certain range (Atkinson, Peacock & Passfield 2007; Liedl, Swain & Branch 1999; Palmer, Noakes & Hawley 1997). In fact, altering the power output and speed within a margin of ± 5 per cent and approximately 2 to 3 per cent, respectively, does not seem to significantly alter oxygen uptake, heart rate and blood lactate responses or perceived exertion during cycling (Atkinson, Peacock & Law 2007; Liedl, Swain & Branch 1999). A running study provides some dissent to this conclusion, however, suggesting that constant pacing is not always beneficial. Billat and colleagues (2006) reported that when runners completed a 10 km run constrained to a fixed pace, they exhibited a higher physiological cost—demonstrated by increased heart rate, oxygen uptake and blood lactate responses— than when they completed the run at the same average speed but were able to pace freely.

However, greater variations in exercise intensity do have a likely adverse effect. Palmer and colleagues (1999) found that the blood lactate concentration and carbohydrate oxidation rate increased during 140 minutes of cycling exercise, when pacing varied significantly (between 40 and 80 per cent of $\dot{V}O_2max$) compared to when it was held constant (at 65 per cent of $\dot{V}O_2max$) during the evenly pace trial. Thomas and colleagues (2012b) reported that during 20 km cycling trials, in which the completion time and total work were matched, even pacing resulted in smaller fluctuations in physiological responses, along with a reduced rating of perceived exertion, compared to a variable pacing strategy. In this study, variable pacing was achieved by changing the power output from 142 to 72 per cent of the average power output achieved during a self-paced time trial the subjects had completed earlier. A 1:1.5 ratio was also used for the two respective power outputs to represent fluctuations that might occur during races in which efforts in the extreme exercise intensity domain (142 per cent of average power output) might be followed by longer periods riding in the moderate exercise intensity domain (72 per cent of average power output, equivalent to below lactate threshold). Theurel and Lepers (2008) compared physiological responses when riders cycled at a constant power output around their heavy-intensity domain (70 per cent of $\dot{V}O_2max$) with a variable strategy that alternated moderate exercise (50 per cent of $\dot{V}O_2max$) with bouts of short, very intense exercise (extreme exercise intensity domain for 10 to 20 seconds). They concluded that varying the power output led to additional muscular fatigue and greater anaerobic energy use. Taken together, all of these experimental findings suggest that even pacing is preferable to variable pacing, at least for cycling time trials, because variable pacing is less energetically efficient, although small fluctuations in power output (± 5 per cent) have a limited physiological effect.

Conclusion

A variety of pacing strategies are evident in sport as a result of the various physiological and psychological stresses placed on athletes during competition. Some sports appear to have established pacing strategies for optimal performance, particularly shorter races in which tactical considerations are limited. However, in middle- to long-distance races, the optimal pacing strategy required to break a world record can be very different to one used during a championship race in which the athletes are interested only in winning. Coaches and athletes therefore need to carefully consider the goal of the competition performance before deciding on the pacing strategy.

Pacing strategies can also be an important consideration in ball and team sports given that physiological fatigue can manifest during multiple-sprint activity (e.g., during Association football). The physiological and psychological research that underpins our current understanding of pacing theory is presented in chapters 3 and 4, respectively. Chapter 5 synthesises this information to provide coaches and athletes with the requisite knowledge to design a pacing strategy for their sports. There is great potential for improvement in the design of pacing strategies as our understanding of pacing theory develops. Presently, coaches lead the way in promoting pacing theory and practice; however, the science of pacing is rapidly developing and in time will provide coaches and athletes with the evidence-based practice they seek.

chapter 3

Physiology of Pacing

This chapter explains the physiological principles and considerations thought to set and regulate the pace at which athletes perform exercise. This area of physiology is often referred to as exercise regulation because it involves a number of regulatory processes that work in tandem to regulate how humans pace exercise. Until recently, the area had not been extensively investigated, possibly because sport scientists tended to focus on the physiological aspects that *limit* exercise performance, rather than on those that *regulate* exercise performance.

It is well established that everyone has a maximal aerobic capacity ($\dot{V}O_2$max) that limits how much energy can be produced from the aerobic energy system. The $\dot{V}O_2$max is much dependent on the person's cardiac output (Basset & Howley 2000; Levine 2008) and factors that affect the conductance of oxygen from the air, through the person's bloodstream and to the muscle's aerobic energy–producing apparatus known as the mitochondria (Wagner 2010). It is also well known that following endurance training, adaptations occur, such as changes in the heart's structure and increases in the number of oxygen-carrying red blood cells, which lead to improvements in $\dot{V}O_2$max (Joyner & Coyle 2008). It is also well established that heart and skeletal muscle adaptations and changes to blood flow resulting from endurance training can improve the rate at which oxygen is delivered during exercise and in so doing improve the efficiency of an athlete's movement (Jones & Burnley 2009; Joyner & Coyle 2008). In addition, a more efficient production and use of energy, following training, is thought to spare carbohydrate use and reduce anaerobic energy production during races, which then reduces the rate of fatigue.

Although we understand a great deal about the aspects of our physiology that limit athletic performance, perhaps surprisingly, much less is known about how the body uses these training-induced, performance-enhancing adaptations in terms of how they affect a change in the athletes' pacing strategy. However, since the early 1990s, when Foster and colleagues (1993, 1994) published groundbreaking scientific articles that discussed how athletes might attempt to manage their physiological resources during races, there has been a marked increase in research in this field. Sport scientists are increasingly investigating the physical and mental effects of variables when athletes are free to pace themselves during exercise. Consequently, a progressively developing, complex model of exercise regulation is beginning to explain how humans pace optimally during exercise.

An early attempt at understanding the physiology of pacing was made by Dr E.B. Turner in a treatise titled the 'Physiology of Waiting and Pace-Making in Competition', which was discussed extensively in an article by Dr Norman Triplett of Indiana University (1898). Triplett suggested that the reason people performed better in paced races than in unpaced races was that they incurred different physiological effects related to physical and mental stresses. Triplett interpreted Dr Turner's data as meaning that

> the man who in a given distance does the greater amount of muscular work, burns up the greater amount of tissue and in consequence his blood is more loaded with waste products and he excretes more urea and uric acid than the man who does a less amount in the same time. The blood surcharged with the poisonous matter, benumbs the brain and diminishes its power to direct and stimulate the muscles. And the muscles themselves, bathed by the impure blood, lose largely their contractile power. [Dr Turner] asserts further that carbonic acid, lactic acid and uric acid are excreted in greater quantities during brain work. Therefore the man racing under conditions to produce brain worry will be the most severely distressed. (Triplett 1898, p. 513)

Triplett put forward the brain worry theory to explain why it was difficult for the leader in an unpaced race to win. His argument was that by having to set the pace of the race, the leader incurred greater 'brain worry' than the followers did. Dr Turner reasoned that the man leading is constantly concerned about whether he is going fast enough to exhaust his adversary and when the adversary means to commence his spurt. Subsequently, the leader's 'nervous system is generally strung up, at concert pitch, and his muscular and nervous efforts act and react on each other, producing an ever increasing exhaustion, which both dulls the impulse-giving power of the brain and the impulse-receiving or contractile power of the muscles' (quote cited in Triplett 1898, p. 515). The article goes on to remark that the rider in a cycle race can ride automatically with the spinal cord providing the nervous command to the muscles (rather like a reflex loop), and so the brain needs to come back into play, to increase muscular output, only when a change in the race pace or race conditions occurs. Then at the end, when the waiting rider approaches the final spurt, 'His brain engages, assuming control again, imparts to the muscles a winning stimulus, while the continued brain work of the leader has brought great fatigue' (Triplett 1898, p. 515).

What is striking about these observations is that, even at the turn of the 20th century, a link was made between the brain and the changes in the body's peripheral physiology and muscular force production during exercise. The brain was thought to be affected by what was happening in the blood as a result of the exercise, a build-up of certain acids that could lead to a reduction in muscle stimulation. Furthermore, the theory of 'brain worry' also recognised the mental aspects of pacing (discussed in chapter 4) and their effect on competitors' effort levels during races.

Peripheral Fatigue

Percy G. Stiles, assistant professor of physiology at Harvard Medical School, wrote in 1920 that 'Muscles that are much used under cerebral control appear to require long intervals of repose. They are capable of spurts so intense as to induce long continued depression' (p. 653). This early description describes the fatigue evident in muscles after 2 to 3 minutes of intense exercise. We now know that fatigue develops progressively during exercise over this time duration, provided that the athlete exercises with near-maximal effort at the start and then maximal effort towards the finish. In fact, during a race lasting around 2 minutes that is being completed at an optimal pace, perhaps to break a world record, the athlete should not be able to accelerate towards the end of the race. Indeed, not only would the athlete be unable to produce an end spurt (or sprint finish), but they would be slowing down as their muscles failed to produce the necessary force to maintain their speed.

Most sport scientists would argue that this represents what is known as peripheral fatigue. This means that the muscle tissue and the junction with the stimulating nerve are fatigued; as a result, further increased activation of the contracting muscles by the brain, known as the central motor drive, does not lead to a subsequent increase in force production. It is proposed that this is due to a shortfall in energy-providing metabolic substrates (adenosine triphosphate, or ATP, and phosphocreatine, or PCr) and the build-up of fatiguing metabolic waste products (hydrogen ions, also known as protons, and inorganic phosphates) in the muscles. These processes render the athlete unable to maintain force production despite the brain either maintaining or increasing activation to the muscles.

Energy Management in Short Competitions

As explained in chapter 2, in shorter athletic contests a combination of anaerobic and aerobic energy production provides the energy for muscle contraction; however, the shorter the event is, the greater the anaerobic energy contribution will be relative to the aerobic energy contribution. This is because fast-twitch muscle fibres are increasingly being recruited to provide the greater force production needed and because oxygen delivery or uptake is increasingly insufficient to produce energy via aerobic energy metabolism at the appropriate rate to match the muscle's increased energy requirements.

A consequence of this proportional increase in anaerobic energy production is an accumulation of metabolites and a reduction in muscle pH (increased acidity), which impairs the muscles' contractile processes and inhibits anaerobic energy production through the process known as anaerobic glycolysis. A further consideration is that because the anaerobic capacity is finite, how it is marshalled across a race (i.e., the pacing strategy) is crucial during short-duration exercise.

The anaerobic capacity is a rather complex physiological concept that involves a number of interacting processes. First, the rate of ATP production from the substrates in the contracting muscles (PCr and glycogen, or carbohydrate, stores) falls at a rate dependent on the type of muscle fibres being recruited. The fast-twitch (Type II) muscle fibres, which contract and produce force more rapidly than the slow-twitch (Type I) muscle fibres, subsequently use ATP more rapidly. In addition, a build-up of fatiguing metabolites during high-intensity exercise can also affect muscle contraction. Although the body has a natural defence called its buffering capacity, this defence is finite and so can only temporarily extend the time it takes to reach a fatiguing level of muscle acidity. Additionally, the ability of the athlete's aerobic system to produce energy quickly (to spare the depletion of the anaerobic capacity) is an important consideration. Also important is the store of oxygen in the muscle (myoglobin) that is used when the athlete is approaching $\dot{V}O_2$max, because at this point the anaerobic capacity will become rapidly depleted. Because all of these factors affect anaerobic capacity, its involvement during exercise relates both to anaerobic and aerobic energy metabolism. The only time the anaerobic capacity would not be used is if the aerobic energy system was supplying all of the energy required. At rest this almost transpires as nearly 100 per cent of the energy being produced comes from aerobic energy metabolism. When athletes exercise at a moderate-exercise-intensity (below the lactate threshold, or approximately 60 to 70 per cent of maximal heart rate) or at a lesser exercise intensity, the anaerobic capacity can remain largely intact because a steady state in aerobic energy production ensues that meets the majority of the energy requirement for the exercise (see chapter 5 for a full explanation).

Foster and colleagues (2003) eloquently described the pattern of energy distribution and power output for high-intensity cycling lasting less than 2 minutes. They concluded that changes within the muscle, such as metabolite accumulation and a shortfall in substrates reducing the availability of ATP, were being monitored and so muscle contractions and hence power output were adapted accordingly to circumvent changes in physiology that would be critical or harmful.

A number of studies have shown that peripheral fatigue limits short-term maximal exercise. For example, Hunter and colleagues (2003) found that the power output of participants during a maximal 30-second cycling test (Wingate test) fell by 45 per cent, yet the brain's electrical activation (the central motor drive) to the rectus femoris leg muscle remained unchanged. This demonstrated that despite the same level of activation, the force production by the muscle had become impaired. Nummela, Vurorimaa and Rusko (1992) reported that, following a maximal 400 m run, the subjects in their study were unable to jump as high as they could before the sprint, demonstrating that muscle contractility was impaired after the sprint. They also found that during the 400 m sprint the subjects had shown increasing muscle electrical activity, demonstrating an increased central motor drive by the brain, presumably to recruit additional muscle fibres to compensate for the falling force production from already contracting muscle fibres as they became fatigued. In another study, participants undertook high-intensity cycling in a state of hypoxia (i.e., the oxygen concentration available was less than normal—11.6 per cent rather than a normal 20.9 per cent). They discovered that force production from the muscles decreased, despite muscle activation increasing, suggesting a progressive reduction in muscle contractility as a result of peripheral muscle fatigue rather than a decrease in the central motor drive (Taylor et al. 1997).

The need to pace exercise lasting only 36 seconds was demonstrated by Ansley and colleagues (2004). They asked participants to exercise maximally for 36 seconds on a cycle ergometer on a number of occasions so they were experienced in doing so. However, on one occasion the subjects were deceived and told that the trial would last only 30 seconds, although it actually lasted for 36 seconds. They found that a significant reduction in power output occurred in the last 6 seconds of the trial, from 30 to 36 seconds, compared to the trials in which participants had been truthfully informed that they would be exercising for 36 seconds. This study demonstrated that in events of only 36 seconds or so, premature peripheral fatigue will take place unless people practise. Prior experience enables them to allocate their physiological resources effectively. Practice is important because the point of fatigue can happen suddenly, catching the athlete unawares. This suggests that the monitoring of the situation by the sensory receptors and the subsequent communication to the brain for interpretation might be a largely subconscious event. Also, a time lag may occur before the athlete is conscious of rapidly developing fatigue in the exercising muscles.

Energy Management in Longer Competitions

As exercise continues beyond 40 seconds, it becomes increasingly important that the human body regulate itself. People simply cannot exercise all-out beyond this time in most sports without suffering significant peripheral fatigue and suboptimal performance (Keller 1974). Therefore, some degree of pacing is needed. The longer the race goes on, the more the aerobic energy system is used. The anaerobic energy system is used only to get up to racing speed at the very start of the race, to produce short surges and to fuel the sprint finish, if required. The increasing use of the aerobic system therefore limits the use of the anaerobic energy system and subsequently the development of peripheral fatigue.

As the aerobic energy system nears its maximal rate during a race, anaerobic metabolism is increasingly used. The depletion of the finite anaerobic capacity leads to the development of fatigue. Hence a well-developed aerobic energy system is increasingly important as the race increases from 40 seconds to a number of minutes. Interestingly during exercise of this duration, metabolites (hydrogen ions and inorganic phosphates), associated with the development of peripheral (muscle) fatigue, appear to reach a certain level at exhaustion. This level is not the same for everybody which suggests that, in terms of peripheral muscle fatigue, there might be an individual critical threshold, during exhaustive, high-intensity endurance exercise that cannot be exceeded (Amman

2011). In races over many hours, the aerobic system is never close to being used at full capacity; hence, the anaerobic system is of little importance. However, athletes have to manage other challenges to their physiology such as heat gain, dehydration, the depletion of the body's carbohydrate reserves and muscle damage. Motivation also becomes an issue in long endurance races.

Athletes have to pace themselves in races longer than 3 minutes to optimise their performance, because they are no longer simply starting fast and slowing down over the race (a strategy known as positive pacing; see table 2.1 in chapter 2 for a review of the most common pacing strategies). Instead, they might set a pace they can maintain throughout the event (even pacing) or even slow down in the middle part of the race so they can increase their pace at the end of the race (parabolic pacing). Parabolic pacing and variable pacing are characterised by tactical surges and then lulls in speed over the course of the event. With these types of pacing, the athlete is clearly racing at a submaximal pace at certain times, which spares the anaerobic capacity so that an end spurt can be produced towards the end of the race through greater activation of the muscles.

Teleoanticipation

To produce a sprint finish (or end spurt), the athlete must have selected the correct starting pace. Recall from chapter 1 that this initial pace is more likely to be optimal if the athlete is aware of the end point of the trial (i.e., the race distance), has prior experience of the course on which the race is taking place and has prepared in training to race over that distance. These factors enable the athlete to anticipate the end point of the exercise and to construct an internal pacing template for the race. This anticipatory process has been called teleoanticipation (Ulmer 1996).

The Triplett (1898) article mentioned earlier alluded to teleoanticipation in its discussion of competitors learning how to pace over repeated trials because they didn't initially 'have proper ideals for speed'. The concept of gaining prior experience, not only of the race distance but also of the course topography and likely racing conditions, is something modern athletes, coaches and sport scientists fastidiously attend to as part of pre-event preparation. Triplett (1898) also observed large differences in individual finishing times in self-paced trials compared to trials in which athletes were being paced or were pacing themselves against others in competition. At the time, these riders would have been relative novices to the distances they were racing over and certainly would not have been undertaking specific training programmes to prepare them, as modern athletes do. Modern athletes are extremely well prepared in comparison.

A study by Skorski and colleagues (2013) demonstrated that highly trained swimmers can create a time trial pace that is similar to their competition pace (i.e., producing a similarly shaped speed profile), except that the race pace is approximately 1 per cent faster throughout because they are highly motivated and tapered at that time. Triplett (1898) recognised the importance of prior experience, stating that an older group of riders who were noticeably better able to pace their competitive races demonstrated 'fewer fluctuations and irregularities (in pacing) and less pronounced fatigue curves at the end (of races)' (p.527). Contemporary studies provide strong evidence that the development of an increasingly precise and consistent pacing 'template' for a race, as Triplett (1898) described, is one of the significant factors that differentiates elite athletes from less gifted athletes.

Clearly, competition experience is a prerequisite for correct pacing during races. Indeed, the extensive and well-constructed training programmes of today's athletes result in modern-day elite-level races being, in general, extremely competitive and consistent in performance levels. This is one reason world records in running, cycling and swimming, for example, are rarely beaten by large amounts anymore.

Role of Afferent Feedback and the Drive Towards Homeostasis

Once a race is underway, it has been suggested that the physiological impact of the racing pace is being continuously monitored by receptors in the body that sense external and internal stimuli. External stimuli that might effect a change in the athlete's pacing strategy would include the tactics of a competitor or a shift in environmental conditions, such as temperature or wind. Internal stimuli are sensed by numerous receptors that pass information about the state of the internal environment of the body through afferent (sensory) nerves to the somatosensory cortex of the brain. For example, changes in the body temperature are sensed by thermoreceptors; changes in glucose concentration, acidity, oxygen pressure and carbon dioxide pressure are sensed by chemoreceptors; changes in muscle fibre strain are sensed by stretch receptors; and changes in pain levels are sensed by nociceptors.

How the brain interprets all this feedback and then creates a response is not yet fully understood. However, during exercise the motor cortex of the brain adjusts electrical activation of the contracting muscles through efferent (motor) nerves, which alter the type, rate and frequency of muscle contraction. This control of muscle fibre activation by the central nervous system is known as the central motor drive. The central motor drive recruits a greater or lesser number of muscle fibres, depending on the physiological reserve remaining and the need to avoid a significant deterioration in performance or actual bodily harm.

The purpose of this feedback loop during exercise is therefore to regulate and restrict developing peripheral muscle fatigue and the associated sensory feedback to an 'individual critical threshold', which is unique to the individual athlete's physiology (Amman 2011). The function of this individual critical threshold might be to avoid potentially long-lasting harmful consequences to the muscle or perhaps even to the heart or the brain.

A fundamental physiological concept is homeostasis, which refers to the body's attempt to maintain a constant internal environment through various processes. This is not actually possible because physiological systems fluctuate constantly as they respond to ever-changing stimuli. Indeed, a degree of variability is likely important for good health because it provides the flexibility needed for making constant adjustments to external stimuli we might not have control over.

Figure 3.1 presents a negative feedback system in which a sensory receptor senses a change in the body's internal environment (e.g., temperature, blood pressure, hormone concentration, concentration of a particular chemical such as glucose). Afferent (moving inwards, towards the brain) nerves inform the control centre, the brain, which then produces an output through efferent (outward moving) nerves to effect a change to address the imbalance and bring the physiological environment in the body back to within a normal range. During exercise significant imbalances can occur, and various homeostatic responses take place to maintain the body's internal environment within tolerable limits to safeguard health.

For example, the body normally has an average internal, 'core' temperature of around 36 to 37.5 °C (96.8 to 99.5 °F), and on a daily basis the temperature might fluctuate by less than 1.0 °C (1.8 °F). However, if the body is exposed to prolonged heavy exercise, illness or extreme conditions of heat or cold, its temperature will change outside of this normal 'homeothermic' range. If your car breaks down and you suddenly find yourself stranded in a really cold environment, miles from human contact and without the car heater or a warm coat, you would suddenly be faced with a potentially dangerous situation because your body would not easily be able to maintain a constant internal temperature. Let's assume you leave the car to walk to get help. A number of things would happen. First, you'd begin to lose body heat because the outside temperature is so much colder than your internal body temperature. Your body would lose heat to the atmosphere by radiation. If there is a wind, then an even more rapid heat loss would

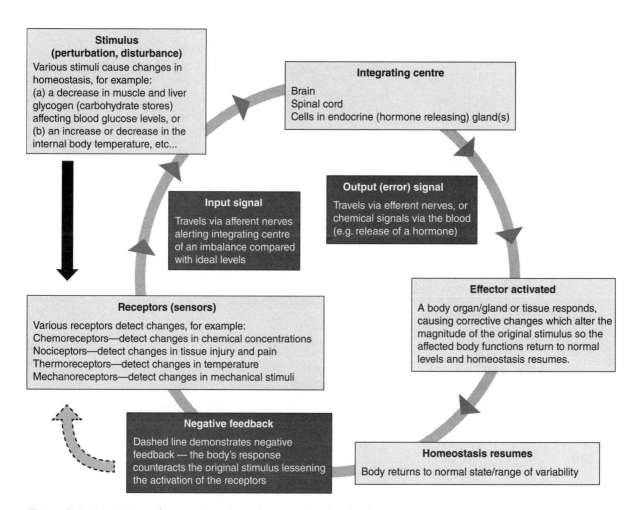

Figure 3.1 Maintaining homeostasis through a negative feedback system.

take place due to convection (i.e., the air molecules that are warmed by their contact with the skin are moved away by the movement of the wind). This is known as the wind chill factor.

The thermoreceptors in the skin and spine would sense a change in external and internal body temperature, respectively, and inform the hypothalamus, an organ at the base of the brain. Receptors in the hypothalamus would also sense a change in the temperature of the circulating blood. As the skin and blood cools down, the hypothalamus would initiate a number of autonomic (involuntary physiological) events designed to bring the body, and subsequently the temperature of the blood, back into normal range (see figure 3.2).

Figure 3.2 illustrates the physiological events that occur when the body temperature increases or decreases, as in the preceding car scenario. As a result of the decrease in body temperature, blood flow changes, because the diameter of the blood vessels (arterioles) near the skin surface is reduced (an effect known as vasoconstriction). This reduces heat loss by directing blood away from the skin surface and towards the central core of the body. Muscles are activated, leading to involuntary muscle contractions, which is essentially a reflex action that produces heat. Fat and carbohydrate stores are mobilised to provide the fuel for the chemical reactions needed to generate the energy required, driven by the changes in neural and hormonal (epinephrine, norepinephrine, thyroxine) responses. Sensory information is also fed back to the somatic sensory cortex, brain stem and insular cortex of the brain which is integrated and interpreted, a behavioural decision is made and a command is sent to the brain's motor cortex, which in turn activates

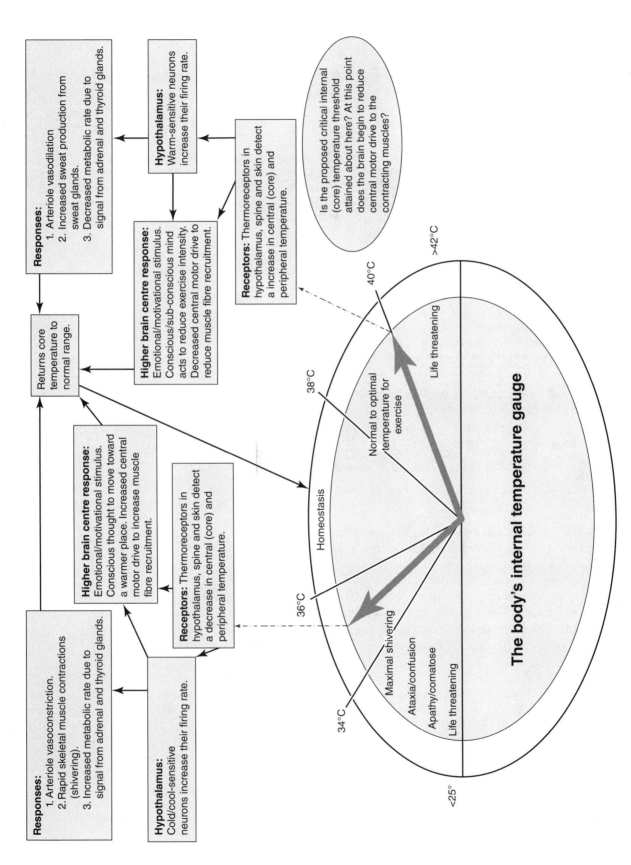

Figure 3.2 Changes initiated by the hypothalamus to restore body temperature to within the normal range and higher brain responses to perceptions of temperature change and discomfort. Note that although some researchers hypothesise that 40 °C (104 °F) is the critical internal temperature threshold, this has yet to be confirmed.

a motor (movement) programme. This motor programme involves an increase in the brain's central motor drive to the muscle fibres of the leg, stimulating them to contract more forcefully to produce a faster walking speed. The purpose of walking faster is not only to reach a warm destination more quickly but also to generate more internal body heat, because only approximately 20 to 30 per cent of the energy generated by chemical reactions in the body actually fuels the muscle contractions, because of a lack of mechanical efficiency. This means that the remaining 70 to 80 per cent of the energy released is dissipated as heat energy, which warms the body. Finally, because additional energy production is needed for the increased muscle contractions to increase walking speed and shivering, the rate and depth of breathing increases to ensure an additional take-up of oxygen for the additional aerobic energy production required.

The brain has good reason to undertake these protective responses: Without them, hypothermia would develop, which could have catastrophic consequences. To safeguard against this, a drop in the body's internal core temperature of a few degrees to a core temperature of around 34 °C (93.2 °F) initiates maximal shivering, increasing heat production approximately two- to fivefold. However, if the body temperature continues to decrease by another couple of degrees, then the brain's ability to control movement becomes affected; known as ataxia, this condition makes it difficult to put gloves on and eventually to walk. At the same time, signs of apathy begin to appear, which affect decision making. Further drops in the body's core temperature can lead to unconsciousness. At this stage the situation is very bleak—if there is any further drop in body temperature, a catastrophic failure inevitably occurs, resulting in death. The heart muscle contracts in an increasingly uncoordinated and inefficient manner associated with ventricular fibrillation, resulting in poorer and poorer blood flow. Subsequently, insufficient oxygen is delivered to the brain and the heart muscle, eventually leading to cell death and complete loss of function.

Central Governor Theory

Homeostasis acts to maintain physiological systems within a normal range to protect the body against a catastrophic failure in one or more of its physiological systems. However, experts also believe that homeostasis plays an important role during exercise. In self-paced exercise, in which the person is freely able to set and change pace, performance is thought to be regulated by the brain to prevent changes in physiological systems that might be detrimental to performance or health (Tucker & Noakes 2009). The idea that the brain regulates exercise is not new; in 1924, Hill, Long and Lupton wrote that 'either in the heart muscle or in the nervous system, there is some mechanism which causes a slowing of the circulation as soon as a serious degree of un-saturation (reduction in blood oxygen levels) occurs'(p 161-2). Hill and colleagues were referring to a 'governor' somewhere in the body that responds to chemoreceptors detecting a shortage of oxygen being delivered to the contracting heart muscle during exhausting exercise. The informed governor then sends an instruction, delivered by the nervous system, to reduce the recruitment of the heart's muscle fibres and subsequently slow down the heart rate and consequently the rate of exercise. Hill and colleagues (1924) believed this would ensure that the mismatch developing between oxygen delivery and oxygen use would be controlled to avoid a catastrophic drop in oxygen delivery to the heart.

A team of sport science researchers from the University of Cape Town, South Africa, took this concept a step further by suggesting that a 'central governor' based in the brain reduces activation of the contracting muscles of the limbs as fatigue develops to safeguard an athlete against prematurely fatiguing (Noakes 2011; St Clair Gibson & Noakes 2004; Tucker & Noakes 2009). These researchers view fatigue as part of a regulated anticipatory response coordinated in the subconscious brain that attempts to preserve homeostasis in each physiological system during exercise, regardless of the intensity, duration or environment of the exercise (Noakes & St Clair Gibson 2004). They suggest that a number of factors regulated by homeostatic mechanisms (oxygen delivery, glucose concentration, temperature increases, metabolite accumulation) as well as psychological factors can affect how the brain's central governor regulates exercise to ensure that a catastrophic deterioration in exercise performance or even catastrophic biological failure leading to a threat to health does not occur. Noakes (2011) proposed that a wide range of factors might affect the pace the athlete sets in a race and that various stimulators from afferent sensory feedback or other performance modifiers affect the brain and how the athlete's pace is set and regulated during a race (see figure 3.3).

Figure 3.3 presents an anticipatory central governor model (St Clair Gibson & Noakes 2004), which means that the magnitude of the brain's central motor drive to the contracting muscles is affected by peripheral feedback from sensory receptors in the skin, muscles, bloodstream and organs as well as the athlete's psychological state, experience of the exercise being undertaken (whether the race distance is novel) and knowledge of the event ahead (e.g., distance, course topography, opposition). All of these factors influence the pace the athlete adopts across a race. During the race the athlete senses the state of the body's fuel reserves, the rate of heat storage, hydration status and many other factors, and the central governor then adjusts the muscle contractions of the exercising limbs accordingly, to maximise performance and minimise failure (Noakes 2011).

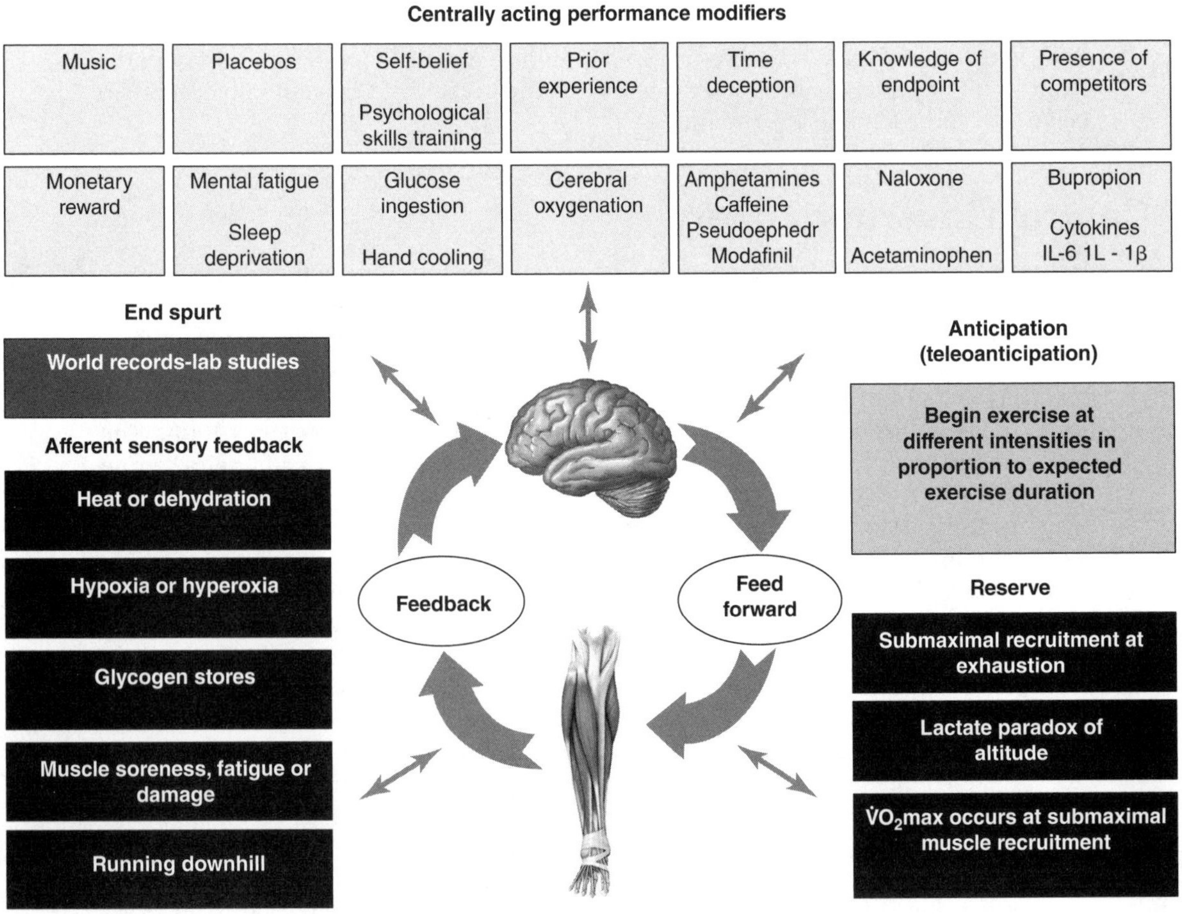

Figure 3.3 Factors that can affect how speed (pace) is set and regulated during a race.

From T.D. Noakes, 2011, "Time to move beyond a brainless exercise physiology: The evidence for complex regulation of human exercise performance," *Applied Physiology Nutrition and Metabolism* 36(1): 23-35. © Canadian Science Publishing or its licensors. Reproduced with permission.

Hot and Humid Conditions

Many athletes compete in races in unusually hot and humid conditions. In this situation, because the ambient air is warmer than the internal body temperature, the athlete gains heat. In addition, as the athlete exercises and produces heat energy internally, further heat gain results, which increases as the exercise intensity increases. Depending on the type of exercise the athlete is undertaking, approximately 70 to 95 per cent of the energy produced for movement is lost as heat energy, which can result in a 25-fold increase in the body's heat production.

As in the previous example of how homeostasis is controlled when a person is exposed to cold weather, the hypothalamus acts to maintain a constant internal environment in hot environments. The hypothalamus senses the increase in skin and body temperature because it is highly sensitive to temperature changes at the skin surface and in the circulating blood. The body's sweat glands are activated after a particular temperature is reached—rather like a thermostat switching on in a house when the room temperature reaches its set point. Blood flow to the skin increases as the nerves increase the diameter of the blood vessels (vasodilation), which provides a supply of filtrate, including water, that the sweat glands use to form sweat. In extreme conditions, 15 to 25 per cent of the circulating blood can be redirected to the skin; however, this compromises oxygen delivery to the contracting muscles.

The sweat glands release sweat onto the skin surface. When it evaporates, heat is lost from the body helping it to cool down. Maximal sweat rates vary among athletes (i.e., from 2 to 3 litres per hour), which is why some athletes are better able to cope with hot conditions than others are. In general, females are less tolerant than males of exercise in the heat because they sweat relatively less and also have a greater percentage of body fat, which hampers heat loss. Someone with a great capacity to evaporate sweat can lose body heat rapidly, but this can compromise endurance performance because the sweat emanates from the blood. Excessive sweating reduces the body's blood volume, which then requires the athlete's heart rate to increase to maintain cardiac (heart) output and blood flow to the muscles. The effect is felt at maximal exercise intensity when the rate of oxygen delivery and the muscles' capacity for aerobic energy production are reduced.

Unfortunately, as the exercise intensity increases, or if the surrounding air temperature increases, the body's heat gain can become greater than its heat loss. This results in a net gain of heat and a rise in internal body temperature during the race, leading to feelings of discomfort as the sensory cortex and insular cortex of the brain receives feedback from afferent nerves regarding the body's increasing heat load. The amount of heat energy required to raise the temperature of the body (known as the specific heat of the human body) is 0.83 kilocalories per kg of body mass per 1.0 °C. This means that a 60 kg (132 lb) athlete would need to gain 49.8 kilocalories before the body temperature would be raised by 1 °C. If that athlete is exercising at a heavy exercise intensity requiring the uptake of 3 litres of oxygen per minute for aerobic energy production, that would equate to approximately 15 kilocalories per minute of energy. If the athlete is exercising with a mechanical efficiency of 20 per cent, which is common in running and cycling, then only 3 kilocalories per minute would be used for mechanical work; the remaining 12 kilocalories per minute would be dissipated as heat in the body. This would lead to a gain of 1 °C in internal body temperature every 4.15 minutes in a 60 kg (132 lb) athlete unless heat could be lost through sweating and convection.

Scientists have proposed that if the core temperature of the body increases above 40 °C, or 104 °F (believed to be the critical internal core temperature), during exercise, the brain will reduce its central motor drive to the contracting muscles, slowing the athlete down (Galloway & Maughan 1997; Nielsen 1996; Nielsen et al. 1990). When exercising intensely in hot conditions, athletes can reach an internal core temperature of 40 °C (104 °F) in events lasting 15 minutes or more, unless the rate of sweat evaporation is sufficient to prevent this. In the example just described, a gain of heat energy of

12 kilocalories per minute would equate to a gain of 720 kilocalories per hour of heat energy. It has been calculated that 0.58 kilocalories of heat energy is lost per millilitre of sweat evaporated. Thus, to lose 720 kilocalories, an athlete would have to evaporate 1.24 litres of sweat per hour, which can happen in a race in hot, dry conditions.

Finally, the humidity of the surrounding air also plays a significant role. The greater the humidity is, the greater the water vapour content of the air is, making it less able to accept water from the evaporation of sweat. This can lead to sweat not being evaporated from the skin, in which case the athlete does not lose body heat. This failure in heat loss becomes significant when the air humidity is high, and athletes will suffer the consequences of the resultant heat gain. In an endurance event under these conditions, the athlete may have to compete at a slower pace to avoid developing a dangerously high internal body temperature and suffering a heat illness.

Endurance Events

To put this thermoregulatory challenge into the context of pacing, hot conditions will probably affect the pace of any athlete undertaking an event that lasts 15 minutes or longer. When athletes race in hot conditions, their core temperature increases and homeostasis is challenged. An increase in core temperature of around 1 to 1.5 °C, to approximately 38.5 to 39.0 °C (101.3 to 102.2 °F), is thought to be a good thing and is one reason athletes warm up prior to races. Scientists believe that this temperature increase speeds up chemical reactions so they work at their optimal rate; for example, to produce energy. However, it is thought that if the core temperature reaches around 40 °C (104 °F), the brain interprets this as a critical temperature and subsequently reduces its central motor drive to the contracting muscles. This ensures that the muscles' force output and heat production decrease, but so will the athlete's race speed.

Long-distance athletes therefore race more conservatively in hot and humid conditions, adjusting their pacing strategy from the outset, presumably to avoid gaining heat too soon during a race and also to limit losing blood volume quickly as a result of excessive sweating. Excessive sweat loss might also reduce blood flow to the skin, compromising heat loss. Taking fluids on board during the race helps to reduce this problem. A number of recent studies have investigated the mechanisms underpinning the conservative pacing strategies exhibited by trained athletes in hot conditions. There is evidence that participants in these studies do not terminate exercise or reduce their speed when they reach the presumed critical core temperature of 40 °C (104 °F), but rather, that they anticipate, either subconsciously or consciously, the potential physiological stress ahead and exercise at a reduced pace well before their bodies reach this temperature!

A long-held principle is that fatigue develops in athletes in long-distance races in hot and humid conditions because of changes in blood flow reducing oxygen delivery to the muscles. A proportion of the blood flow having been directed to the skin and in addition, high rates of sweating lead to a loss of blood volume that further reduces oxygen delivery to the muscles for aerobic energy production. These events can increase anaerobic energy metabolism and the accumulation of fatiguing waste products (lactate ions and potassium ions), leading to peripheral fatigue. However, Tucker and Noakes (2009) argued that peripheral fatigue is not the major issue; rather, the major issue is the rate of heat storage the brain senses, which results in runners and cyclists choosing a more conservative pace early on when exercising in hot conditions compared to cool conditions. They also contended that this occurs *before* the core temperature is significantly raised to a critical level or oxygen delivery is sufficiently compromised to result in any associated accumulation of waste products leading to fatigue.

Evidence for this argument comes from a study by Tucker and colleagues (2006), in which they asked well-trained cyclists to complete a 20 km time trial in temperatures of 35 °C (95 °F) and 15 °C (59 °F), respectively. They found that the pacing strategy of the participants in the hotter condition changed early in the trial, despite their demonstrating rectal temperatures, heart rates and feelings of perceived exertion similar to those they demonstrated in the cooler trial. In the hotter trial, the participants demonstrated a reduced power output profile. In both temperature conditions, the participants exhibited a sprint finish, suggesting that the brain was regulating efforts in both trials to ensure that a capacity was left in reserve at the end.

In a similar study, Tatterson and colleagues (2000) also observed that participants in a 30-minute cycling time trial reduced their power output after only 15 minutes of exercise at 32 °C (89.6 °F), but not when they exercised in a temperature of 23 °C (73.4 °F). Marino, Lambert and Noakes (2004) noted that African runners paced themselves in a similar fashion in both cool and hot conditions; however, larger Caucasian runners could not, probably as a result of their larger size, which leads to a greater rate of heat storage.

These studies suggest that a reduction in self-paced exercise performance might occur before body temperature reaches critically high levels and that a centrally mediated mechanism, at the brain level, reduces muscle activation to avoid a rate of heat storage that might lead to a critical core temperature before the end of the exercise bout. This mediator, or central governor, in the brain has been proposed to protect the body from harm and from a catastrophic deterioration of performance during races (Noakes 2011).

Other Variables That May Affect Pacing

As sport science researchers have become increasingly interested in the many factors that might affect how humans pace their exercise, they have begun to design increasingly sophisticated studies to elucidate which factors are most critical and the physiological mechanism or mechanisms responsible. This section highlights some of the findings to date and explores the important role the brain plays in exercise regulation.

Oxygen Content   A number of researchers have manipulated the oxygen content of the air athletes take in during exercise to demonstrate that the brain senses this and alters muscle activation accordingly. Tucker and colleagues (2007) found that increasing the oxygen content of the air to 40 per cent (hyperoxia) allowed cyclists to exhibit higher power output during a 20 km time trial than they did when cycling while breathing air with a normal oxygen content of 20.9 per cent. The authors concluded that the greater oxygen availability enabled a higher degree of force production because more muscle fibres were activated. Peltonen and colleagues (1997) found that muscle activation, measured using integrated electromyography (iEMG) at seven muscle sites, decreased during a 2500 m rowing ergometry trial when the oxygen content of the air breathed by the rowers was reduced to 15.8 per cent (hypoxia). They also observed a reduction in force production and an impaired 2500 m performance. Amman and colleagues (2006) demonstrated that subjects in a controlled laboratory altered their pacing strategy within 60 seconds of the oxygen content of the surrounding air changing, and that muscle activation, as indirectly measured by iEMG, reduced in proportion to the reduction in the oxygen content (i.e., the degree of hypoxia) of the surrounding air. Importantly, the reduction in muscle contraction occurred before a catastrophic failure in oxygen delivery occurred, indicating an anticipatory response.

Sprint Finish   The phenomenon of athletes speeding up towards the end of endurance races has also been suggested as an indication that an anticipatory central governor must be operating. The fact that athletes are running at their fastest when they should be most tired seems to indicate that they have been conserving energy by exercising submaximally during the middle portion of the race (Noakes 2011). Tucker and Noakes (2009) suggested that because power output and muscle activation increase at the end of endurance exercise trials in conditions of both hyperoxia and hypoxia, the typical reduction in pace in the middle of short-term endurance trials may not solely be due to peripheral fatigue. They suggested that it must be due to a central governor that allows for a capacity to be retained, which then allows for an increase in muscle fibre recruitment and power output towards the final stage of the exercise trial.

Dietary Factors   Tucker and Noakes (2009) reviewed a number of dietary intervention studies that manipulated the availability and use of carbohydrate and fat during exercise. They concluded that the influence of a central governor on pacing strategy changes was difficult to determine because of the variability of participants' responses. However, they did cite a study by Rauch and colleagues (2005) that revealed that a pre-trial high-carbohydrate diet increased the carbohydrate stores in the exercising muscles of cyclists, compared to cyclists who had a normal diet. The high-carbohydrate group also demonstrated a better 1-hour time trial performance. The researchers reported that the cyclists on the normal diet demonstrated a lower power output than those in the high-carbohydrate group did, from the onset of the time trial. They suggested the presence of an anticipatory response, because it was too early in the exercise bout for carbohydrate levels in the muscles to have become depleted. Indeed, the reduced power output in the normal diet trial had begun during the first minute of exercise! At the end of the 1-hour trials, similar muscle carbohydrate levels occurred in both groups, which the researchers suggested was due to exercise regulation to ensure a critical level of muscle carbohydrate stores at the end of the bout. This implies that the carbohydrate levels were monitored by chemoreceptors and that afferent nerves sent information back to the brain to interpret the fuel usage rate and set a muscle activation rate to ensure sufficient fuel for the remaining part of the trial.

Feedback Manipulation   Markus Amann (2011) suggested that the central nervous system (brain and spinal cord) processes afferent feedback from the contracting muscles and then regulates the remaining exercise by adjusting central motor drive to the contracting muscles. This ensures that peripheral fatigue develops only to a level termed the individual critical threshold, beyond which the associated sensory feedback would not be tolerable. This hypothesis was put forward for high-intensity, whole-body endurance exercise, such as cycling for 5 km. Amman and co-investigators have conducted a series of studies challenging their hypothesis. In one study, Amman and Dempsey (2008) studied the effects of around 10 minutes of severely fatiguing, moderately fatiguing or no fatiguing exercise prior to a 5 km cycling time trial. They found that the greater the level of pre-existing fatigue experienced by the participants prior to the 5 km time trial was, the greater was the subsequent reduction in the activation of their vastus lateralis leg muscle and the slower was their speed in the 5 km time trial that followed. This 'dose-dependent' reduction in the electrical activation of the leg muscles suggested that a reduction in the central motor drive of the participants was proportional to the level of the pre-existing fatigue. The researchers also found similar levels of peripheral fatigue at the end of each 5 km time trial, measured using femoral (leg) nerve stimulation tests, suggesting that the participants' muscle fibres had attained a similar level of impairment in terms of their ability to produce force by the end of the trial. The researchers concluded that the central nervous system had adjusted the level of central motor drive to account for the level of pre-existing fatigue to ensure that a similar level of peripheral fatigue was reached by the end of each trial.

To put these findings into a real-world context such as a cycling time trial, it would appear that the more a cyclist is fatigued prior to the start of a cycling time trial, the greater the reduction in the cyclist's race pace would be—and the change in pace would be evident from the outset of the race. The athlete's brain seems to adjust the pacing template (or algorithm) from the start of the time trial, based on the level of pre-existing fatigue, to set a rate of central motor drive that allows the athlete to complete the trial without prematurely fatiguing. Interestingly, in the Amman and Dempsey (2008) study, the participants demonstrated an end spurt in each of the 5 km trials starting at about the same point (3.5 to 4 km), albeit to varying degrees depending on the level of pre-existing level of fatigue. This finding demonstrates that in each trial participants maintained a physiological reserve well beyond the midpoint of the trial, allowing the central motor drive to then be increased during the last 20 to 30 per cent of the 5 km trial. Evidence for the increase in the central motor drive came from the increases found in the electrical activity of the participants' leg muscles, measured by iEMG.

In a later study, Amann and colleagues (2009) used fentanyl, an opioid analgesic, injected in the lumbar spine (L3/L4) to selectively block afferent nerve feedback from the muscles (it would not affect the brain's central motor drive to the contracting muscles). The subjects completed one 5 km cycling time trial with fentanyl and then another with a saline placebo injected instead. With the fentanyl blocking the normal sensory feedback, a greater power output was exhibited by the study participants at the start of the trial, and subsequently a greater degree of peripheral fatigue ensued as compared to the placebo trial, suggesting that the central motor drive was appreciably more active. The researchers concluded that blocking the afferent feedback allowed participants to exercise beyond their normal individual critical thresholds.

Assorted Interventions   Further evidence that a central governor exists to regulate the pacing strategy has been critically reviewed by Noakes (2011). This review cites evidence from many studies to support the concept of a central governor model in terms of how exercise performance is affected by various challenges and interventions, including drugs that act on the central nervous system, placebos, deception of time and distance covered, self-belief, the presence of other competitors, mental fatigue, sleep deprivation, monetary reward and music. Because these challenges and interventions affect predominantly the central nervous system, they point to a central governor controlling exercise regulation. In addition, Noakes cites other studies that demonstrate that an end spurt is possible because a reserve in skeletal muscle recruitment is available at the end of exercise, and that afferent feedback and anticipatory control influence exercise performance and the end spurt. The interested reader is referred to this article for further details of the studies involved.

Is the Central Governor Fallible?

The anticipatory central governor model theory has been widely debated and criticised on a number of levels (Hopkins 2009; Levine 2008; Shepherd 2009). Some have argued that athletes will push themselves to exhaustion during significant races such as the Olympic Games and risk not only a catastrophic deterioration in race performance but also their health (Hopkins 2009). For example, American football players have died from hyperthermia while exerting themselves on the field, and endurance runners have suffered myocardial fibrosis during ultra-distance races such as the Comrades Marathon (Shepherd 2009). It has been argued that these clinically dangerous events provide evidence that a central governor might not exist, or at least if it does, that it cannot control exercise exertion effectively in all situations.

A study by Amann and colleagues (2007) suggests that the central governor model is conservative in terms of exercise performance in the presence of a life-threatening situation. They reported that when participants cycled to exhaustion while breathing in a reduced level of oxygen, they were unable to exercise beyond approximately 2 minutes. However, when they exercised to exhaustion breathing in normal levels of oxygen, they could last for around 10 minutes at the same fixed power output (333 ± 9 W). What was surprising about the study was that at exhaustion the participants in the reduced oxygen trial demonstrated only two-thirds of the level of peripheral fatigue that participants in the normal oxygen level trial demonstrated. This suggests that the participants terminated their exercise in the low oxygen trial with a reserve remaining, likely in their anaerobic capacity. The researchers concluded that this rather conservative level of exhaustion might have been due to the threat of a shortfall in oxygen to the brain (cerebral hypoxemia) being a higher priority than the afferent feedback from the muscles. As a result, the brain chose to reduce its activation of the muscles (i.e., central motor drive) prematurely. Indeed, when the researchers added in supplemental oxygen at higher-than-normal levels (i.e., 30 per cent oxygen content in the air rather than the normal 20.9 per cent) after exhaustion was reached by the participants in both trials, they observed that the participants could not exercise anymore when they had just finished the normal oxygen trial but they could do so having just completed the low oxygen trial. Indeed, the participants then exercised until they reached the same level of peripheral fatigue as did those in the normal oxygen trial at exhaustion. This confirmed that a reserve had been present following the low oxygen part of the trial and that afferent feedback from the muscles had been prioritised to a lower degree than afferent feedback from chemoreceptors informing the brain about low oxygen levels.

If a central governor does exist, then it is clearly fallible. For example, even experienced athletes exhibit misjudgements in race pacing. This is particularly evident in races lasting between 30 seconds and a few minutes. In races of this duration, the pace is often positive, meaning that the athlete sets off at a fast speed and then slows down over the race. An infallible central governor would anticipate fatigue ahead of time and reduce muscle activation progressively to avoid a catastrophic deterioration in performance and optimise performance. However, it is common in short, positively paced races for a sudden, rather 'catastrophic' drop-off in speed to occur as a result of a miscalculation of pace. This would surely not occur if a central governor were solely acting. In fact, if the central governor were infallible, it would precisely sense, through afferent feedback from chemoreceptors, the rate at which peripheral fatigue was developing at the contracting muscles and command the fatiguing muscles to reduce their activity *before* fatigue had developed to such an extent that a dramatic fall in the racing speed occurs leading to a suboptimal performance. In reality, athletes often suffer significant fatigue in races because of incorrect pacing. Therefore, it seems quite possible that peripheral fatigue can develop so rapidly that a central governor cannot *always* react sufficiently quickly to adjust the athlete's pace prior to a catastrophic deterioration in performance.

It would appear that there can be a delay in the brain receiving and interpreting feedback from the sensory receptors, which leads to the brain delaying an amendment to the pacing strategy. In short-distance events, this can result in the adjustment in pace, through a reduction in central motor drive, coming too late to stave off significant fatigue and circumvent a poor performance. Evidence of this comes from a recent study by Henslin-Harris and colleagues (2013). They had participants undertake three 3 km cycling time trials. In one trial the participants breathed in normal air, in a second trial they began to breathe air with low oxygen content 3 minutes before the trial started and in the third trial they began to breathe in air with low oxygen content just as they began the time trial. Interestingly, the cyclists demonstrated the same starting pace in all three trials despite the low oxygen levels in two of the trials, and only after approximately 40 seconds of exercise did the power output decrease in the two low oxygen trials compared to the normal oxygen trial. This demonstrates that there was a delay, when the exercise began, before afferent feedback from carotid bodies (containing chemoreceptors) close to the heart's arteries informed the brain of low oxygen levels and led to a reduction in muscle activation to produce a more conservative pace.

Perhaps another explanation for the occasional catastrophic deterioration in performance is that the athlete is so motivated or emotional during a competitive race that the central governor is somehow overruled perhaps by a deeper, more primitive part of the brain. Even in longer events in which peripheral fatigue does not develop rapidly, athletes can terminate a race prematurely as a result of overwhelming symptoms of exhaustion. Some even collapse some distance before the finish line. It is certainly reasonable to assume that the feedback provided by afferent nerves from sensory receptors is assimilated at various levels of the spine and brain to elicit homeostatic control resulting in changes to movement. However, it is also likely that strong psychological drives in athletes result in a catastrophic failure to pace correctly, which then leads to a loss of muscle function (force production and coordinated contraction) and a poor race performance or even a non-finish. In extreme circumstances an abnormally high level of effort by an athlete can manifest in the athlete collapsing during the race. In some cases athletes suffer significant health threats as a result of exercise. The potential drivers for such an event might be a pre-existing clinical condition; however, this could also indicate a loss of homeostasis and physiological function, perhaps brought about by psychological drives that compel the athlete to override the controlling influence of the central governor (St Clair Gibson et al. 2013).

Conclusion

Some general agreement is emerging among sport scientists that the pacing strategy is organised in an anticipatory manner, in part to optimise performance but also to prevent large homeostatic disturbances during the exercise (de Koning et al. 2011). That said, in all-out races and sometimes in short races, peripheral fatigue develops and limits further exercise seemingly independently of the central governor's control. In agreement with the central governor model, de Koning and colleagues (2011) used the analogy of the body being rather like a race car in which the driver (the brain) monitors various gauges (such as the internal temperature gauge illustrated in figure 3.2) to see how the car is running. However, depending on the length of the race, the driver may monitor one gauge more than another. In the human body, the anaerobic capacity and oxygen delivery gauges might be critical in events lasting from a few seconds to 40 minutes or so, whereas the core temperature and heat storage gauges might be more critical in hot races that last 15 minutes to a number of hours. The carbohydrate availability gauge would be monitored closely in long-distance events of 90 minutes or more. Motivation and muscle damage gauges would become increasingly important in multistage races taking many days to complete.

A person's rating of perceived exertion (RPE) might be a surrogate for most of these gauges when the afferent feedback is integrated by the conscious brain (de Koning et al. 2011). The RPE at a particular point in time has been suggested to reflect the disturbance to homeostasis, because homeostasis becomes increasingly difficult for the body to maintain as a race progresses and this coincides with the RPE rising. Consequently, the athlete's RPE is a reflection of what the athlete is experiencing during the exercise. However researchers are now also suggesting that RPE might reflect what the athlete feels he should be experiencing as well. Hence, if the RPE is high but there is still a long way to go, the athlete will slow down; conversely, if the RPE is below expectations, the athlete may well speed up. Based on this principle, a hazard score has been put forward, which is simply the RPE at a given moment multiplied by the race distance remaining (de Koning et al. 2011).

In a study of cyclists and runners, de Koning and colleagues (2011) demonstrated that changes in racing velocity mirrored changes in the hazard score: participants accelerated when their hazard scores were low and decelerated when they were high. The mental side of pacing is therefore clearly significant, and there is no doubt that athletes can even choose to ignore their afferent feedback and hazard score if sufficiently motivated and emotional. However, this often leads to a large change in homeostasis, a catastrophic misjudgement of pace and a significant loss of performance in a race. Therefore, overriding the central governor should, perhaps, happen only at the very end of the race; otherwise, fatigue will ensue prematurely, and the athlete will slow down too much before the end.

chapter 4

Psychology of Pacing

Richard J. Keegan, PhD

This chapter offers a unique and forward-looking overview of the psychological factors in the pacing of sport. It illustrates the relevance of mental factors to pacing, outlines the key considerations in the current literature, reviews the neuropsychology of pacing and examines the psychological techniques and strategies that may assist athletes in pacing. The cutting-edge nature of this area means that the conclusion is a resounding 'we don't know enough about this yet to offer concrete, guaranteed advice'. However, two very meaningful implications emerge. First, researchers have a tremendous opportunity to describe, test and understand the complex ways psychology and physiology interact in determining an athlete's pacing. Second, athletes and coaches who are willing to try some of the techniques that are coming to light may be able to gain a (legal) competitive advantage while the rest of the world tries to catch up. Key considerations in the psychology of pacing are explained, and the most promising options for athletes wishing to improve their pacing are presented.

Whether one believes that fatigue is a purely physical phenomenon, a mental experience or both, it is almost impossible to conceive of a model of pacing that does not involve some form of psychological input. The accumulation of metabolites in muscles or, for example, a slight change in the pH of the blood as carbon dioxide accrues causes the sensation of pain. This signal is interpreted by the athlete (e.g., as tolerable, intolerable, catastrophic), who then chooses how to respond (e.g., stop, carry on, ease off).

Let's consider a real-life example. As a sport psychologist, I once worked with a high-performing amateur cyclist who had been unable to train properly because of work commitments. His concerned family questioned his ability to participate in a long-distance endurance race. His response was noteworthy: 'I'll be fine; I know how to suffer better than anyone'. It was a striking sentiment. When questioned further, he explained that he knew his lack of fitness would take him to the 'place of suffering' earlier than others, but that he could 'live' there longer than anyone. As a result, he expected to be near the front of the peloton as they approached the finish, at which point he felt it would be anybody's race.

Many blogs by endurance athletes in cycling, swimming, triathlon and other endurance sports speak about how deliberately seeking, experiencing, managing and even enjoying suffering is a necessary component of success in the sport. According to this approach, pain signals reach the brain, and how you interpret them and respond will ultimately determine how successful you can be.

AT A GLANCE　**Tapping What's Left in the Tank**

Consider the following example of pushing through physical discomfort. As part of an Introduction to Sport Psychology workshop, I regularly ask for three brave volunteers to participate in a game. I make a point of warning them that it will involve some physical exertion. I inform the volunteers that the game is quite simple: Participants are to do the absolute maximal number of press-ups they can do. To be sure that 100 per cent effort has been put forth, I challenge participants to look me in the eye and promise they can't possibly do any more, adding, 'I'm a psychologist, so I'll know if you're lying!' I really push them on this point, and many are then able to do a few more. After establishing that none of the three participants could *possibly* do another press-up, I tell them, 'Well, I guess I forgot to say—the winner is the person who can do 10 more press-ups from *this point on!*' In five years of conducting this demonstration, I have never had participants perform fewer than 25 additional press-ups among them (nor have I been forcibly ejected from the building—yet!). With the right motivation, a simple act of willpower allows athletes to overrule the message from their muscles that they are 'spent'.

So we have some nice examples of how psychology pertains to pacing and fatigue, but what does the literature say? How can thoughts and emotions override physical sensations of exhaustion, or manage the body so that exhaustion never occurs?

We also have an important lesson emerging from these examples, which is that the subjective experience of fatigue (in particular) and pacing (more generally) involves the management of the pain, discomfort and negative emotions or feelings generated when we push our bodies to perform at or beyond their maximum. Studies examining 'mental toughness' in sport (Clough, Earle & Sewell 2002), as well as websites and interviews with elite athletes, suggest that accepting and even embracing such suffering is a vital aspect of learning how to pursue sporting excellence. Viewing such suffering as undesirable, and to be avoided, is not an attitude displayed by elite athletes.

Another key element of the psychology of pacing is the accuracy of one's perceptions: Athletes frequently believe that they have tried just as hard, and suffered just as much, as on any other day, and yet their performance may have been diminished. This chapter examines both the way we perceive bodily sensations around fatigue and pacing, and the ways psychology can help to manage the body to ensure peak performance when it really matters.

Central Versus Peripheral Fatigue

For a long time, the research examining fatigue (the point at which performance declines involuntarily) has been dominated by physiological interpretations: usually based on the belief that the mind is powerless to control fatigue once it occurs. In this view, the mind is cast as a passive observer of events. The perspective that fatigue occurs in the muscles has resulted in the term *peripheral fatigue*, and for over 50 years one very influential experiment effectively won the argument that fatigue is peripheral.

Merton (1954) attempted to distinguish between *central* and *peripheral* fatigue by inducing exhaustion in a muscle group through repeated maximal voluntary contractions (MVCs). At this point, as performance dropped off, electrodes were used to stimulate the muscles during contraction. Interesting hypotheses were offered. One was that if the electrical stimulation increased the force of contraction, the muscles, exhausted from the MVC test, must have been receiving less stimulation (and once more stimulation was provided directly via the electrodes, the strength of the contraction would increase). This hypothesis lent credence to the theory of a central influence. If, however, the contraction force remained depleted, then the hypothesis was that the fatigue must be in the muscle itself (i.e., the muscles were so fatigued they simply could not contract again, even with a direct stimulation), which supported the peripheral fatigue theory. The stimulation did not alter the performance of the muscles, and so peripheral fatigue was supported. This study convinced many people that physiology holds the key to fatigue.

However, two vital caveats must be highlighted. First, the Merton study has not been consistently replicated. In fact, when researchers use techniques such as magnetic resonance imaging (MRI) and electromyography (EMG) to assess which parts of a muscle are activated during exercise, voluntary recruitment seems to be limited to 85 to 90 per cent for strength tasks, with electrical stimulation being needed to recruit the remaining power (Herbert & Gandevia 1996). Likewise, Tucker and colleagues (2004) and Amann and colleagues (2006) reported a 35 to 50 per cent limit to the voluntary recruitment of the active muscle mass being recruited during prolonged exercise. During maximal exercise this increases to only about 60 per cent (Albertus 2008; Sloniger et al. 1997a, 1997b). Second, and very important, we almost never push ourselves to absolute exhaustion during sport; rather, we pace ourselves and (unavoidably?) ease off well before a catastrophic failure occurs (Tucker 2009).

A contrasting viewpoint was offered by Marcora, Staiano and Manning (2009), who asked participants to undertake a fixed-load exercise-to-exhaustion test on a standing cycle, after either viewing a neutral video (*The History of Ferrari: The Definitive Story*, Boulevard Entertainment 2006) or undertaking a mentally fatiguing computer task (the AX-CPT; Carter et al. 1998), which placed heavy demands on attention and working memory. Participants who were mentally fatigued by the computer task were unable to maintain exercise as long as those who watched the video, and they rated their perceived exertion (RPE; Borg 1982) as much higher throughout the task (even quite early on), relative to the control group. This reduced performance and increased perceptions of exertion occurred despite the fact that their physiological markers were either unchanged (oxygen uptake) or reduced (heart rate, blood lactate) relative to their pre-test. In this case, mental fatigue led to impaired physical performance, even though there was no physiological reason for this impairment. These findings suggest an important role for the central regulation of exercise and pacing. At the very least, someone who is tired after a long day at work or poor sleep may not be able to produce a personal best performance (even though she may feel as though she tried just as hard as on any other day).

The reality, of course, is that making a distinction between the mental and the physical (dualism) is quite misleading (Edwards & Polman 2012). Real-life physiological performance does not involve stimulating muscles with electrodes without any brain to manage or interpret the signals, nor can a brain drive muscles to contract maximally once they contain an imbalance of the necessary metabolites. There does not appear to be any particular region of the brain devoted solely to regulating fatigue and pacing (the following section will outline several), and there does not appear to be an all-knowing but subconscious central governor acting independently of consciousness (Hill, Long & Lupton 1924; Noakes 1997). Likewise, with sufficient direction and training, a person can become aware of many aspects of how to perceive and manage fatigue, and this may actually be an important aspect of learning how to pace oneself. Arguably, if we were to accurately pin down a central governor for pacing exercise, it would be the whole brain, and it would need to be a brain attached to a body from which it can receive and process signals, store memories of sensations and their meaning, send responses and record the consequences of each action or inaction (e.g., relieved or increased discomfort). Although some of the effects of fatigue occur in the muscles and some occur in the brain, the totality of the system they form, and its oversight by conscious thought and decision making, appear to be inseparable when we consider the pacing of sporting performances.

Neuropsychology of Fatigue

The world of neuroscience was shaken up recently when a detailed analysis by Button and colleagues (2013) demonstrated a strong tendency to 'over-interpret' signals from MRI and CAT scans as indications that certain brain areas have specific roles. In particular, issues were raised about the use of small samples and the way equipment is set up and subsequently interpreted—particularly after a dead salmon (used to calibrate a machine) returned a signal (Bennett et al. 2010)! More realistically, brain regions are often involved in several tasks, often seemingly unrelated, and a signal in the scanner can indicate activation, inhibition, increased blood flow, and more, and so each observation needs to be interpreted cautiously. Notwithstanding these caveats, we can cautiously suggest that the brain areas discussed in the following section and neural processes do appear to be associated with pacing and fatigue.

Brain Mapping

Sitting on either side of the central sulcus (a fold in the brain that spans from ear to ear) are areas of sensory cortex and motor cortex that either perceive or stimulate their respective body areas. These two brain regions appear to correlate directly to particular body areas, although more brain tissue is devoted to sensing and controlling the hands and face (mouth and tongue) than to any other regions, because of the complex tasks they perform. The sensory cortex receives and processes signals from the body, including the muscles, and the motor cortex (which consists of several smaller areas) sends signals to the muscles (sometimes termed the central motor drive). However, the ability of these areas to either perceive or stimulate their respective muscles groups appears to be moderated (both inhibited and encouraged) by processes occurring elsewhere. Located centrally, between the spine and cortex, the thalamus acts as a kind of relay station. The insular cortex, two areas of cortex located on either side of the brain in deep folds underneath the temple, appear to be responsible for monitoring sensations of exertion. The anterior cingulate cortex, an area deep inside the frontal lobe, on the inner surface of the central fissure (a front-to-back split between the two hemispheres of the brain), is linked to motivation, attention and error detection (Williamson et al. 2006).

Using a pedalling task and functional magnetic resonance imaging (fMRI), Mehta and colleagues (2009) found *all* of the preceding areas to be involved during normal exercise. However, regarding the decision to terminate exercise as a result of fatigue, Hilty and colleagues (2011a) found increased activation of the insular region immediately prior to termination. Following this, Hilty and colleagues (2011b) found evidence for increased communication between the insular and the motor cortex during fatiguing exercise, suggesting perhaps that the insular cortex may inhibit the motor cortex's attempts to 'drive' the fatiguing muscles. In a study of the key difference between athletes and non-athletes, Paulus and colleagues (2011) reported that marked activation of *both* insular regions and the anterior cingulate gyrus suggests a clear response to an unpleasant task. However, trained athletes demonstrate a much lower response in the right insular cortex, which may be related to their ability to push themselves harder or longer (most likely an adaptation following training).

The most recent attempt to model the pacing process suggests that physical fatigue (and pacing) may be regulated by the balance between separate inhibitory and facilitatory systems influencing the motor cortex. Tanaka and Watanabe (2012) proposed an *inhibitory* neural pathway that connects the spinal cord, thalamus, somatosensory cortex, insular cortex, anterior cingulate cortex and movement control areas; as well as a *facilitatory* pathway that connects the limbic system, basal ganglia, thalamus, frontal cortex, anterior cingulate cortex and movement control areas. In their model, motivation stimulates the facilitatory system, but not the inhibitory one. Notably, several of the areas that appear to be active in pacing and fatigue are also central to motivational processes, including the anterior cingulate cortex and the ('orbito') frontal cortex (Reeve 2009). This evidence suggests that properly motivated athletes may be able to drive this facilitatory pathway to either outstrip or at least match the inhibitory influences (from fatigue and pain), and thus produce improved power or endurance, or both.

Neurochemical Activation

It is clear that (neuro)chemicals are involved in pain, motivation, fatigue and pacing. These substances can sit between nerves in the brain or body and either transmit signals or amplify, inhibit or even block signals. As an example, chemicals known as endorphins (often released during exercise) can prevent the transmission of pain signals, thereby reducing the experience of pain. The release of endorphins is thought to be responsible for the 'runner's high' that results from long, strenuous exercise (Boecker et al. 2008).

Boosting   AT A GLANCE

Endorphins also play a role in the controversial practice of 'boosting' employed by some Paralympic athletes (Karlsson 1999; Marsh & Weaver 2004). Technically termed induced autonomic dysreflexia, the practice refers to the process of causing trauma to a paralysed limb—through electric shocks or deliberately breaking small bones, for example—to benefit from the body's response, including increased endorphins, adrenaline and blood pressure (Magnay 2012). The practice is extremely dangerous and can cause strokes or heart attacks (Valles et al. 2005), but it illustrates one way knowledge of neurological responses can be (ab)used in sport.

Returning to motivation and the idea of willpower, a key line of research suggests that tasks requiring willpower consume a limited resource of glucose in the brain—for example, by showing that blood glucose drops after tasks requiring effortful self-control, and that this drop leads to subsequent failures in the task (DeWall et al. 2008; Gailliot et al. 2009). In particular, these authors found that glucose supplements can boost self-control and willpower (reviewed by Hagger et al. 2010). However, recent studies have questioned this by showing that using but not consuming carbohydrate 'mouth rinses' can also boost self-control in tasks requiring persistence and willpower (e.g., Molden et al. 2012). This suggests that the taste may fool the body into allowing more glucose into the brain, without necessarily needing to eat or drink it (Beedie & Lane 2012). Alternatively, it may be that the pleasurable experience of a sweet drink releases a chemical called dopamine in key motivation-linked areas of the brain (Painelli, Nicastro & Lancha 2010). In truth, most (if not all) athletes drink glucose- or carbohydrate-containing drinks before, during and after competition, so this may not be an area in which a competitive advantage can be easily gained.

Given that the experiences of pain, discomfort and exhaustion are important in the study of fatigue and pacing, it is worth noting that the release of (neuro)chemicals in the brain is highly relevant to these sensations. For example, in sufferers of depression, chronic pain, headaches or migraines and chronic fatigue (among others conditions), imbalances in these chemicals are often involved (e.g., Fitzgerald & Carter 2012; Shabbir et al. 2013). As such, feelings of fatigue or pain may be unnecessarily strong and unpleasant when the brain regions that process this information are incorrectly excited or inhibited by imbalances in these chemicals. The science of studying these influences is incredibly complex. and so real-life implications remain elusive. However, we do know that sleep deprivation (e.g., Bettendorff et al. 1996) and poor diet (Chang, Ke & Chen 2009; Lopresti, Hood & Drummond 2013) can also cause similar imbalances. Hence, athletes must focus on sleep and nutrition to support not just their physical capacity, but also their mental faculties.

Neurodoping

A very recent development in neuropsychology is the use of noninvasive stimulation techniques such as transcranial direct current stimulation (tDCS) and transcranial magnetic stimulation (TMS) to provoke activity in certain brain areas. For example, in TMS a powerful electromagnetic coil is positioned over the brain, which when quickly switched on and off stimulates the neurons in that region. The technique can be used to make people move an arm involuntarily or slur their speech in the same way that inserting a metal electrode into that region might do. These effects can also be used to catalyse (i.e., speed up) learning in sports, such that athletes may be able to learn the meaning of their physiological signals more quickly (Davis 2013).

Davis (2013) noted that studies demonstrating improvements in time to fatigue, response time and tremor suppression are highly relevant to sport. One study demonstrated that cyclists who received just 20 minutes of tDCS on the insula region obtained a 4 per cent improvement in peak power output (Okano et al. 2013). This technique is very difficult to detect and does not involve introducing synthetic chemicals into the body, yet it still seems to be inconsistent with the spirit of sport. The occurrence of side effects also remains relatively unknown, because only small groups of vetted participants are usually involved in these studies. As such, it represents a new and unique challenge for governing bodies to define and regulate.

Overall, however, neuroscience may not be of interest to healthy athletes who eat and sleep well, who are unwilling to effectively torture themselves (boosting) and who cannot afford (or are unwilling to risk) 'zapping' their own brains. Athletes and coaches may find the following sections, which outline specific psychological techniques for monitoring and managing pacing in sport, more useful.

Subjective Assessments and Expectations

To make the subjective experience of exercise more objective, Borg (1982) suggested a scale for recording participants' rating of perceived exertion (RPE). The most common methods of measuring the RPE are Borg's 6–20 Category Scale (1998) and the Category-Ratio-10 scale (CR-10; Borg 1982). In these scoring systems, athletes are asked to indicate their perceptions of exertion on scales ranging from 'no exertion at all' to 'maximal exertion' and to consider their overall experience, rather than focusing on one particular area or feeling.

As summarised by Eston (2012), RPE involves the collective integration of afferent feedback from cardiorespiratory, metabolic and thermal stimuli to enable people to evaluate how difficult an exercise task feels at any point in time. Although it links reliably to physiological measures such as core body temperature (Hampson et al. 2001; Rasmussen et al. 2004), RPE is moderated by psychological factors and situational factors such as duration (Pires et al. 2011), temperature (Crewe, Tucker & Noakes 2008) and altitude (oxygen availability) (Johnson et al. 2009). RPE measurements at low-to-moderate levels of exertion are a good predictor of maximal performance in various activities involving both aerobic and anaerobic energy-producing pathways (Coquart et al. 2012; Davies, Rowlands & Eston 2008).

Parfitt, Evans and Eston (2012) recently used RPE alone to guide an exercise programme. Participants were asked to limit their exertion to 'moderately hard' (RPE 13/20). A 17 per cent increase in $\dot{V}O_2$max was observed over the self-paced eight-week treadmill training programme, yet the average exercise intensity produced was quite reliable: 61 per cent of $\dot{V}O_2$max in week 1 and 64 per cent of $\dot{V}O_2$max in week 8. Participants were unaware of treadmill speed, heart rate or any other measures of intensity, and so this study offers meaningful evidence that RPE is a useful indicator of training intensity and effectiveness.

Although these studies capture the use of RPE as a summary function of all the physical and mental perceptions feeding back to the brain, there is also evidence that RPE relates to expectations and feeds forward in terms of planned future exertion based on knowledge of the end point of an exercise challenge or race. During prolonged submaximal exercise to exhaustion, RPE rises in direct relation to the total exercise duration (Horstman et al. 1979). As such, the *rate* at which RPE increases should be (and frequently is) a strong predictor of when participants will voluntarily cease the activity (Al-Rahamneh & Eston 2011; Eston 2012; Faulkner, Parfitt & Eston 2008; Marcora & Staiano 2010). Likewise, knowing exactly when the exercise will end has been shown to affect RPE progression and changes (Swart et al. 2009). Moreover, deliberately deceiving participants about the end point disrupts the linear increase in RPE (as well as causing irritation, anxiety or discomfort) even in the absence of increased heart rate or oxygen uptake (Baden et al. 2005; Eston et al. 2012). Hence, there is a strong argument that RPE is based on the athlete's expectations of duration and difficulty—a kind of template derived from experience (Tucker 2009) that is constantly being negotiated and renegotiated in light of the ongoing experience.

Two's Company?   AT A GLANCE

To examine the effects of pacemakers, teammates and chasers in running, Bath and colleagues (2011) looked at the use of a second runner who would run in front of, behind or alongside the subject. Impact on 5 km time, heart rate and rating of perceived exertion (RPE) were measured, and subjective assessments of pace were gathered. They noted no differences between the time, heart rate and RPE scores obtained when running with the second runner and when running alone, regardless of the position of the second runner. However, despite the identical performances and RPE scores, all 11 participants believed that they had run faster with the second runner, and 9 of the 11 found running with the second runner to be easier.

This ongoing anticipatory process known as *teleoanticipation* (introduced in chapters 1 and 3), involves constantly comparing existing knowledge about the expected end point and previous experiences of exertion to determine current effort levels. The training of teleoanticipation arguably forms the first psychological strategy for improving pacing. Deliberately working on teleoanticipation involves explicitly building a good knowledge base of various exercise intensities and the associated experiences and effects they produce. To inform teleoanticipation, athletes must build an awareness of their personal limits and the associated experiences and sensations. This might include deliberately going under and over the preferred pacing strategy to test their limits—even if this were to involve occasionally pushing too hard and recording a poor time or result (preferably not at meaningful competitions!). In addition to changes in intensity or duration, athletes may wish to experience various conditions such as hot and cold temperatures, high and low altitude or high and low humidity.

Athletes' knowledge of their capabilities under various circumstances is extremely valuable and, most likely, hard-won. It is not something you can buy or be told in a class, because the information is deeply personal: Only you can experience what it feels like when your body undergoes each specific challenge. A mountaineer should not attempt Everest with psychological tricks alone (i.e., no training or conditioning). Along the same lines, the following discussion of such strategies is provided with a view to complementing, not replacing, substantive training efforts.

Why do so many athletes struggle inexplicably at their first big events (e.g., Olympics, World Cup), despite having trained for them? Many have no frame of reference in their internal template as to how this level of competition should feel. As a result, they may be fooled into trying too hard or underestimate the mental exhaustion caused by excitement, media, the need to manage tickets for family, and so on. This may be the reason many athletes are encouraged to participate in big events when they are young and still developing, rather than wait until they are completely 'ready'—just to get the experience.

Psychological Effects and Strategies

When considering the relationship between body and mind in managing fatigue and pacing, we must also consider psychological influences. This area includes a mixture of effects such as the placebo effect and priming, which can be quite difficult to self-manage, and strategies such as self-talk and mental imagery, which are often deliberately deployed by athletes to boost performance. This section presents an overview of these effects and strategies, including their possible links to fatigue and pacing.

Placebo Effect

No discussion of the psychology of fatigue and pacing, which involves perceiving and managing pain and discomfort, would be complete without a consideration of the placebo effect. Put simply, when patients are given substances with no pharmacological effects (such as sugar or saline), yet are manipulated into expecting some benefit (e.g., pain relief), they frequently experience the expected benefit even though the pill or injection used could not possibly have generated that benefit. The patient generates the benefit, often through very complex mechanisms (Benedetti et al. 2005). There is no placebo effect if the patient does not expect some sort of treatment or benefit: Expectation is key (Colloca et al. 2004).

Placebo effects can be very strong. Kirsch and Sapirstein's 1998 study showed that placebo groups showed 200 per cent improvement in depression symptoms over non-treatment groups, although placebos are not as effective as drugs in treating depression. Nobody is immune to the effect, although certain conditions are more responsive than others. Hence, although a placebo effect cannot cure cancer, it appears to be highly effective in reducing pain and affective imbalances such as depression and fatigue.

Perhaps most interesting, the pain-reducing effects of a placebo can be blocked with naxolone, a drug that blocks opioid receptors, which indicates that a placebo can trigger the body to release its own endogenous opioids (Amanzio & Benedetti 1998; Colloca & Benedetti 2005; Levine, Gordon & Fields 1978). To be clear, the pain-reducing effects of a placebo—a psychological intervention—can be blocked via a drug that prevents opioid receptors from being stimulated by the endogenous opioids that were released as a result of the placebo. This clearly suggests that the placebo stimulated the production of endogenous opioids.

These reductions in pain perceptions may allow an athlete to persist at higher levels of exertion for longer or to produce more powerful one-off efforts (Beedie 2007). One very famous example comes from Vogt (1999), who (in an ethically questionable situation) tricked French cyclist Richard Virenque into believing that he had taken a stimulant by injecting him with vitamin C. Other examples include skin-contact patches, various types of bracelets and wristbands, some forms of alternative medicines and even certain taping techniques.

Nocebo Effect

The 'nocebo' effect is the opposite of the placebo effect; it occurs when a person's belief causes negative effects. Perhaps the most famous illustration of a nocebo effect is the story of Vance Vanders' near-death experience.

The story goes that late one night in a small Alabama cemetery, Vanders 'crossed' the local witch doctor, who cast a spell, including the use of an unpleasant-smelling liquid, and told him he would die in a month.

At home that night, Vanders felt ill and went to bed early, and his deterioration began. Three weeks later, emaciated and 'circling the drain', he was admitted to hospital. Doctors were unable to find a cause for his symptoms. Vanders was dying. In desperation, his wife told the doctor, Drayton Doherty, of the incident.

The next morning Doherty called the family to Vance's bedside. He told them that he had lured the witch doctor back to the cemetery, fought with him and forced him to explain how the curse worked. The witch doctor said that he had rubbed lizard eggs into Vanders' stomach. One of them had hatched and was eating Vanders from the inside out. Doherty said he had forced the man to provide him with the remedy. *The entire story was fabricated.*

Doherty then summoned a nurse, who had been asked to prepare an injection that would make Vanders vomit (an emetic). While Vanders was vomiting, Doherty slipped a toy rubber lizard into the bucket. 'Look what has come out of you, Vance!' he shouted. 'The voodoo curse is lifted'.

Vanders did a double-take, lurched backwards into the bed and then drifted into a deep sleep. When he woke the next day, he was alert and ravenous. He quickly regained his strength and was discharged a week later.

Adapted from H. Pitcher, 2009, "The new witch doctors: How belief can kill," *New Scientist* 202(2078): 30-33.

The problem with placebos is that, although the device or treatment itself is not doing what it says (some would require new laws of physics to work as advertised!), the athlete may be getting some benefit from the effect it generates. Do we allow the misperception to persist and thus risk undermining science and ethics, or do we play kill-joy and inform the athlete that any benefit he feels is entirely a result of the placebo effect, thereby preventing the beneficial effects from happening? Different practitioners have different answers to this question, and there may not be a universally correct answer. However, it may be worth considering what the consequences would be if an athlete or team discovered the ruse.

Priming and Conditioning

In 1996, Bargh, Chen and Burrows asked volunteers to make sentences out of apparently random lists of words. However, one list contained words we associate with old age (e.g., *grey, shuffleboard, Bingo, cane*), whereas the other list was neutral. Participants who had thought about 'elderly' words subsequently took much longer to walk down the hall to the elevator, despite (when asked) being totally unaware of any effects or instructions to do so. Although it remains unclear exactly what causes this (often replicated) result (Doyen et al. 2012), the lesson in terms of pacing is that athletes can easily be influenced unconsciously into changing how they behave.

Subliminal messaging has been a key theme in advertising for many years (Dijksterhuis, Chartrand & Aarts 2005) and has been linked to improvements in academic performance, memory and learning capacity (Chakalis & Lowe 1992; Cook 1985; Parker 1982). It is possible, therefore, that an athlete primed to overcome pain or discomfort would be more likely to do so than one primed to feel weak or fatigued. Priming may also play a role in placebo effects. Ader and Cohen (1975) used the Pavlov's dog paradigm to associate a flavoured drink with the effects of a drug that suppresses immune responses (used for organ transplants or to reduce inflammatory diseases such as arthritis). After conditioning, blood titres testing for antibodies showed that the drink alone with no drug could suppress the immune response. In applied settings, athletes and coaches should give careful consideration to priming.

How many times do we hear athletes express sentiments such as 'It's gonna be hard today; it's gonna hurt'? What if, through priming, this becomes a self-fulfilling prophecy? Given that priming can be quite deceitful, how far should coaches be prepared to go in using it with athletes? Should they splice images and words conveying strength or endurance into athletes' favourite movies? Is it more realistic to examine the way they behave and speak around their athletes, and to make sure every possible cue they send conveys belief and strength? In the absence of strong studies examining priming in sport pacing, the current best advice may be for coaches to at least consider how their behaviour and language may be priming. Coaches, athletes and psychologists should at least ensure that they are doing no harm to athletes' chances.

Attentional Strategies: Association and Dissociation

Research has identified a key distinction in the way athletes process the feelings of discomfort and pain associated with fatigue and pacing, particularly in endurance events (Goode & Roth 1993; Morgan 1978; Morgan & Pollock 1977). They may either focus on the physical sensations their body generates (e.g., breathing, burning sensations), termed *association*, or they may attempt to divert attention away from these stimuli, termed *dissociation*. Dissociation tactics may include using music to distract or focusing on external surroundings. Morgan (1978) asserted that successful marathon runners would be more likely to use associative strategies because they are more likely to be in tune with their breathing, temperature, hydration, pain level and so on. Martin, Craib and Mitchell (1995) supported this notion by showing that those deploying associative strategies also had the most economical running styles. This means that those who habitually attend to internal stimuli may be better at detecting and reducing discomfort, and thus able to run faster for longer.

Tammen's (1996) findings suggested that elite runners were more likely to use associative coping at higher running speeds than when running slowly. Schomer (1987) also suggested that runners may use dissociative strategies early in a race and use associative strategies later on. However, many successful marathon runners do habitually use dissociative strategies, particularly during training (Masters & Ogles 1998).

Aitcheson and colleagues (2013) examined the contents of thoughts reported by recreational runners at various running speeds and levels of RPE. At low speeds and low RPE, runners reporting thinking about 'personal problem solving' and 'conversational chatter' (dissociative thoughts). However, at higher speeds, and higher RPE, runners reported thinking about 'pace monitoring', 'feelings and affect' and 'body monitoring' (associative thoughts—see figure 4.1). This is another good example of how attentional strategies can vary depending on the pace or level of exertion. It is also an example of the power of self-talk, one of the four classic mental skills strategies outlined later in this chapter.

Overall, where there is a danger of fatiguing too early and 'hitting the wall' (i.e., at longer distances and at higher speeds), associative strategies would appear to be useful for managing and avoiding this risk (Morgan & Pollock 1977). In the absence of conclusive evidence for or against associative and dissociative strategies, athletes should be encouraged to develop both and to keep careful tabs on which works better in specific situations. As an extension of the earlier discussion of teleoanticipation, athletes must become their own scientists.

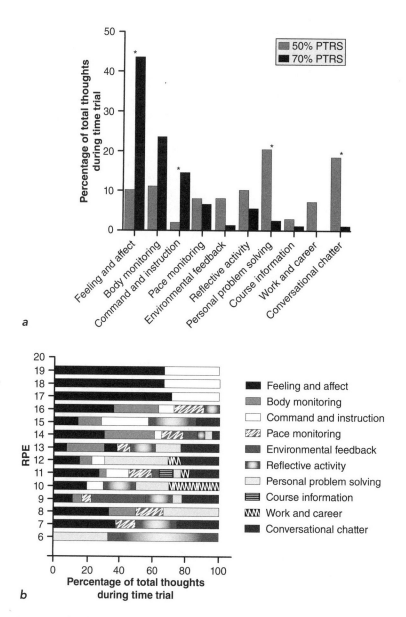

Figure 4.1 Graphs displaying the thoughts reported by runners *(a)* at different running speeds and *(b)* at different RPE.

PTRS = Peak treadmill running speed

Republished with permission of Ammons Scientific, from C. Aitchison, L.A.Turner, L. Ansley, K.G. Thompson, D. Micklewright, and A. St. Clair Gibson, 2013, "Inner dialogue and its relationship to perceived exertion during different running intensities," *Perceptual & Motor Skills: Exercise & Sport* 117(1): 11-30. Permission conveyed through Copyright Clearance Center, Inc.

Mental Skills Training

Four broad categories of intervention have, to a large extent, dominated sport psychology to the point that many believe they are all sport psychology has to offer (Gardner & Moore 2006). These strategies are imagery (Cumming & Ramsey 2009; Holmes & Collins 2001), self-talk (Hardy 2006; Hardy, Oliver & Tod 2009), goal setting (Burton & Naylor 2002; Kingston & Wilson 2009) and arousal control (Murphy, Nordin & Cumming 2008), and each is devoted a chapter in almost all sport psychology textbooks. The following sections briefly review why each intervention could conceivably be applied to pacing.

Imagery   Imagery involves creating an inner experience that mimics real life, using a combination of senses (Cumming & Ramsey 2009). It may be deliberate and purposeful, but it may also include unstructured daydreaming. Explanations of how imagery might work include the psychoneuromuscular theory (e.g., Suinn 1980)—which states that imagery produces low-level activation in the muscles and generates feedback and improved awareness—and several variations of symbolic learning theory (e.g., Ahsen 1984) –which states that imagery allows the person to form important associations; and, for example, practise timings or the ordering of events. An athlete's ability to form clear and vivid images and to control the outcomes of imagery, as well as issues such as the speed of imagery (slowed down or sped up), the environment in which imagery occurs (e.g., relaxed or at pitch-side) and even the degree of accuracy of the athlete's learning (improved technique or understanding) have all been shown to influence the effectiveness of imagery (Cumming & Ramsey 2009; Holmes & Collins 2001).

There is nothing to suggest that imagery could not be used to manage pacing—for example, by mentally practising key accelerations during a race (notably without getting tired!) or by replaying certain experiences of fatigue so as to understand them better for future reference. This area is ripe for research attention and, in the meantime, a promising area for athletes to explore with the goal of eking out any available competitive advantages.

Self-Talk   Self-talk refers to the internal voice (although it may also refer to utterances spoken aloud) that often narrates or interprets events as they occur (Hardy 2006; Hardy, Oliver & Tod 2009). Researchers examine the contents of self-talk (positive or negative, motivational or instructional, and so on) as well as the frequency (some negative thoughts may need to be reduced or prevented to boost confidence). Explanations of self-talk are often varied, although priming and attentional cuing (discussed earlier in this chapter) are two strong candidates for explaining why self-talk works. In the press-ups example given earlier, as well as the wall-squat (or 'ski-hold') test, subjects quickly experience the urge to give up, yet if they deliberately steer their thoughts towards persistence and feeling strong, the impulse to give up is less likely to win out. Hardy, Oliver and Tod (2009) considered these explanations cognitive mechanisms, but also offered motivational (e.g., persistence or desire), behavioural (e.g., instructional cuing) and affective (e.g., mood or emotion) theories for explaining the observed effects of self-talk.

Realistically, self-talk may well operate through various mechanisms to achieve various outcomes. As mentioned, there is reason to believe self-talk could be used to manage pacing; for example, by managing feelings of exertion or discomfort or by cuing key technical or tactical instructions. Also as noted previously, researchers, athletes and their coaches could all stand to benefit from exploring self-talk in relation to pacing.

Goal Setting   Goal setting is a relatively common practice in sport, and psychologists tend to focus on managing how goals are set rather than on persuading athletes to use them. A goal can be defined very simply as something a person is trying to accomplish—that is, the objective or aim of one's actions (Locke et al. 1981). Under this definition, goals may be unconscious, and so goal setting should involve deliberately and explicitly setting meaningful goals that one wishes to pursue.

In principle, goal setting should involve prioritising objectives and avoiding distractions by steering behaviour towards suitable, rather than unsuitable, pursuits, by producing improved training and practice and (done properly) by increasing self-esteem through the gradual accrual of multiple personally meaningful successes. In this respect, like self-talk, goal setting may work through cognitive, motivational, behavioural and affective channels to help people achieve multiple desired outcomes (Kingston & Wilson 2009).

As applied to pacing, athletes may pursue outcome goals (placings, selections—i.e., in relation to competitors) by focusing on specific performance goals (times, scores—i.e., independent of competitors) and ultimately by deploying process goals (e.g., split times, training intensities or even specifying how to feel at a certain point). Generally, the most beneficial goal-setting programmes are

- a good mix of outcome, performance and process goals;
- split into short- and long-term goals (ideally with short-term goals building towards the long-term goals);
- set by (or in collaboration with) the athlete;
- pitched at a suitable degree of difficulty; and
- as specific or precise as realistically possible (e.g., not just 'more confident' but a rating of confidence improving 'from 6 out of 10 to 9 out of 10').

Arousal Control   Arousal control is the term used to describe psyching up or calming down, although much research in this area focuses on relaxation and avoiding overarousal (Edwards & Polman 2012). Arousal can be manipulated physically (e.g., by lying down rather than running up the stairs, or by breathing fast and hard rather than slow and deep) and psychologically (e.g., by remembering calm moments or by using self-talk to get angry). Note the use of other mental skills to achieve arousal control, which is itself viewed as a mental skill.

Perhaps the most basic theory of arousal is the inverted U, which depicts an athlete as underaroused, overaroused or 'just right' (Yerkes & Dodson 1908). Hanin (1980) adapted this theory into the IZOF model (individual zones of optimal functioning). This model considers the athlete's personality and the nature of the sport, but still ultimately invokes a simple inverted-U model. Liebert and Morris (1967) specified different roles for cognitive versus somatic arousal (or 'anxiety'), with an inverted U for physical arousal but a straight negative relationship between cognitive anxiety and performance. Perhaps the simplest way of viewing arousal control in sport and pacing is the matching hypothesis put forward by Davidson and Schwartz (1976). This hypothesis states that the arousal level for each performance should match the requirements of the task as opposed to the situation (e.g., if performance during training is optimal when calm, then the athlete should seek the same state of arousal even in the presence of a roaring crowd).

Numerous techniques are available to control arousal, especially down-regulation, including various types breathing (e.g., diaphragmatic breathing: in for 5, out for 10), progressive muscle relaxation (PMR; Jacobson 1930), imagery and self-talk, and physically lying down (or bouncing around, depending on what is necessary). Anecdotally, many athletes believe that 'nervous energy' can undermine pacing, because the nerves of a big event may render them 'pre-tired' or 'emotionally spent'. This belief would be consistent with Marcora and colleagues' (2009) findings, reported earlier, that mental fatigue can lead to faster physical fatigue. The specific arousal control requirements of various sports remain relatively poorly understood, and so there is tremendous scope for researchers and athletes to explore how best to use arousal control for pacing in various contexts.

Each mental skill, or strategy, can be used to pursue multiple aims (e.g., performance, confidence, motivation, pacing) and through multiple mechanisms. For example, imagery, self-talk and goal setting could be used to pursue these aims by influencing cognition, behaviours, motivation, confidence or emotions. To a large extent the mechanism will depend on the desired outcomes.

Given the broad applicability of these mental skills, a clear case can be made for applying them to pacing and for researchers to explore this link.

Biofeedback

An emerging technique in sport psychology is biofeedback, which usually involves communicating objective data to athletes in the form of information from electromyograms (EMG), electroencephalogram (EEG), heart rate (HR), heart rate variability (HRV), core body temperature or breathing rates/volumes (Paul, Gargh & Sandhu 2012). By viewing these data, preferably within the performance context or as close as possible to maintain relevance, athletes can appraise their subjective perceptions (e.g., realising that a particular level of discomfort or RPE was occurring well before maximal HR was reached).

Likewise, athletes can learn to associate particular signals and feelings with a given pace, or become better able to judge their sprint finish based on how their subjective perceptions link to their physiological states. Given that one key aim of training, from a pacing perspective, is to build awareness to inform teleoanticipation, biofeedback seems highly likely to support this process. In effect, it should be possible to say to a training athlete: 'OK, you are definitely in the desired performance zone. This is how it feels. Remember it and try to reproduce it during the race'. To date, biofeedback remains relatively untested, but it holds strong promise to assist athletes in understanding their pacing strategies so they can achieve maximal performances.

Conclusion

The psychology of pacing includes many areas of controversy, challenge, opportunity and threat. The debate about the roles of central versus peripheral fatigue in pacing (or more likely, their complex interplay), as well as the effects of training on these mechanisms suggests the need for careful research to realise progress in this field. Likewise, recent developments in cognitive neuropsychology necessitate comprehensive programmes of research to reach a complete and robust understanding of how the brain regulates pacing. Further still, the mechanisms behind psychological effects such as placebos, as well as the effectiveness of strategies such as imagery and self-talk, also require careful consideration. Research in all of these areas must do substantially more than simply establish correlations (relationships), which can never truly indicate causal links. As each of these phenomena becomes better understood, our ability to support athletes—both amateur and elite—will be enhanced. However, additional questions will undoubtedly be raised regarding which statistically significant findings generate genuine benefits to athletes and which can realistically be applied in sport settings (within the rules and reasonable ethical boundaries).

Overall, pacing is an area of sport research that is only beginning to receive the attention it deserves. Within that broader category, the psychology of pacing remains at a relatively immature stage of development. Although this state of affairs may disappoint those seeking concrete guarantees of performance enhancements, it is also an exciting time for researchers and athletes alike. Opportunities to produce meaningful research papers as well as notable improvements in athlete performance are available. As such, those willing to invest time and effort in exploring the area should be richly rewarded.

chapter 5

Adapting Pacing Strategies

Over the last 20 years, sport scientists have begun in earnest to try to understand the mechanisms that determine how a pacing strategy is generated in the brain and then applied and adapted during a race. Much has been discovered about how the body is regulated during exercise and how information concerning the physiological status of the muscle and the blood are fed back to the central nervous system for the brain to regulate the exercise intensity and the pacing strategy that emerges. Applied sport scientists and sport coaches are interested in this research to help athletes improve their performance. This chapter addresses the complex nature of pacing strategies and reviews findings from research studies on the psychophysiology (the interaction between psychology and physiology) of pacing that have implications for improved competition performance.

It is reasonable to suggest that anything that improves human performance would presumably influence the pacing strategy. Unfortunately, all potential performance-enhancing interventions cannot be covered in this single chapter. Therefore, the focus here is on the training, nutritional, environmental and psychological aspects that might affect the selection and use of the commonly used pacing strategies outlined in chapter 2. The examples in this chapter demonstrate how particular pacing strategies might be manipulated to improve performance. An understanding of the underlying psychophysiology of pacing allows coaches and athletes to manipulate the pacing strategy in whatever manner is most appropriate and complementary to the competitive event and the athlete.

Factors That Affect Strategy Selection

The pacing strategy an athlete selects determines the rate at which muscular work and the energy required to fuel that work are distributed across the event. Of course, the type of event has a direct bearing on the work distribution and therefore on strategy selection. The type of event also has a somewhat more indirect bearing on strategy selection as well, in that it determines an athlete's proximity to other competitors. Other influences on pacing strategy selection include genetics, life experiences, equipment and environmental conditions at the venue.

Many sports involve individuals racing against each other with only small margins separating them at the finish, making the pacing strategy critical. In some sports the race takes the form of a time trial and the athletes set off at regular time intervals (e.g.,

90-second intervals during the time trial stage in the Tour de France), allowing them to adopt their own pacing strategies.

In events such as swimming, rowing and 100 to 400 m running sprints, athletes compete in separate lanes—or, as in the 4000 m individual pursuit in cycling, on opposite sides of the track. In these situations the athletes might set out with the intention of adopting their own pacing strategies; however, because the competitors are in view of each other during some parts of the race, some might amend their pacing strategies based on the appearance and actions of their competitors.

In lengthy events, athletes compete over a set distance alongside their competitors and might change their positions relative to each other throughout the race. In this situation the pace of the race may be dictated by the tactics of others. However, athletes in long-distance events often state afterward that they 'ran their own race', suggesting that they competed with a particular pacing strategy in mind throughout the race or that they set out running at a pace they could comfortably manage and then, at a certain point, sped up to attempt to win the race or gain a further place.

When world records are attempted, the race may have a pacemaker, or a series of pacemakers, to 'tow' the athletes along in their slipstream, to reduce the air resistance and conserve the energy of the fastest athletes for the later stages of the race. The towed athletes conserve their energy until they feel the pace is no longer sufficient, at which point they overtake the pacemaker to attack the world record. This tactic represents a manipulation of pacing called drafting, which is commonly used in sports in which air resistance is significant in terms of energy cost. Because of the high speeds in cycling, drafting behind other riders saves significant amounts of energy and lowers the drafting riders' heart rates dramatically. Figure 5.1 depicts drafting perhaps at its most striking in the cycling road race peloton or 'flying ball'.

Genetic make-up, training and competition history undoubtedly help to shape an athlete's preferred pacing strategy. All of us begin life as unique individuals with our own genetic make-ups (or genotypes), with the exception of identical twins. The environment and the exercise activity we experience determine how our genotypes respond over our lifespans, creating what is known as our phenotypes. Even identical twins adapt differently if they are exposed to different environments and training practices.

Environmental and physical conditions such as climate, altitude, wind, course topography and terrain at the competition venue also affect the pacing strategy of an event. The impact of these factors on human physiology has been well researched, but not specifically in terms of how they influence pacing.

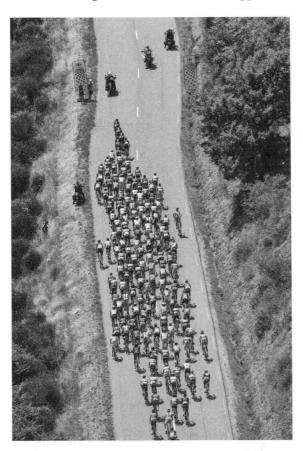

Figure 5.1 The road race peloton (or flying ball) is a great example of cyclists using drafting techniques to their advantage.

© Nico Vereecken/Photo News/Panoramic/Icon SMI

Only a few studies have directly examined how these factors affect pacing. For example, sport scientists are beginning to explore how pacing strategies can be altered by manipulating the oxygen content of the inspired air (to simulate altitude) or by varying the air temperature and humidity using environmental chambers.

This brief discussion demonstrates why the question of which pacing strategy is optimal for a particular sport or event on a given day is actually an extremely complex one. Nonetheless, athletes and their coaches often start a competition with a pacing strategy in mind, as part of their overall race tactics, based on their experiences of previous competition successes and failures. Indeed, elite athletes and their coaches often develop a pacing plan months in advance of a competition, mapping out the specific phases of the event (start phase, pickup phase, midphase, finishing phase), which then informs the performance goals and the subsequent training practices needed to execute the pacing plan. The pacing plan might be adjusted further on the day of the event to meet the particular challenges presented, in response to changing environmental conditions or the tactics of competitors.

An understanding of pacing and its inclusion as part of competition preparations is critical to being a successful competitor. Individual performance differences among athletes are often small, and the correctness of the pacing strategy—a factor that, unlike genetics, is within the control of the coach and athlete—may be the factor that determines success or failure.

Considerations for Sprints

The rate of energy use is a key consideration in short distance events. All-out exercise requires a high limb-movement frequency to maximise power output, which means that rapid muscle contractions are needed primarily from the fast-twitch muscle fibres. Each muscle contraction requires energy from the breakdown of adenosine triphosphate (ATP). ATP is a molecule that, when split apart, releases energy to power physiological functions, including muscle contractions and the related brain and nerve activity. An important consideration, however, is that ATP is supplied at different rates by different metabolic pathways and sources, known as substrates. The substrates are carbohydrate, fat and protein; the metabolic pathways are the anaerobic energy pathway, which does not require oxygen to function, and the aerobic energy pathway, which does require oxygen to function. ATP itself is stored only in tiny amounts and so can supply energy for muscle contractions only in the first second or so of exercise, when the ATP turnover rate in contracting muscle cells might increase 100-fold (Jones & Burnley 2009). To avoid a catastrophic fall in ATP and almost instant exhaustion, ATP must be resynthesised from the breakdown of substrates to allow muscle contractions to continue. The body regulates ATP stores so tightly that they remain around 60 to 70 per cent intact even during exhaustive exercise. The consequence of having no ATP available for muscle contraction would be rigor (as in rigor mortis!), so you can see why the body regulates its concentration so well!

During all-out sporting events, the production of ATP is primarily from anaerobic energy metabolism using two substrates stored in the muscle: phosphocreatine, a protein present in small amounts that is rapidly used up during all-out exercise, and glycogen, a form of carbohydrate stored in larger quantities that is sufficient to last the duration of an all-out sprint event.

In events lasting around 30 seconds, anaerobic energy metabolism provides the majority of the ATP contribution for muscle contraction (approximately 75 per cent). The remaining 25 per cent comes from aerobic energy metabolism, which produces ATP by breaking down muscle glycogen and fat but requires oxygen to do so. As a result, ATP is produced more slowly, in fact 50 to 70 per cent more slowly. In addition, a time lag exists before aerobic energy production ramps up at the start of exercise, because the extra oxygen required takes time to be delivered via the lungs and bloodstream to the working muscles. The aerobic energy contribution is therefore of less importance than the anaerobic metabolism in sprint events, although its importance increases as the race length increases.

In longer races, the initial lag in ATP production at the start of exercise is less important, because the muscles require energy at a reduced rate as a result of the slower speed and because the rate of ATP use is more closely matched with the slow rate of aerobic ATP production. In events lasting, say, 2 minutes, the ATP contribution would be more like 55 per cent anaerobic energy contribution and 45 per cent aerobic contribution.

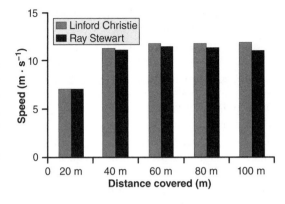

Figure 5.2 Speed and distance data for two athletes in the 1992 Barcelona Olympics 100 m final.

Clearly, the rate of ATP production is critical in all-out events to provide the energy at the highest rate possible for fast-twitch muscle fibres to contract. If there is a shortfall in the rate of ATP production, fatigue will occur. Because these muscle fibres will not contract sufficiently to maintain force production, the athlete will slow down.

Figure 5.2 demonstrates that even elite sprint track and field athletes cannot sustain maximal sprinting speed through the end of a 100 m race, although the athlete who can achieve the highest peak speed and maintain it for the longest will win.

Part of the reason sprinters cannot maintain their speed during races lasting only a few seconds is that they deplete their phosphocreatine stores. The rate of ATP production from phosphocreatine breakdown is approximately twice that from the breakdown of glycogen; however, because only a small store of phosphocreatine exists, it is rapidly depleted and reduces to very low concentrations within 10 seconds during all-out exercise. The production of ATP from phosphocreatine actually reaches its peak in about 1 to 3 seconds; thereafter, its ability to resynthesise ATP falls dramatically with each second, until after 30 seconds (if the sprint race takes that long) the production rate would be only a few per cent of its peak rate. It has been demonstrated that the rate of ATP production during the anaerobic breakdown of glycogen (known as anaerobic glycolysis) also falls significantly, by approximately 50 per cent, after only 20 to 30 seconds of exercise. Substrate depletion is therefore a cause of fatigue in all-out pace events, because the capacity for anaerobic energy metabolism to maintain its highest rate of ATP resynthesis to power muscle contractions is limited to only a few seconds.

Crucially, the rate of ATP production affects the rate of muscle contraction during sprinting. During all-out sprinting, fast-twitch muscle fibres are required to contract at their maximal rate, and they rely heavily on anaerobic energy metabolism to supply the ATP to do so. However, a shortfall in ATP supply versus demand occurs during sprinting, leading to a reduction in force production from the fast-twitch muscle fibres, so the athlete slows down.

The type(s) of muscle fibres that are contracting during exercise play a critical role in the rate of force production and the development of fatigue. Type I muscle fibres, also known as slow-twitch muscle fibres, are fatigue-resistant fibres because they are supplied with ATP from aerobic energy metabolism. Type IIA muscle fibres are fast-twitch muscle fibres, supplied with ATP from both anaerobic and aerobic energy metabolism. However, these muscle fibres fatigue more rapidly than Type I muscle fibres during high-intensity exercise because of their partial reliance on anaerobic metabolism. Indeed, the rate of production of ATP from anaerobic metabolism significantly decreases over 25 seconds of all-out exercise in Type IIA fibres leading to a significant decrease in their ATP concentration. Type IIX muscle fibres are another form of fast-twitch fibre. They contract and develop tension two or three times faster than slow-twitch fibres do, but fatigue rapidly because anaerobic ATP production provides the majority of ATP to these fibres. During sprint exercise their ATP concentration falls dramatically after only 10 seconds of all-out exercise.

Figure 5.3 depicts how the concentration of ATP typically diminishes over 25 seconds of maximal exercise in fast-twitch (Type II) and slow-twitch (Type I) muscle fibres of the exercising limbs. These data are from Karatzaferi, Sargeant and colleagues (Karatzaferi et al. 2001; Sargeant 2009), who conducted a series of laboratory-based studies with participants pedalling with maximal effort at 120 rpm on an isokinetic cycle ergometer for 10 seconds in one trial and for 25 seconds in another. The participants had muscle fibre fragments taken from their quadriceps (front thigh) muscle, by needle biopsy, before and after each bout of exercise to determine the concentration of ATP in the various muscle fibres types. The wiggly line drawn on figure 5.3 demonstrates the reduction in power output from one of the participants in the studies. The vertical axis on the right-hand side of the figure indicates that an approximate decline in the power output of 20 per cent and 40 per cent was observed after 10 and 25 seconds, respectively. This deterioration in performance coincides with a significant fall in the ATP concentration of the fast-twitch fibres (see the left-hand vertical axis). This is due to their rapid use of ATP during contractions, which outstrips supply from the anaerobic energy metabolism as the phosphocreatine stores become depleted and ATP production from glycolysis is reduced. Interestingly, the ATP concentration in the Type I (slow-twitch) muscle fibres suffers only a modest (10 per cent) reduction after 25 seconds. Clearly, the drop in power output is largely due to the reduced ability of the fast-twitch fibres to contract.

It is therefore not surprising that athletes in all-out, short sprints (e.g., the 100 m in track and field or match sprint in track cycling) attempt to boost their muscle phosphocreatine stores by adopting high-protein diets or taking supplements containing creatine. This practice is legal, although the evidence in the scientific literature remains unclear about whether such nutritional strategies can improve performance in a single all-out sprint or in multiple-sprint sports (e.g., team sports requiring repeated all-out sprinting). However, in activities that involve sprinting or cycling, performance is generally improved, and participants in controlled studies have been shown to store more phosphocreatine in their muscle following supplementation (Bemben & Lamont 2005; Lemon 2002).

There is also evidence that a high-carbohydrate diet can improve the ability to undertake repeated sprinting activity, presumably as a result of a boost in muscle glycogen levels. Balsom and colleagues (1999) demonstrated that subjects on a high-carbohydrate diet cycled at a higher pedal rate and had a subsequent higher power output than those on a low-carbohydrate diet. They also completed 295 six-second sprints, whereas those on the low-carbohydrate diet completed 111.

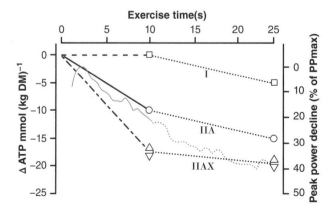

Figure 5.3 Decline in ATP concentrations in muscle fibres and the loss of power output during 10 and 25 seconds of maximal isokinetic cycling exercise.

Reprinted, by permission, from C. Karatzaferi, A. de Haan, W. van Mechelen, and A.J. Sargeant, 2001, "Metabolic changes in single human fibres during brief maximal exercise," *Experimental Physiology* 86(3): 411-415.

Considerations for Events Lasting 40 Seconds to a Few Minutes

An all-out pacing strategy has been calculated to be optimal for up to 291 m (~40 seconds) of running (Keller 1974). However, in events such as cycling and speed skating, all-out efforts have been calculated to be possible for events lasting as long as a minute (1000 m cycling and speed skating; van Ingen Schenau, de Koning & de Groot 1990). This is due to an enhanced ability to maintain speed despite reduced power output in these sports. The important point here is that the decision to adopt an all-out, or positive-pace, strategy depends not only on the physiology of the athlete but also on the biomechanics of the event

As explained in chapter 2, the ability to maintain kinetic energy is an important consideration, and this is easier in some sports than in others. Important factors such as the surface the sport takes place on, whether the sport is predominantly water or air resisted, the equipment used (e.g., skates on ice) and the topography and climate of the competition course all play a part in the pacing strategy. For example, Foster and colleagues (1993) noticed that 1500 m speed skaters slowed down less in the 1988 Calgary Olympiad than in the 1992 Albertville Olympiad despite a faster first 700 m. They attributed this to the lower air friction, lack of wind gusts and superior ice surface at the indoor venue in Calgary.

Figure 5.4 shows how in cycling it is possible to maintain almost 90 per cent of the peak speed achieved just after the start to the end of a 1 km trial, despite being able to produce less than 25 per cent of the peak power! This is because of the large amount of kinetic energy developed at the start. This example demonstrates that an all-out strategy is possible even in an event lasting around 60 seconds in some sports. In contrast, in the 1.5 km event depicted on the same graph, a positive pacing strategy was adopted by recreational standard riders who took approximately 120 seconds to complete the event. Their speed dropped proportionately more than that of the riders in the 1 km trial, although they maintained their power output to a much greater extent (approximately 57 per cent of peak power output). In the 1.5 km example, a reduced starting power and greater maintenance of power over the event would indicate a reduced use of the

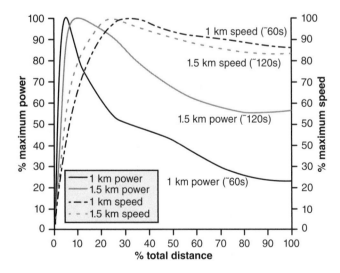

Figure 5.4 Power and speed patterns during cycling events of approximately 60 seconds and 120 seconds.

Data from C.R. Abbiss and P.B. Laursen, 2008, "Describing and understanding pacing strategies during athletic competition," *Sports Medicine* 38(3): 239-252 and C. Foster, J.J. de Koning, F. Hettinga, et al., 2003, "Pattern of energy expenditure during simulated competition," *Medicine & Science in Sports & Exercise* 35(5): 826-831.

Type IIX fibres in comparison to the 1 km event, but a greater use of Type IIA and Type I muscle fibres (refer to figure 5.3). Because Type IIA and Type I muscle fibres fatigue more slowly than Type IIX muscle fibres, maintenance of a greater proportion of the peak power was possible. However, the starting power, kinetic energy and speed were much decreased, greatly reducing the average speed.

In track and field, athletes complete the first 50 m more slowly in a 400 m race than they do in a 200 m race. This demonstrates that they have to pace the early part of the race to avoid premature fatigue; yet, despite doing so, they inevitably slow down in the last 50 m of a 400 m race (Tucker, Lambert & Noakes 2006). Treadmill running and cycle ergometry studies have also demonstrated that an all-out strategy often results in a loss of approximately 50 per cent of peak power output after around 40 seconds (Foster et al. 1994). Athletes report that in events lasting 30 seconds or more, they are acutely aware that fatigue is developing and that they cannot maintain their speed. This also means that they consciously consider slowing down. Therefore, an important question for the competing athlete is: *At what point (time duration) should I make the transition from all-out pacing to positive pacing?* The answer is likely to be somewhere between 20 and 60 seconds depending on the sport (e.g., swimming versus cycling). Importantly, as the duration of an event increases, the loss of kinetic energy becomes less important than the energy cost associated with aerodynamic and hydrodynamic resistance. Additionally, the initial rate of acceleration becomes less important, and the athlete's speed endurance becomes more important.

Sport science lecturers often use a Wingate anaerobic test, involving a 30-second maximal sprint on a stationary cycle ergometer, to teach undergraduate students about anaerobic energy metabolism. One of the criteria for a successful test is to achieve peak power within 3 to 5 seconds of the start. This is done to check whether the students are truly attempting an all-out effort from the outset! Many sport science students dread this test because of the discomfort and acute fatigue they experience, which accompanies a massive drop-off in their power output in the last 10 seconds or so of the test. The temptation for the experienced participant in a Wingate anaerobic test is to 'positively pace' the test—that is, start fast, but not maximally, and then pace the test in a controlled manner to avoid prematurely fatiguing and the resulting considerable discomfort! Clearly, exercising all-out for 30 seconds or more requires tremendous commitment and motivation, which is one reason coaches do not ask sprint athletes to undertake maximal 30-second efforts too often in training.

One culprit implicated in the fatigue and discomfort experienced when exercising intensely for 40 to 60 seconds is the increase in the acidity within the muscles as a result of the high, and prolonged, rate of anaerobic metabolism. Scientists use the measurement of blood lactate as an indication of anaerobic energy production in the muscle because it generally mirrors muscle lactate production and so gives an indirect yet reproducible indication of when an increased energy contribution from anaerobic glycolysis occurs. This also gives valuable information about whether aerobic energy production is meeting the energy requirements of the contracting muscles.

At rest the blood lactate value is less than 1 mmol/L (or 18 mg/dL). Elite 400 m track and field athletes produce values of 20 to 25 mmol/L of blood lactate, which suggests a considerable change in their acid–base balance. Athletes who produce high concentrations of lactic acid may actually feel pain and be physically sick. In very short events (<15 seconds) there is not sufficient time for lactic acid levels to accumulate to this degree, so it is events lasting 40 seconds or more that are particularly painful, distressing and fatiguing. It is no wonder that 400 m track and field sprinters, 1 km track cyclists and 500 to 1000 m speed skaters talk about pacing so much during their post-race interviews. When their pacing is well judged, they can finish with good form; however, when they go out too fast, they prematurely fatigue and seemingly feel as though they are unable to do anything about it. This is somewhat true because, despite their brains sending down increasing messages (motor commands) to their muscles to contract, the muscles can no longer maintain force production and dramatically reduce their work output at this point.

An intervention that might improve the ability to maintain speed and so allow for a more aggressive pacing strategy is bicarbonate supplementation. Scientific studies report that sodium bicarbonate (or sodium citrate) supplementation prior to a prolonged bout of high-intensity exercise boosts the buffering capacity of the muscle by enlarging the bicarbonate pool, which can stave off fatigue temporarily in events lasting from 40 seconds to 7 minutes. However, because health risks are associated with sodium bicarbonate loading, athletes are advised to consult with a qualified sport nutritionist before undertaking this practice (Carr, Gore & Dawson 2011; Carr, Hopkins & Gore 2011).

Role of Aerobic Energy Production

In races lasting 1 to 2 minutes, athletes often demonstrate a positive-pace strategy that involves a fast but not all-out start. Events of this duration require athletes to exercise at an intensity termed by physiologists as the extreme exercise intensity domain. This means that they reach the finish line before their cardiorespiratory system has reached its absolute maximal operating capacity, or $\dot{V}O_2$max (although they are rapidly approaching it).

$\dot{V}O_2$max is the maximal rate oxygen can be taken from the surrounding air and delivered to the cells in the muscles to produce ATP via aerobic metabolism. Thompson and colleagues (2003) found that the heart rates of well-trained swimmers were at 98 per cent of maximum at half-distance (70+ seconds or so) in a 200 m breaststroke event lasting just over 2 minutes. What this tells us is that because the heart rate was close to its maximum halfway through the race, the oxygen uptake would have been close to its maximum as well. Therefore, a high rate of oxygen intake and delivery to the muscles is critical to meet the energy requirements of races lasting beyond 60 seconds.

Is it important for athletes to have a high $\dot{V}O_2$max in positively paced races lasting around a minute or so? The answer is yes, because it provides a large capacity for taking up oxygen and producing ATP. The ability to increase the rate of oxygen uptake during the race determines how close the athlete's oxygen uptake will be to its maximal capacity by the end of the race. However, more important, it determines the rate of aerobic energy production. The greater the oxygen uptake is per second, the more ATP is produced from aerobic energy pathways for muscle contractions. In addition, the requirement for energy provision from anaerobic sources is reduced, leaving more anaerobic energy capacity available across the rest of the race, which will enhance the athlete's speed endurance. Sport scientists increasingly recognise that an athlete's ability to take up oxygen for aerobic energy production, termed oxygen uptake kinetics, affects the rate of both aerobic and anaerobic energy transfer. This in turn affects the blend of substrate use and subsequently has a profound effect on the tolerable pace in events lasting beyond a minute or so (Burnley & Jones 2007).

Because an athlete's oxygen uptake needs time to increase at the start of a race, energy for initial movement has to come predominantly from anaerobic energy pathways. The rate at which this occurs is important because anaerobic metabolism capacity is thought to be limited. Sport scientists contend that if more of the anaerobic capacity is used at the start of a race, less is available for a sprint finish, and vice versa. For example, if athlete A possessed a relatively slow rate of oxygen uptake at the start of a race but a similar maximal capacity for oxygen uptake ($\dot{V}O_2$max) and anaerobic capacity compared to a fellow competitor, athlete B, then the anaerobic capacity of athlete A would be depleted earlier in the race than that of athlete B. The implication would be that towards the end of the race, athlete B would have relatively more anaerobic capacity left for powerful muscle contractions. In a positively paced race, this means less of a decline in finishing speed, compared to athlete A. Of course, this is a simplistic view because sport performance is multifactorial, but the principle is important. From a training perspective, it demonstrates why the ability to take up oxygen and produce ATP via oxidative phosphorylation (aerobic metabolism) is important for speed endurance during a positively paced race.

Training Implications

Low-intensity endurance and interval training have both been found to improve the rate of oxygen uptake (Jones & Burnley 2009). This has positive implications for athletes training for a race of a couple of minutes' duration, because this adaptation would conserve their anaerobic capacity and reduce the rate of depletion of the muscles' phosphocreatine and glycogen reserves at the start of the race. A further benefit is that metabolites (e.g., hydrogen ions and inorganic phosphates) associated with fatigue and the stimulation of anaerobic glycolysis would accumulate more slowly. Similarly, athletes who improve technically (either biomechanically or through advancement in equipment design) and become more economical would use less force and energy for the same speed during races and potentially reduce their anaerobic energy cost. These improvements would allow them to sustain a higher speed over a race because more energy would be provided proportionately from aerobic metabolism for muscle contraction. Therefore, getting the balance right, in training, between maximising the aerobic and anaerobic capacities is crucial for an event lasting a few minutes.

To put some of this into a sporting context, let's consider the 800 m race in running, the 100 m race in swimming and the 1 km time trial in track cycling. In races of this duration, a curious contest often occurs when athletes with more of a sprint background compete with athletes with more of an endurance background and the two are on an almost equal footing in terms of race performance. Why is this? What enables this battle to emerge, aside from drag and biomechanical factors, is the individual nature of the athletes' physiology, which can be more developed in some areas than others. The sprinter might possess a greater anaerobic capacity and complement of fast-twitch muscle fibres, but slower oxygen uptake kinetics and so a lower rate of aerobic energy production. Meanwhile, the endurance athlete demonstrates a faster oxygen uptake at the beginning of exercise and so a greater rate of aerobic energy production and a better running economy as well as a greater aerobic capacity, but might possess a reduced anaerobic capacity. The differences in physiology will be apparent in the pacing strategy. For example, in the 1 km track cycling event, the sprinter-type rider will go out fast and try to hang on, thus demonstrating a more aggressive positive-pace strategy. A greater muscle mass and complement of fast-twitch fibres will afford a faster acceleration and higher peak speed in the early stages but lead to a more marked deterioration in speed as the race progresses. The endurance-type rider does not have the absolute strength of the sprint-type rider and so takes longer to accelerate the large-fixed gear at the start and will also not achieve as high a peak speed. However, as a result of superior aerobic energy metabolism, he will demonstrate greater speed endurance. The 1 km event is exciting as a spectacle because the race unravels towards the end as the two riders with differing physiological characteristics converge on a similar time at the finish!

In a laboratory cycling-based study, Jones and colleagues (2008) showed that a fast-start strategy can speed up oxygen uptake kinetics during the transition from rest to high-intensity exercise, compared to an even-pace or negative-pace strategy. In this study, the positive-pace strategy required the participants to set off with a mean power output 10 per cent greater than they would use for an even-pace trial, until the midpoint of the trial, whereupon they would switch to a power output 10 per cent below the mean power output for the even-pace trial. A negative-pace trial was also undertaken, which was simply the reverse of the positive-pace trial. Interestingly, the participants were able to continue exercising well beyond 120 seconds in the positive-pace trial, but not in the negative- or even-paced trials. The authors concluded that the speeded-up oxygen uptake kinetics, as a result of the fast start, facilitated aerobic energy metabolism and spared the anaerobic capacity, which participants were then able to use towards the end of the trial.

Further supporting evidence for adopting a fast-start strategy comes from a study by Hulleman and colleagues (2007), who observed that the faster subjects in a series of 1500 m cycling time trials adopted a more aggressive early pace. As an aside, 200 m breaststroke swimmers have been shown to positively pace in national and international standard competitions. They demonstrated a 7 per cent reduction in midpool swimming velocity from lap 1 to lap 4 (Thompson & Haljand 2000), providing further evidence that an aggressive positive pacing strategy is metabolically beneficial in events lasting 2 to 3 minutes.

The initial pace of a positively paced race appears to be critical with regard to oxygen uptake kinetics. Laboratory-based cycling studies have found that 2000 m events lasting approximately 3 minutes are even-paced, whereas 1500 m events using a fast start (Foster et al. 1993, 1994) are positive-paced. Therefore, at around 2 to 3 minutes, athletes (cyclists at least) tend to change from positive pacing to even pacing.

Considerations for Middle-Distance to Longer Distance Events

Generally, in prolonged middle-distance to long-distance races, athletes demonstrate a preference for even pacing. This is because, in comparison to short events, the initial acceleration phase is relatively less important to the race outcome; the key consideration is speed maintenance, particularly in time trial races or races run at close to world-record pace. In events of this duration, even-paced race strategies seem to relate well to mathematical models and indicate that the race speed is determined by the maximal constant force an athlete can exert along with the resistive forces experienced (Abbiss & Laursen 2008).

One such mathematical model, the critical power model, is particularly relevant for events taking from 3 to 45 minutes or so to complete. Critical power refers to an exercise intensity termed severe by exercise physiologists. It first occurs at a power output (and speed) similar to that which elicits the maximal lactate steady state, which is the highest workload at which blood lactate will stabilise (not continue to rise) during exercise. Exercising just above critical power results in endurance athletes using up their anaerobic capacity; additionally, the oxygen uptake and heart rate can no longer maintain a steady state and so continue to rise until the maximal oxygen uptake ($\dot{V}O_2$max) is attained. Fatigue will occur soon afterwards (within 1 or 2 minutes). The gradual rise in oxygen uptake observed when someone exercises above critical power is called the slow component and can be seen developing with time (see figure 5.5).

The slow component is important because it is telling us that even if there is no further increase in race speed, the athlete's oxygen uptake (and heart rate) will continue to rise until it reaches its maximum, and exhaustion will occur soon after. Clearly, then, the greater the power output or speed is at which this happens, the more likely athletes will be to succeed in endurance races because they can tolerate a higher speed for longer. Long-distance athletes therefore perform training sessions at speeds around their critical power to improve their racing economy.

Why does the slow component develop? It is thought that it signals the recruitment of inefficient fast-twitch muscle fibres, which means there is an additional oxygen requirement and also that the anaerobic capacity is being exhausted. In the context of a race, then, the slow component is associated with a race speed at which the power output cannot be sustained without the recruitment of fast-twitch muscle fibres. The faster the race speed is above the speed associated with reaching the critical power, the greater the requirement for fast-twitch muscle fibre activation will be and hence the greater the slow component will be. Not surprisingly, the greatest increases in the slow component (perhaps more than 20 per cent of the total oxygen uptake, or 1 litre per minute; Burnley, Doust & Jones 2005) are observed when athletes are exercising above their critical speed throughout the event. Crucially, because fast-twitch fibres are being increasingly recruited, the anaerobic capacity is being increasingly used and, consequently, diminishes.

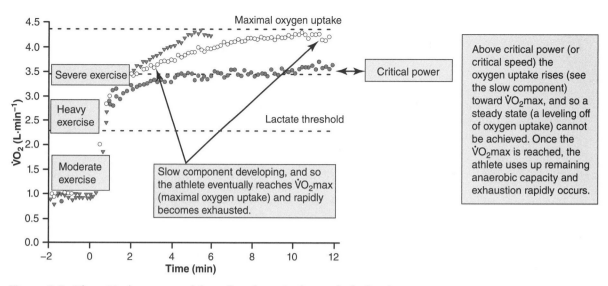

Figure 5.5 The critical power model predicts the point beyond which exhaustion is certain to set in.

From M. Burnley and A.M. Jones, 2007, "Oxygen uptake kinetics as a determinant of sports performance," *European Journal of Sport Science* 7(2): 63-79. Adapted with permission of Taylor & Francis Ltd.

An athlete exercising just above critical power (i.e., the severe exercise intensity domain) will gradually reach $\dot{V}O_2$max and experience fatigue within 30 to 45 minutes depending on fitness level (Burnley & Jones 2007). However, an athlete exercising at the top end of this exercise domain (e.g., 95 per cent of $\dot{V}O_2$max, or approximately 95 to 98 per cent of maximal heart rate) will attain $\dot{V}O_2$max within 10 minutes or so. In events lasting approximately 13 to 30 minutes (e.g., 5 and 10 km running), the aerobic metabolism might contribute as much as 80 to 90 per cent of the total energy turnover, mainly using glycogen (carbohydrate) as the energy source. The anaerobic metabolism will contribute the remaining 10 to 20 per cent of the energy needed. If athletes competing in long-distance races conducted in the severe exercise domain can meet the energy cost of the exercise for most of the race using aerobic metabolism, the anaerobic capacity will be largely spared. The anaerobic capacity remaining at the end of the race can then be used to help sustain a long finishing surge or to sprint right at the end of the race. This increase in speed at the end of a race is termed an end spurt in scientific studies, but is called a sprint finish by everyone else!

In endurance races run at or near severe exercise intensity, minimising variations in pace (i.e., even pacing) is important to avoid fully using the aerobic capacity too early in the race and subsequently being unable to produce a long surge or a sprint finish at the end. In long-distance races in which medals rather than world records are at stake, athletes possessing superior oxygen uptake kinetics and higher speeds at their critical power compared to their competitors frequently accelerate to force the other competitors toward their $\dot{V}O_2$max so they expend their anaerobic capacity prior to the end of the race. When this happens, race commentators often say that an athlete is trying to run the sprint finish out of the opposition.

In the example illustrated in figure 5.6, athlete A possesses a superior ability to take up oxygen at the start of exercise compared to athlete B, and can also exercise at a higher exercise intensity (87 per cent of $\dot{V}O_2$max) before attaining critical power. Athlete B attains critical power at only 83 per cent of $\dot{V}O_2$max. These subtle but important physiological differences mean that, by pacing strategically, athlete A can tire athlete B while maintaining a relatively comfortable physiological state for himself, at least until the final stages of the race. Note that athlete A surges twice, at 4 and 10 minutes into the race, forcing athlete B to exercise well above his critical power. This pacing strategy serves to tire athlete B and to deplete his anaerobic capacity. Then, at 14 minutes into

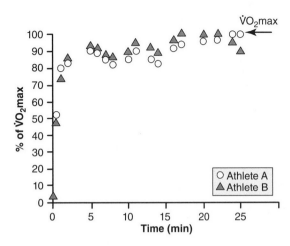

Figure 5.6 Frequent increases in pace during a longer event can draw a competitor out of his even pacing strategy and into his critical power zone, depleting the anaerobic capacity reserves required for a sprint finish.

the race, athlete A increases the pace again, but this time he holds the pace steady. This causes athlete B to reach his $\dot{V}O_2$max well before the end of the race. After a few minutes athlete B suffers overwhelming fatigue and discomfort, leading him to reduce his running speed to avoid a catastrophic drop in performance. Conversely, athlete A maintains his speed throughout, reaching his $\dot{V}O_2$max just prior to the end of the race. Having conserved his anaerobic capacity to some degree, he can use up what is remaining in the final stages of the race and win the race comfortably.

A further example is provided in figure 5.7, which depicts a competitive amateur cyclist who had a power meter fitted to collect his power output data during a road race. The cyclist's performance was retrospectively analysed by calculating his critical power (CP) and W' (W prime) to establish the point at which he was using up his finite anaerobic capacity. W' is the finite work capacity available above the critical power, and it incorporates anaerobic capacity. Figure 5.7 highlights how W', and hence anaerobic capacity, is used up when the rider surges during the race. This happens because the surges in speed require the rider to produce power outputs well above his critical power. Each time this happens, the anaerobic capacity is depleted to some degree; and because the rider does not spend sufficient time riding below his CP, the anaerobic capacity is not regenerated sufficiently. This imbalance leads to the finite W' being severely depleted (at point 4 in the figure), and at this point the rider is unable to stay with the leading group in the race.

Padilla and colleagues (2000) observed that during a 1-hour cycling record attempt in which the goal was to achieve the maximal distance possible, the rider's speed deviated little from the target speed of 53 km/h (33 mph). At such high speeds, aerodynamic resistance is high, and by even pacing (i.e., avoiding needless accelerations and decelerations), the rider could be as economical as possible. The rider would have also been making sure that he was cycling at just around his critical power until the closing stages of the record attempt, whereupon he would have attempted to sprint. Frequent speed fluctuations are not desirable in long-distance record attempts because they can lead to crossing far into the severe exercise domain. This produces a large slow component and uses up the finite anaerobic capacity, culminating in premature exhaustion. By even pacing, the athlete might exercise at, or just above, critical power for much of the event, keeping a sustainable pace at a high average speed.

It has been suggested that elite cyclists can exercise efficiently for an hour in the severe exercise domain (85 to 90 per cent of $\dot{V}O_2$max) by sharing power production among their individual muscle fibres. The assumption is that these cyclists stave off fatigue by rotating their slow-twitch muscle fibres so that at times some are contracting while others are resting. This adaptation, developed through hours of endurance training,

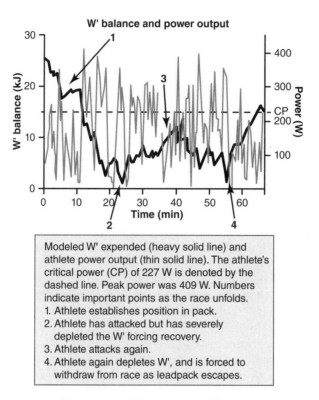

W' balance and power output

Modeled W' expended (heavy solid line) and athlete power output (thin solid line). The athlete's critical power (CP) of 227 W is denoted by the dashed line. Peak power was 409 W. Numbers indicate important points as the race unfolds.
1. Athlete establishes position in pack.
2. Athlete has attacked but has severely depleted the W' forcing recovery.
3. Athlete attacks again.
4. Athlete again depletes W', and is forced to withdraw from race as leadpack escapes.

Figure 5.7 Using up anaerobic capacity (W') during a cycling road race.

Reprinted, by permission, from P.F. Skiba, C. Weerapong, A. Vanhatalo, and A.M. Jones, 2012, "Modeling the expenditure and reconstitution of work capacity above critical power," *Medicine & Science in Sports & Exercise* 44(8): 1526-1532.

would have the benefit of reducing the relative power production of each muscle fibre and would spread the energy cost and mechanical stress of the exercise among the million or so fibres in each of the four quadriceps muscles (Coyle 1995; Coyle et al. 1988). This power sharing among slow-twitch muscle fibres could mean that 20 to 25 per cent more of them are used (than if no rotating occurred), which would reduce the need to recruit inefficient fast-twitch fibres and so delay the appearance of the slow component (Joyner & Coyle 2008).

Perhaps contrary to the previous discussion, which suggests that an even pace race should be started conservatively, a recent study found that a brief, fast start might be beneficial for optimal performance when cycling for 5 minutes. In a cycling ergometer–based study, Aisbett and colleagues (2009) found that an all-out start for 15 seconds at a power output of 754 W, followed by 45 seconds of cycling at around 375 W, produced a better overall performance over a 5-minute trial than a lower but more sustained fast start did (60 seconds at a power output around 470 W). The same amount of work was completed by the riders during the first minute of both trials; however, the investigators found that the take-up of oxygen by the riders was greater in the first quarter of the brief, all-out-start trial. They concluded that the all-out start speeded up the rider's oxygen uptake at the beginning of the trial and that this was the reason the participants' improved their performance, rather than the time saved due to the initial rapid acceleration, because the greater oxygen uptake would have spared the rider's anaerobic capacity.

Stone and colleagues (2012) had well-trained cyclists undertake a 4000 m time trial on a cycle ergometer on a number of occasions to establish personal best performances. The riders were then asked to return to the laboratory on two further occasions to compete against a computer-generated avatar, on a video screen placed in front of them, which they were told would represent their personal best performance. A second avatar that represented their real-time performance was also shown on the screen, and so in effect they could see themselves racing against their personal best avatar. On one occasion they competed against the avatar, which was set to complete the trial at the average power output of their previously established best performance, and they were informed of this. However, on another occasion they were led to believe that the avatar was still set to simulate their best performance, but it was actually programmed to ride with an average power output that was 2 per cent higher!

In the deception trial, riders managed to beat the avatar, which meant that they cycled 1 per cent faster over the 4000 m trial than they had managed when they had established their personal best time! However, in the other trial, in which the avatar was set at their best average power output, they beat the avatar but by a smaller amount and were significantly slower than they were in the deception trial. Measures of power output and expired gas analysis were computed to determine the aerobic and anaerobic energy contributions in each trial. The researchers found that in the deception trial the additional power output to defeat the avatar came from the anaerobic energy system during the last 10 per cent of the race. They concluded that athletes might maintain an anaerobic reserve that they tap into only when they are highly motivated and believe they can complete the task ahead of them.

In a follow-up study, Stone (2012) had another group of riders perform the same two trials as well as an additional deception trial in which the avatar was programmed with a mean power output 5 per cent greater than the average power for the personal best trial. In the second deception trial the riders were unable to keep up with the avatar and dropped back to similar performances to their personal best trials. However, the original finding of an improved performance in the 2 per cent deception trial was reproduced. Hence, a limit to the anaerobic reserve seems to exist between 2 and 5 per cent.

During the same study, a second group undertook the same three trials except that they were informed about the 2 per cent and 5 per cent increases in average power output of the avatar they were racing. In this informed group, performances were not significantly different to the personal best trial, and in the 5 per cent trial participants actually demonstrated a trend toward a poorer performance. Notably, in the 5 per cent trial, when the personal best avatar passed the real-time avatar at half-distance, the riders appeared to evaluate the distance remaining, as well as their current state of discomfort, and make a decision to reduce their pace.

Self-belief and motivation are clearly critical factors when trying to access the anaerobic reserve. In a sporting context, coaches might be able to encourage athletes to tap into their energy reserves in training or competition by deceiving them about their split times. However, this ethically dubious practice is risky because any suspicion or knowledge of deception on the part of the athletes could erode their trust in the coach, which could have catastrophic consequences for their relationship.

Considerations for Longer-Term Endurance Events

It is well known that elite long-distance runners possess a higher running speed at their lactate threshold and gas exchange threshold as a result of training adaptations that improve oxygen delivery and consequently aerobic energy production in their muscles. These adaptations mean that athletes can exercise at relatively high exercise intensities while still using fat stores as the predominant fuel source, sparing the glycogen stores and allowing them to increase their race pace in the later stages. These elite athletes can maintain a high speed with a relatively even pace for a prolonged period of time. For example, when the world records for the marathon and 100 km were set by Paul Tergat (2:04:55) and Takahiro Sunada (6:13:33), the variation in their speed over the race course was minimal (coefficient of variation = 1.2 and 3.2 per cent), demonstrating incredible running economy and consistency in pacing.

However, although an even pace would seem to be the most appropriate pacing strategy, positive pacing has also been observed in events of considerable duration. In long-distance events, the athletes' physical and mental capacities dictate their pacing strategy. Often, the pace is more stochastic early in the race, as the leaders surge and then slow down to engender discomfort in lesser athletes, who in response exercise above their critical power and incur additional energy costs. The less fit or mentally resilient competitors often let go after the midway point and return to their natural pace for the distance remaining (Foster et al. 2012).

Evidence suggests, however, that as athletes improve their performance or gain competition experience (usually after at least three events), they are more willing to risk a faster early pace (Foster et al. 2012). The decision to let go or surge involves subconscious and conscious processes in the brain that are based on athletes' prior experience, afferent (sensory) feedback and perceptions concerning their current physiological status, the distance remaining and feelings of discomfort and motivation. De Koning and colleagues (2011) developed a hazard score for long-distance events that is simply the rating of perceived exertion (RPE) multiplied by the distance remaining in the race. They postulated that this score could discriminate whether athletes let go or surge and so might predict their pacing behavior; however, experimental results to date have shown it to be more predictive of group rather than individual behaviour (see chapter 1 for more detail).

As stated in chapter 2, the likely fatigue mechanisms in events of up to 4 hours will be carbohydrate (glycogen) depletion and hyperthermia (if exercising in hot conditions) with muscle damage and a loss of central drive and motivation also implicated, particularly in events beyond 4 hours (Burnley & Jones 2007). During 100 km running races, fatigue is often observed after about 50 km, as a result of glycogen depletion, because these races are run at approximately 65 per cent $\dot{V}O_2max$, and it has been estimated that glycogen depletion occurs after 40 to 50 km of running at this intensity (Karlsson & Saltin 1971). When marathon runners hit the wall, generally at 32 km into the event (~75 per cent race distance), their glycogen stores are significantly depleted and, consequently, the energy for skeletal muscle contraction must come mainly from fat oxidation.

There appear to be large inter-individual variations in response to low blood glucose concentrations (hypoglycaemia, an abnormal decrease in blood sugar); some athletes are unable to continue exercising when hypoglycaemia occurs (Christensen 1939; Coyle et al. 1983, 1986). However, studies with highly trained participants have found that some people can demonstrate a remarkable resistance to hypoglycaemia. In this instance, the ability of these athletes to maintain their speed depends on their rate of muscle carbohydrate (glycogen) depletion.

It is possible to increase muscle glycogen stores by 40 per cent before endurance exercise through carbohydrate feeding strategies. Scientific studies have demonstrated that carbohydrate loading prior to races reduces the risk of hypoglycaemia and improves the ability to undertake heavy exercise (exercise around the lactate threshold), which might be extended from 2 to 3 hours, or 3 to 4 hours (Coyle et al. 1983,1986; Sherman & Costill 1984). However, taking in carbohydrate during ultra-distance events might become less effective once the athlete begins to suffer significant levels of muscle damage. Researchers have speculated that an alternative explanation for the reduction in running speed and subsequent positive pacing observed in ultra-distance races might be muscle damage, discomfort and fatigue (Lambert et al. 2004; Nicol, Komi & Marconnet 1991). Studies that have specifically investigated muscle damage have also found that the transport of glucose to the muscle is slowed when the muscle is damaged, which might mean that taking a carbohydrate supplement during a ultra-distance race to elevate muscle carbohydrate content becomes less effective as the race progresses.

Exercising in the heavy-intensity exercise domain for prolonged periods can lead to a risk of hypoglycaemia and ketosis (excessive accumulation of ketone bodies in body tissues and fluids caused by a deficiency in the metabolism of carbohydrate, as can occur when carbohydrate stores are depleted). Even trained marathon runners can make pacing mistakes and suffer losses of coordination and even collapse as a result (St Clair Gibson et al. 2013).

A compounding issue when running a marathon is that a gradual rise in the body's internal temperature leads to increases in blood flow distribution to the skin to help with heat loss. However, this indirectly creates a greater need for oxygen uptake, and in turn, further aerobic energy production adds to the body's internal heat gain! When this is further exaggerated by hot atmospheric conditions, it is not surprising that a positive pacing strategy is often observed in marathons. Athletes have to slow down both to conserve carbohydrate reserves and to limit thermoregulatory stress.

Motivation is an important factor in ultra-distance events because such races provide plenty of time for athletes to ponder how tired and uncomfortable they are. During exercise in hot conditions, the internal body temperature increases over time as heat storage occurs from internal metabolic reactions and the external environment. If less heat is lost than gained, the body temperature will not be able to stabilise and will rise. Thermoreceptors in the skin and blood will sense the increasing body temperature and communicate it to the hypothalamus. The hypothalamus, which is situated just above the brainstem, regulates body temperature loss by increasing blood flow to the skin and stimulating sweat glands to increase their sweat rate, and it is highly sensitive to temperature changes in the circulating blood. As the athlete becomes hot, the hypothalamus senses it, and subsequently the athlete may decide, consciously or subconsciously, to slow down to reduce metabolic heat production and consequently body temperature. Of course, the general wear and tear of long-distance events also adds to the overall feelings of discomfort, as would a developing awareness of thirst as dehydration develops.

Hydration status is a major consideration in endurance events that take hours to complete, because it can be difficult to consume sufficient fluid to compensate for the loss of body water from the evaporation of sweat from the skin and from the upper part of the lungs, which occurs as a result of breathing large volumes of dry air. High sweat rates can result in a loss of 1.8 litres of fluid per hour from the body but can be much greater in elite athletes who have spent two to three weeks acclimatising to hot conditions in preparation for a hot race. To 'protect' their racing pace, athletes develop a hydration strategy, often with the help of a sport nutrition expert, to ensure that they take fluid on board at regular intervals and in sufficient quantities to avoid significant dehydration. In long-distance races in hot conditions, an adequate hydration strategy is critical for maintaining race pace. Maintaining an adequate fluid balance in the body helps to optimise performance by creating an adequate sweat rate (and thus heat loss) and adequate blood flow to maintain oxygen delivery to the muscles.

Environmental Considerations for Middle-Distance and Long-Distance Events

Endurance capacity, or the ability to continue exercising for as long as possible at a particular work rate, is reduced in hot compared to temperate conditions (Galloway & Maughan 1997). It has also been reported that exercise performance, or the ability to complete a set distance in the fastest time, is also adversely affected by hot conditions. Marathon running performance, for example, has been reported to reduce by 2 to 3 per cent when the wet bulb globe temperature (a widely used heat stress index that estimates the effect of temperature, humidity, wind speed and solar radiation on humans, and is derived from a formula that includes temperature readings from a wet bulb, dry bulb and black globe) exceeds 20 °C (68 °F) (Ely et al. 2007; Trapasso & Cooper 1989). Marathon running conditions have been suggested to be optimal at an air temperature of 12 to 13 °C (53.6 to 55.4 °F) with a predicted 40-second decrement in race time expected for every additional 1°C (1.8 °F) rise (Foster & Daniels 1975). There is evidence that an increasing internal body temperature due to exercising in hot conditions leads to enhanced muscle glycogen (carbohydrate) use as muscle temperatures and hormone levels become elevated. However, a reduction in carbohydrate stores might not be the primary cause of fatigue when endurance athletes exercise in the heat, because muscle glycogen stores have been observed to remain high even when athletes have felt compelled to stop exercising (Hargreaves 2008).

Fascinatingly, some recent studies have demonstrated that humans might anticipate the effect of exercising in hot conditions and choose, either subconsciously or consciously, to exercise at a reduced pace early in the exercise bout, even before their internal body temperature has become significantly increased or indeed before any other physiological responses would suggest that they are physically stressed! For example, Tatterson and colleagues (2000) observed that participants undertaking a 30-minute cycling time trial at 32 °C (89.6 °F) air temperature reduced their power output after only 15 minutes, but this did not happen when they exercised in a temperature of 23 °C (73.4 °F).

Tucker and colleagues (2006) reported similar findings when they asked well-trained cyclists to complete a 20 km time trial in temperatures of 35 °C (95 °F) and 15°C (59 °F). They found that the power outputs of the participants were reduced in the hotter condition despite the participants having similar internal body (core) temperatures in both trials (~39 to 40 °C, or 102.2 to 104 °F). In both temperature conditions, the participants exhibited a sprint finish, suggesting that the brain was regulating their efforts so that some capacity was left in reserve at the end. However, in the hot condition, the reduced power output was suggested to demonstrate that a more conservative regulation by the brain had occurred. Interestingly, some elite athletes attempt to cool their extremities prior to a hot race by using ice vests or water baths, by drinking an ice slurry, or by using a combination of these methods, to delay the rise in their core temperature during the race. Perhaps this also deceives the brain's regulatory mechanisms at the start of the race, allowing the athletes to undertake a more aggressive early pace.

Levels and colleagues (2013) compared 15 km cycling time trials in 30 °C (86 °F) heat, in which participants undertook a variety of pre-exercise pre-cooling strategies. In one trial they completed a normal 10-minute warm-up prior to the time trial; in another they undertook 30 minutes of scalp cooling as well as the warm-up. On another occasion they drank an ice slurry prior to the time trial, and finally, on another occasion they had the ice slurry and also undertook 30 minutes of scalp cooling. The researchers observed no differences in overall trial performance time, although the participants' core temperatures were slightly lower in the ice slurry trials just before beginning the time trial, and they reported feeling cooler.

Stevenson and Thompson (2002) asked well-trained cyclists to complete a 4000 m self-paced cycle ergometer time trial in a laboratory with a temperature of 20 °C (68 °F). They then asked the riders to return on three other occasions (see figure 5.8). On one occasion they completed the same trial in the same conditions (CON trial). On another occasion they did the same again but this time they were slightly dehydrated (by 2 per cent of their body weight) before completing the time trial (DEH trial). On a final

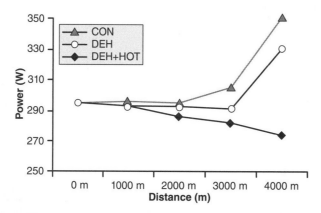

Figure 5.8 Effect of heat and dehydration on pacing in 4 km cycling time trials.

2 per cent DEH = slight dehydration (e.g., a 70 kg [154.3 lb] person losing 1.4 kg [3 lb], which would primarily be water loss (1.4 L).

Adapted from R.D.M. Stevenson and K.G. Thompson, 2002, "Hypohydration, heat and 4000m cycling performance," *Journal of Human Movement Studies* 43(5): 363-375.

occasion they were dehydrated again but completed the time trial in a higher laboratory temperature of 30 °C (86 °F) (DEH + HOT trial). For the last three trials, the pacing was controlled to the halfway point (i.e., 2000 m) by asking the riders to pace the ride based on information presented on a small screen mounted on the handlebars. The screen showed their average power output, distance covered and time taken as they rode, and they were asked to cycle at the average power output of the very first time trial.

The participants accurately paced the first 2000 m based on the information provided in all the trials. At the halfway point, however, the information screen was covered up so they had to self-pace the rest of the trial. Figure 5.8 shows the pattern of pacing over each of the trials. The researchers found no difference among the trials for oxygen uptake or blood lactate responses, suggesting similar aerobic and anaerobic energy contributions under each condition. Also, ear temperature, as a measure of body temperature, rose similarly among the trials. However, the rating of perceived exertion was significantly greater in the 2 per cent dehydration plus 30 °C temperature time trial (DEH + HOT trial), and performance was also reduced in this trial. Significantly, a reduction in power output began in this trial soon after the pacing information was withdrawn from view, and no sprint finish was produced either.

It would appear that the brain sensed the additional temperature conditions in the 30 °C (86 °F) trial, but acted on that information only when the pacing information was taken away. Therefore, it is possible that the pacing information distracted the participants from the additional heat load and discomfort they were experiencing up to the midpoint of the trial. Some sport scientists believe that the brain can sense only a limited amount of information during exercise; they call this a finite sensory channel capacity (Sporer & McKenzie 2007). If this is true, then during exhaustive and prolonged exercise there might be a danger of information overload. Because the brain cannot simultaneously process and discriminate among the numerous distress-related cues (e.g., rising internal temperature, low blood glucose concentration, muscle fatigue, the position of competitors) from the afferent sensory nerves, this could lead to poor decision making.

The experiment described earlier might suggest that because the brain is somewhat conservative (as suggested by the central governor theory outlined in chapters 3 and 4), it will elect to reduce the exercise intensity early in hot racing conditions. However, if appropriate information is provided to athletes during the event, they might elect to exercise at a faster pace and potentially improve their performance.

Providing athletes with objective data might improve their confidence and allow them to filter sensory information more effectively to make better use of their physiological resources. Long-distance athletes often wear heart rate monitors to guide them, and many receive objective data in real time from a plethora of technological tools developed by sport equipment manufacturers such as power output data from power meters (for bikes); core temperature information from temperature-monitoring pills; environmental data from air temperature, humidity and wind speed monitors; distance travelled and course location from GPS systems; and competitor positions from video screens. A word of caution is in order, however. A Grand Prix Formula 1 team that explored providing an array of information on displays projected onto drivers' helmet visors found that the drivers were unable to process all the information on the display without being danger-ously distracted from their high-speed driving! Although this is an extreme example, the inability of the brain to process all the information available to it, particularly as fatigue sets in, means that a decision about what information to provide should be made in advance of hot races.

Variable pacing can be a good strategy for any number of environmental conditions such as temperature, humidity, altitude, wind speed, wind direction, gusts of wind, uphill and downhill sections, change of surface, transitions from exercising in water to air as in a triathlon, wave formation, the tightness of a bend or perhaps simply when drafting behind someone to conserve energy. For these reasons the coach and athlete 'walk the course', sometimes well before the competition, to gain knowledge of the environment so they can devise a variable pacing strategy. The Great Britain sailing team was rumoured to have begun collecting environmental information at Qingdao International Marina some four years prior to the Olympic Games in Beijing! The Great Britain and Australian cycling teams collect race course data well in advance of road and mountain bike races using GPS, radio telemetry data from the bikes and even camera goggles giving a rider's-eye view of the course.

To date, very few researchers have investigated the effect of external factors on pacing to determine the most effective pacing strategies. It is logical that a variable (fluctuating) pacing strategy would be appropriate to counter changeable conditions during outdoor races. Using mathematical modelling techniques, Swain (1997) demonstrated that it is better to increase power output on uphill sections and reduce power output on downhill sections, rather than maintain a constant power output throughout a 10 km time trial. Cangley and colleagues (2010) had competitive male cyclists complete an undulating 4 km course using a variable power output and a constant power output and concluded that the variable strategy saved around 11 seconds on average. Another study in which experienced 10,000 m runners completed three laps of a 3.2 km (2-mile) hilly course revealed that those who varied their pace more as a function of the gradients they experienced demonstrated a more consistent oxygen uptake, which the researchers believed to be advantageous (Townshend, Worringham & Stewart 2010). The researchers also believed that optimising time on the flat sections after hills offered the greatest gain in terms of minimising the race time on an undulating course.

To investigate the effects of headwinds and tailwinds, Atkinson and Brunskill (2000) conducted a laboratory-based experiment in which seven riders, in the first trial, completed a self-paced simulated 16.1 km (3.8-mile) time trial on a flat course with a headwind for the first half and a tailwind for the second half (trial 1). The riders then completed another trial (trial 2) over the same course but this time their work rate was held constant, with the riders maintaining a power output set at the average power output for their self-paced trial (trial 1). Finally, the riders completed a third trial in which the work rate for the first half of the trial (headwind section) was set at a power output 5% greater than their average power output for trial 1, while for the second half of the trial (tailwind section) the work rate was set at a power output 5% less than their average power output for trial 1. This meant that the mean power output was the same for all the trials. The researchers discovered that the constant and variable strategies yielded better performance times than the self-paced trial, in which they believed the riders had initially set off too fast in the first few kilometres. The variable pacing strategy produced slightly faster times than the constant-pace trial did, and also led to reduced physiological responses and ratings of perceived exertion. They concluded this was due to the riders spending more time in the headwind section relative to the tailwind section and so the distribution of the power output in the variable trial was better suited to improving performance under these conditions.

Finally, variable pacing occurs during long-distance races, particularly during the middle portions, irrespective of environmental conditions, when athletes repeatedly surge to tire their fellow competitors. Surges are preceded by 'taking a breather' by hiding in the pack to conserve energy. The tactic of suddenly changing pace is not done randomly, but often when fellow competitors have completed their turn at the front and are fatigued. It is thought that by taking a breather, long-distance athletes exercise below their severe exercise intensity domain (refer to figure 5.5), thereby regenerating their anaerobic capacity. These metabolic changes allow them to produce short, rapid changes of pace later in the race. This is a good tactic, because changing pace rapidly is a way of both physically and mentally fatiguing the opposition. For example, when athletes manage to 'jump' the leaders and take the lead by surprise, they have difficulty closing the gap because they have already been exercising in their severe exercise intensity domain for some time and may have little anaerobic capacity left in reserve. This is also why many elite athletes like to draft behind other competitors until the latter stages of a race; conserving their anaerobic capacity enables them to launch a sustained sprint at the end.

Variable pacing is less evident in short and middle-distance races because the exercise intensity usually remains well above the severe exercise intensity domain (i.e., above critical power) throughout the event and so phosphocreatine cannot be resynthesised. Short bursts of acceleration have to be well judged in short and long-distance events because the anaerobic capacity will decrease on each occasion, which will adversely affect the sprint finish.

Finally, in a study of 100 km ultra-distance runners, Lambert and colleagues (2004) observed that, although all the runners were unable to maintain their early speed over the course of the event, the faster runners tended to start the race faster and thereafter maintain their initial pace for longer with only small fluctuations. Therefore, variable pacing, as a strategy, may be less applicable to ultra-distance events than to long-distance events, perhaps because ensuring economical movement and managing diminishing energy reserves by not changing pace frequently is more important in ultra-distance events.

Conclusion

A number of key considerations affect the pacing strategy of particular events. Table 5.1 presents a comprehensive, although not exhaustive, list of factors to consider when designing a pacing strategy. Athlete and coach testimonies suggest that a pacing strategy should be a key part of a training programme. By breaking down the competition performance into specific components (eg. start, middle, finish), a coach or athlete can design a training programme that achieves the desired pacing profile. For example, if the athlete cannot accelerate to a required peak speed in an all-out pacing race, then the pacing plan is not achievable. In this case the training emphasis should be on developing sufficient power output at the start of the race by focusing on strength and power development and technical aspects. A middle-distance athlete who wants to inject a fast pace with 600 m to go must develop speed endurance along with the ability to accelerate rapidly up to speed at that point in a race. The importance of this tactic is that it can surprise the opposition and gain a second of time on them which, at the elite level, would be an arduous gap to close. Finally it is important to note that as the athlete adapts through training then their pacing strategy will also evolve.

To maximise training, athletes and coaches need to know the performance requirements for each part of the pacing profile. Peter Elliott (1500 m Olympic silver medallist in athletics, Seoul 1988) determined that 24 seconds was the target time for the 200 m starting phase of an 800 m race to put him in the right tactical position for the rest of the race. He trained for this by running as fast as he could in sprinting sessions against a specialist 400 m runner. However, he realised that this was leading to injuries, because he was always trying to run faster than 24 seconds during repetitions to beat the 400 m runner. At this stage, he decided that this was unnecessary because he needed to run 24 seconds only in the starting phase, and he could already do it. He then amended his training and spent more time on the other aspects of the pacing profile. This anecdote tells us that elite athletes and their coaches have to truly understand their event, and also be flexible.

The ability to be flexible, especially on the day of competition when conditions might change (e.g., the time of the event, weather, opposition), and remain confident comes from experience, trusting the advice of support providers (coaches, sport scientists and medical staff) and knowing that planning and training have been meticulous. The experience gained from training and competition gives the athlete a library of pacing templates to use in any competition setting. The sensory feedback from the body to the brain during training guides the athlete during the competition. It provides the confi-

Table 5.1 Checklist for Developing an Appropriate Pacing Strategy and Related Training Programme

1	**Event duration**
2	**Prior experience** of the event and pace judgement.
3	**Current fitness level** (aerobic, anaerobic, power development) and training emphasis of previous macrocycle(s) (physiological and technical improvements).
4	**Nutritional strategies** (e.g., creatine, bicarbonate or carbohydrate supplementation).
5	**Warm-up (prior to exercise)** to stimulate aerobic metabolism and spare the anaerobic capacity.
6	**Drag considerations:** Is the event predominantly air resisted or water resisted? What equipment is available to reduce resistance (e.g., skin suits)?
7	**Surface:** Frictional resistance (e.g., ice, wooden boards, synthetic track). Equipment available to reduce resistance (e.g., tyre pressures, lower-rolling-resistance tyres, ski wax) or improve traction (e.g., tyre tread, running spike length).
8	**Course conditions:** • Topography of the course (e.g., slope gradients—undulating, hilly or mountainous) • Duration of uphill, downhill and flat sections.
9	**Climatic considerations:** • Heat and humidity • Altitude • Wind speed, direction and chill
10	**Opposition:** Is there a pacemaker? Is the main threat a front runner or a sprint finisher or someone who mixes the pace up?
11	**Event goal:** Is a record or championship at stake? **Major championship or event:** Develop a strategic race plan with various scenarios (e.g., slow start and sprint finish, slow start with a sustained high-speed finish or fast pace throughout with frequent surges). **World record attempt:** Develop a strategy specific to the athlete's physiology and event requirements (e.g., calculate the correct starting pace and the appropriate pacing strategy throughout).
12	**Psychological status:** Can the athlete consistently execute the pacing strategy in training and competition? Consider the following: • Emotional state • Confidence level • Motivation • Mental toughness • Executive function—can the athlete make good decisions during a race? • Feedback to focus on during the race

dence that comes from knowing that the effort ahead is within the realm of previous efforts and is possible.

Paul Manning (gold medallist, cycling team pursuit, Beijing 2008) recalled that the GB team pursuit riders would adapt their pace when they were the last team to race in qualifying, because they would know their competitors' times at that stage. That being the case, Paul states, 'You still keep it [the qualifying round] in the realms of the right speed and cadences so you do not drop too far off the pace'.

part II

Pacing Applications for Sport

chapter 6

Swimming

Due to the highly resistive properties of water, pacing is arguably more critical in swimming than in many other sports. Swimming is mechanically inefficient, because only 6 to 18 per cent of the energy created from metabolism is actually converted into the muscles doing gainful work (Holmer 1974b; Pendergast et al. 1978). Therefore, an increase in swimming speed increases energy expenditure substantially. Swimmers who fail to pace properly suffer poor race performances as a result of a rapid onset of fatigue, which results in a loss of stroke power, coordination and speed. This is due to the high metabolic cost of swimming against the highly resistive medium of water and the additional drag caused by the swimmer becoming less streamlined and subsequently dropping deeper in the water (often at the hips) as fatigue ensues. It is a catch-22 situation at this point, in which the more fatigued the swimmer becomes, the greater technique deterioration becomes. This further increases drag and results in an increased metabolic energy cost and an even greater rate of fatigue!

Another consideration is that, in swimming, the stroke frequency (number of strokes per minute) dictates the number of opportunities to breathe. As the swimmer fatigues, the temptation is to breathe more often, perhaps every stroke rather than every other stroke, which negatively affects streamlining and may result in greater drag and energy expenditure. In a fatigued state, the swimmer has to slow down to a speed at which it is possible to finish the race in reasonably good form without any hope of winning it—damage limitation! Clearly, technique and physiology have to be very much in tune in swimming, and pacing strategy has a massive impact on both of these areas.

In physics, mechanical efficiency relates to the actual work output divided by the ideal work output. If mechanical efficiency is 0.25 (or 25 per cent), then around 75 per cent of the energy used will eventually become heat. This definition reveals the inefficient nature of swimming, in which actual work output ranges from 6 to 18 per cent. In comparison, the mechanical efficiency in cycling is much greater at 18 to 24 per cent (Coyle et al. 1992).

The higher the standard of swimming competition, the more difficult it is for swimmers to improve their race performances. It has been calculated that a true improvement in elite swimming performance requires a 0.4 per cent or greater reduction in finishing time (Pyne, Trewin & Hopkins 2004), based on the premise that a swimmer's race time varies slightly from race to race for many reasons (e.g., time of the race, motivation, time of year, pool conditions). An analysis of Olympic, World Championship, Commonwealth, and European Championship finalists revealed that an achievable change in lap time could result in a 0.4 to 0.8 per cent improvement in finishing time depending on stroke, sex and event (Robertson et al. 2009). Many international coaches agree that potential finalists at a major championship who improve their race performance by 1 per cent are highly likely to medal, because an improvement of 0.5 per cent or less would be a realistic possibility for most swimmers in an Olympic year. Achieving such a small, but critical improvement in overall time (e.g., a 1-second reduction in finishing time in a 200 m freestyle race corresponds approximately to a 1 per cent improvement) may not seem like much, but it could be enough to lead to victory.

However, even if a swimmer is in the right physical condition to make such an improvement, there is still the matter of getting the pacing strategy just right. As highlighted earlier, starting a race too fast often results in the rapid development of fatigue and a dramatic loss of speed. Setting off too conservatively, on the other hand, can lead to a significant gap between a swimmer and the race leader. This gap is difficult to close if the lead swimmer has paced correctly, because the energy cost required to increase swimming speed will be significant and, again, could easily lead to premature fatigue. An extensive analysis of international competition lap times has revealed that races are often won in the middle portions, in which gaps open up that cannot then be closed (Robertson et al. 2009).

Key Factors in Determining a Pacing Strategy for Swimming

Pacing patterns differ according to the distance of the event and the stroke. Despite coaches giving swimmers split times to pace to as part of normal pre-race preparations, data on the implications of pacing strategies in swimming are hard to come by. Choosing the most appropriate pacing strategy is an extremely complex question for the coach of a swimming team, because strategies may be needed for athletes competing in up to four swimming strokes over varying distances. Moreover, in the 200 m and 400 m individual medley events, swimmers undertake all four strokes in one race!

The Olympic Games swimming programme includes the following events:

- 50 m (freestyle only)
- 100 m (all four strokes)
- 200 m (all four strokes and a medley event)
- 400 m (freestyle and a medley event)
- 800 m (women's freestyle only)
- 1500 m (men's freestyle only)
- Marathon over 10 km (a new event introduced in 2008, swum in open water)

Stroke

The stroke is important because each one has its own mechanical efficiency that influences how quickly the swimmer fatigues and determines how effective and feasible it is to change the stroke rate (or frequency) during a race. It has been reported that the breaststroke is the least efficient of the strokes, whereas the freestyle is the most efficient (Holmer 1974b). For example, at the same swimming speed, it has been reported that the breaststroke requires an additional 1.2 litres of oxygen per minute, or approximately 5 extra kilocalories of energy per minute than the freestyle (Holmer 1974a). In fact, the breaststroke is three times less efficient than the freestyle (Pendergast et al. 1978). This is partly because the speed of the breaststroke swimmer fluctuates markedly during each stroke cycle, whereas the freestyle swimmer's speed varies to a much lesser degree.

During the breaststroke, the peak velocity might be around 1.8 metres per second following completion of the leg kick, but it may fall to 0.2 metres per second during the leg recovery phase (D'Aquisto et al. 1988). The need to violently accelerate during each stroke of the breaststroke contributes to its relative inefficiency compared to the other strokes (Thompson & Haljand 1997a). The breaststroke swimmer actually produces more propulsion during the leg kick than the freestyle swimmer does. However, the opposite is true for the arm pull, and over the whole stroke cycle this makes the breaststroke less effective in terms of overall propulsion.

The butterfly is also less efficient than the freestyle and backstroke events. Craig and Pendergast (1979) calculated that a 45 to 50 per cent change in swimming speed occurred during the butterfly and breaststroke stroke events, compared to only a 15 to 20 per cent difference for the freestyle and backstroke events. Perhaps unsurprisingly, butterfly swimmers demonstrate relatively little variation in their stroke rates during races, presumably to avoid losing their rhythm and to maintain relatively efficient propulsion. Butterfly swimmers place a greater emphasis on maintaining as great a stroke length as possible to limit the number of stroke cycles they complete during a race. Swimming speed is equal to the *stroke length multiplied by the stroke rate,* and if stroke length can be maintained over a race, the stroke rate does not have to increase greatly to compensate.

As previously discussed, because it is problematic in both the breaststroke and butterfly to increase the stroke rate, maintaining the stroke length is particularly important in these events. In the 200 m butterfly events of the 1995 European Swimming Championships, the stroke length was observed to fall by 8 to 12 per cent, whereas the stroke rate fluctuated by only 1.5 to 4 per cent (Thompson & Haljand 1997b). The purpose of this strategy is to keep the power output of the arms from having to increase over the race to such an extent that excessive local muscle fatigue developed (Chollet et al. 1996).

In comparison to the breaststroke and butterfly, the freestyle and backstroke (the 'crawl strokes') are much more efficient. This is demonstrated in a comparison of drop-offs in competition lap times during elite 200 m races. In the crawl strokes, lap times may fall by only approximately 0.4 second, from lap 2 to lap 4, whereas in the breaststroke and butterfly, a drop-off of closer to 1.0 to 1.2 seconds is more common (Robertson et al. 2009). The greater efficiency of the crawl strokes means that the stroke rate (or frequency) can be increased to a much larger extent than it can in the other two strokes. This has a number of important implications for the pacing strategy of crawl swimmers. First, it allows for greater flexibility in terms of race strategy because there is a greater potential to increase pace during a race, possibly on a number of occasions. It also means that the swimmer can compensate for the greater loss in the stroke length by increasing the stroke rate to a greater extent. For example, Craig and Pendergast (1979) reported that the stroke length of butterfly swimmers may decrease by 15 to 18 per cent during racing, whereas freestyle and backstroke swimmers lose up to 30 per cent of their stroke lengths. However, the crawl swimmers can increase their stroke rate to compensate to a much greater extent. Thus, the initial pace a swimmer adopts early in a race may be more critical in the breaststroke and butterfly events because of the relative inefficiency of these strokes and because changing pace during racing is much less feasible than it is in the crawl strokes.

Early Swimming Research

AT A GLANCE

Scientific investigation into swimming is thought to have begun with a series of studies by Lijestrand and Strenstrom (1919) and Lijestrand and Lindhard (1919). They calculated oxygen consumption from expired air collections taken while swimmers were paced by a rowing boat in a lake and also while tethered to a mooring, effectively swimming in place! They collected expired gases by asking swimmers to breathe through a mouthpiece connected to tubes that led to a large collection bag stowed on the boat. This system must have been extremely cumbersome for the swimmers, especially when attempting to swim at a maximal effort.

Distance

Maglischo (1993) reported that successful swimmers in 100 m events pace positively (i.e., fast start, slower finish), whereas those in the 200 m and 400 m events adopt a more evenly paced strategy. Some swimmers in the longer events were able to achieve an end spurt (faster finish) in the final lap or so, suggesting that they were able to conserve some of their finite anaerobic energy for the final stage of the race. A recent study of 264 elite national and international 400 m freestyle competitions revealed that a fast start followed by an even pace was common in races, although some competitors managed end spurts to achieve a parabolic pacing profile (Mauger, Neuloh & Castle 2012). In the longer events (800 m and 1500 m), swimmers generally pace evenly.

It has been postulated that sprint races are decided in the final 25 m of the 50 m event and the final 50 m of the 100 m event. In the 200 m and 400 m events, the competitive advantage is gained in the second 50 m and 100 m laps, respectively, and that gain is often largely maintained over the remainder of the race (unpublished observations from the Australian Institute of Sport; Robertson et al. 2009). It has also been reported that there is a poor relationship between final-length mid-pool swimming velocity and finishing time in the 200 m breaststroke event, which means that the race was decided earlier on and the eventual winner is not necessarily the fastest finisher. This demonstrates a fine line between pacing success and failure in this particular event (Thompson & Haljand1997a; Thompson & Haljand, 2000, Thompson et al. 2000).

In a large-scale competition analysis of over 155 national and international swimmers per event, Thompson and Haljand (2000) reported that in breaststroke events the mid-pool swimming velocity decreased significantly over each consecutive 50 m of a race; the first length was swum 6 to 7 per cent faster than the final length in both male and female 100 m and 200 m events. The drop in swimming speed in the final three lengths of the men's 200 m was attributed to the onset of leg fatigue. Across breaststroke events the researchers found that the stroke length deteriorated on each subsequent length, indicating that fatigue was developing. Although the swimmers attempted to compensate by increasing their stroke rate, this proved to be insufficient (and inefficient), and the swimming velocity fell. Interestingly, the swimmers demonstrated a consistent reduction in stroke rate in the second 50 m lap of the 200 m breaststroke events, presumably to conserve energy after the fast start. However, the distance per stroke still decreased, which further indicates the inefficiency of breaststroke swimming. The strategy of increasing the stroke rate during a race to compensate for a reduced stroke length (or distance per stroke) is common in the other strokes and events, too; however, it is most effective in maintaining swimming velocity in the crawl strokes (Arrelano et al. 1994; Chengalur & Brown 1992; Kennedy et al. 1990; Wakayoshi et al 1992).

Figure 6.1 shows the usual variations of pacing patterns among strokes and events. Across events there is clear evidence of positive pacing in the 50 m and 100 m, and it is probable that swimmers in the shorter events adopt an all-out strategy of swimming maximally throughout and risking a catastrophic performance failure by inducing acute peripheral (muscle) fatigue prior to the end. This is a risky strategy because being able to finish strongly in the final 25 m of the 50 m event is critical for success. In the 200 m events, subtle changes in lap times clearly occur after the first length; swimmers often swim the second length (assuming a 50 m pool) faster than they do the third and fourth lengths.

In contrast, in an in-depth analysis of 16 swimmers over nine competitions in the men's 200 m freestyle, Robertson and colleagues (2009) observed that elite swimmers generally managed to increase their swimming speed slightly in the final length (by 0.1 second compared to the third length). These findings demonstrate how subtle the pacing strategy can be in swimming and also that the loss of swimming speed in 100 m to 200 m events is most obvious in the least efficient strokes, the butterfly and breaststroke.

Arguably, coaches need to consider the subtlety of pacing strategies and the impact of them, because even a small change in racing speed will have a marked effect on the swimmer's physiology. This, of course, also has repercussions for the individual medley events.

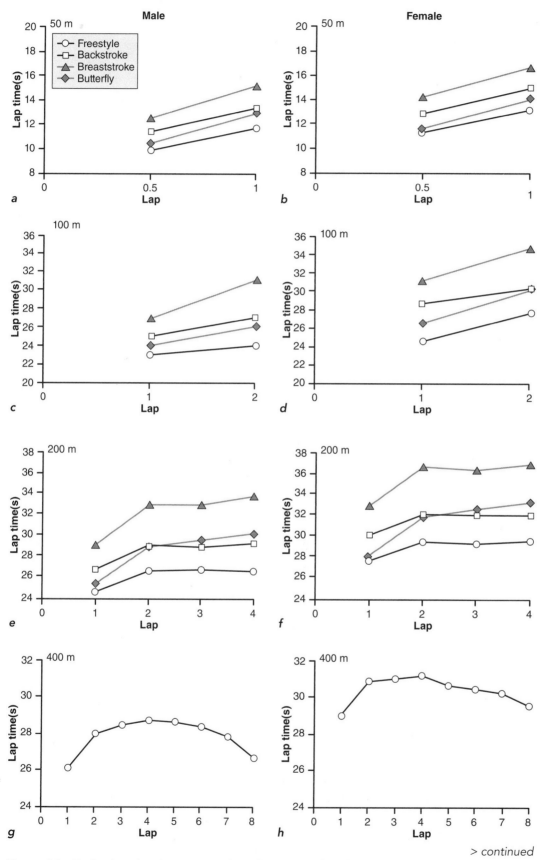

Figure 6.1 Pacing in swimming across various distances and strokes.

> continued

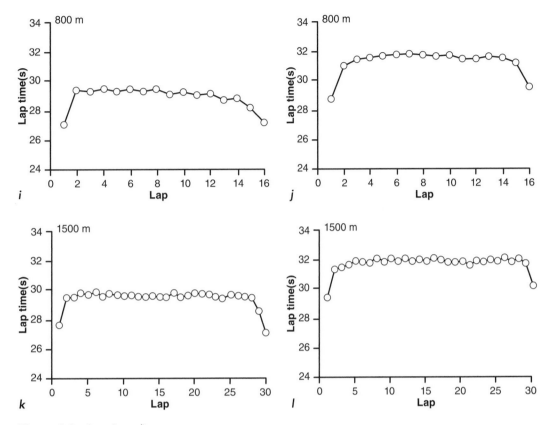

Figure 6.1   (continued)

Physiological and Performance Effects of Pacing

Researchers have suggested that a greater blood lactate is elicited in the 200 m events than in the 100 m events (Madsen & Lohberg 1987; Vescovi et al. 2010). This may seem strange given that the 100 m event is swum at a faster speed and with a more aggressive pacing strategy (positive pacing). However, the longer duration of the 200 m event may nonetheless result in a greater proportion of the anaerobic capacity being used or a greater lactate accumulation occurring as a result of a prolonged imbalance between lactate appearance and lactate removal. The tendency in the 200 m events towards more even pacing compared to the 100 m events perhaps reflects the need to marshal the anaerobic capacity more sensitively in this event by avoiding too fast a start, which would deplete the anaerobic energy reserves too quickly. However, by still starting relatively quickly (using a positive pace), the 200 m swimmer will maximise the efficiency of the oxygen uptake kinetics at the start of the race by using slow-twitch Type I muscle fibres as much as possible, rather than fast-twitch Type II fibres. As a result, more of the swimmer's force will come from aerobic energy production, reducing the early reliance on anaerobic energy production seen at the beginning of exercise as the body's cardiorespiratory system gets up to speed. This conserves anaerobic capacity for use later in the race.

Robertson and colleagues (2009) reported that international freestyle swimmers competing in 100 m, 200 m and 400 m events tended to adopt similar pacing strategies from race to race. Slower swimmers completed slower lap times, often by a consistent amount, over the course of the race. It would seem from this analysis that if you were to bet on the leading swimmer midway through a freestyle race, you would win the bet most of the time! In addition, swimmers who achieved faster times had most likely consistently reduced their lap time across laps in such a way that *the pacing pattern was the same*; the time for each lap had improved by a small but similar margin.

Skorski and colleagues (2013a) reported that a group of competitive freestyle swimmers demonstrated highly reproducible pacing profiles in time trials, which were similar to the pacing profiles the swimmers exhibited during races, except that during the races, they swam each section faster. In another study, Skorski and colleagues (2013b) observed that the pacing of elite 200 m swimmers from lap to lap was very consistent, differing by only 1 to 2 per cent generally. However, in the backstroke and butterfly, greater variability occurred in the last 25 m or so, presumably as a result of fatigue. Also, breaststroke swimmers generally showed greater variability in pacing than did those performing other strokes. Taken together, these findings demonstrate that well-trained swimmers possess a robust pacing template.

Robertson and colleagues (2009) argued that because swimmers appear to adopt similar pacing strategies to each other and from race to race, it was their fitness rather than their pacing strategy that had to improve to achieve faster lap times across the race. This is a reasonable argument; however, even if a swimmer's fitness does improve, the pacing strategy would still need to be perfected, either in training or over a series of races, to achieve a personal best time. As noted in previous chapters, athletes rely on prior experience as well as ongoing feedback to judge the pace of a race. This is why practising paced efforts in training and then in competition is important to realise the swimmer's potential.

The causes of improved lap times and race performance have not been extensively researched. Given that sophisticated measurements are required to detect small improvements in performance, few coaches have the equipment necessary for answering these questions. The accurate capture of changes in start times, midpool swimming velocity, stroke rate or length and turning times requires sophisticated pool-side cameras, calibrated lane markings and video frame–counting techniques. Unfortunately, the measurement error inherent when hand-timing with stopwatches (0.3 to 0.4 second; Thompson et al. 2002) is simply too great to provide sufficient accuracy.

A study using sophisticated measurements to compare the race performances of 36 elite swimmers over two 200 m breaststroke races revealed that the improvement in finishing time (~1.90 seconds) was largely due to an improvement in mid-pool swimming velocity in each lap. This suggests that either the swimmers' fitness or their technique had improved (Thompson, Haljand & Lindley 2004). The researchers suggested that the improvement in swimming speed was primarily due to a higher stroke rate, although stroke length improved as well. In addition to the stroke changes, the swimmers' turning times also improved, accounting for approximately 0.5 second of the improvement. The dive start and swim to 15 m and the finish phase in the last 5 m of the race explained a further 0.3 second of the improvement. This demonstrates the importance of coaches adopting a holistic view of race performance and the pacing strategy. The improvement in turning performance in the preceding study was quite likely due to a faster approach speed into the turn. However, the turn had to be executed properly with good (or improved) technique. Also, because turns are highly susceptible to fatigue (Thompson et al. 2003, 2004a,b), improved fitness likely played a significant role, too.

Only a few research studies have looked specifically at the effect of changing pace during swimming. In a study that manipulated stroke rate rather than swimming velocity, Swaine and Reilly (1983) found small but significant changes in oxygen uptake and minute ventilation (the volume of air breathed per minute) when small changes were observed in stroke rate during high-intensity freestyle swimming simulations on a swim bench.

In another study, swimmers were asked to swim with a fixed stroke rate at 92 per cent, 95 per cent, 100 per cent and 107 per cent of the average stroke rate they had demonstrated for a 200 m breaststroke time trial. The stroke rate was paced using a programmable audible pacing device placed close to the ear in a swimming cap so the

ATHLETE'S PERSPECTIVE: Pacing in Swimming

Chris Cook
50 m, 100 m and 200 m GB international breaststroke swimmer, 50 m and 100 m gold medallist, Commonwealth Games, 2006

In the 100 m, I would build as the race progressed based on the stroke rate, beginning with 17 strokes and then coming back (second 50 m) with 21 strokes. When I broke my PB (personal best time), I actually managed 16 and then 20 strokes.

I knew with these stroke rates that I could hit 28 (seconds) low or maybe a 27 high on a good day for the first 50 m. My PB for the 50 m is 27.7 seconds, which I did with 23 strokes, so I was much less efficient swimming (less distance per stroke) in the 50 m than in the 100 m and found only a bit more speed.

Pacing is so important. People have different strengths. My competitors were generally taller than I am (they would be over 6 feet [183 cm] tall and 8 to 10 kg [18 to 22 lb] heavier), so they could shoot through the water from the dive and start faster than I could. This meant I was often behind early in the race, but my coach (Ian Oliver) and I decided to work on getting more distance per stroke so I could catch up and pass my competitors as the race progressed. By doing this, I would try to exploit the weakness of my competitors, to capitalise on their slowing down at the end while I would be maintaining good speed for longer and overtake them.

I remember in the 100 m of the semi-final of the Commonwealth Games in Melbourne that the aim was to take it out easy, but I misjudged it and went out faster than planned. In the tank (the pool) I go by feel; I cannot compute numbers. That race I swam very fast, and I was worried afterward whether that would affect my performance in the final. There were external pressures, and I was concerned I could not reproduce that performance in the final. However, by the final I had put it behind me and took confidence in knowing that I was a talented racer. I knew that nobody was better prepared than I was, and I won the race.

For the 100 m breaststroke, to break the world record, a swimmer would need to go out in a 27 (-second) point at the 50 m mark and bring it home in a 30 point and would have to maintain composure throughout. If you achieve a 28 point and then a 30 point, then you are fast, but if you make small errors and go out in, say, 28.6 and come back in 30.6, then you are nowhere—the margins are just so small.

Breaststroke is all about rhythm; if you are shoulder to shoulder with someone, it is difficult either for the other swimmer to keep from adopting your rhythm or for you to not adopt his! Competition is so tight in the world now that it is rare for someone to win at the highest level from behind. The minute barrier has been broken numerous times now—many swimmers finish races strongly in the last 15 m now and do not die away at the end.

Breaststroke is a uniquely difficult event technically, and even in a world-class final, the eight swimmers standing on the blocks will all have very different techniques. Today, physical conditioning is key; no one has a poor technique at the elite level, and there are incredible athletes such as Brenton Rickard, who is extremely tall (well over 6 ft 5 in.[196 cm]). I used to work on getting power gains out of the water, using gym conditioning, to make me as powerful as possible for the start and to propel myself through the water as well as larger swimmers.

For the 200 m breaststroke event, I would adopt an 18-month build-up in terms of the pacing strategy. For the 100 m, I would build from September on a 9- to 10-month build-up. I would need to get long course training in, and would work on getting good times through the first 25 m using a low number of strokes. The training would be tough throughout, and it would take time to become efficient to get the speed we wanted. It was surprising to see how late in the cycle the speed would suddenly develop. You cannot develop a pacing strategy that holds you back; you have to go with how you feel and adjust expectations. Going by how you feel is, however, a sort of uncharted territory! But when you get the right feeling, then you think you can pretty much do anything; you rehearse and rehearse so that a lot of what you are then doing becomes largely subconscious—you feel incredible!

My pacing strategy has developed over time. My coach and I have tried to change it at certain periods; at one point we worked on getting out quicker, but I ended up dying! We tried this strategy because the UK group were so strong at that particular time that I would be on the back-foot (behind) after the start. However, from a young age I realised that I finished better than most. I was a strong finisher and could hold my stroke well even when I was in real pain. I realised that having control and coming home fast was my strength, and so we used that as the pacing strategy.

Pacing is a critical component of racing. If you go out slightly too fast, then you lose composure and come back slow; if you go out too slow, then you might finish strong but have too much to make up to win the race. At times in my career, I knew that if I could get to the first 50 m right, even if I had lost 0.5 m on my competitors, I would pass them in the second 50 m to win.

swimmer could match each stroke cycle with a signal from the pacing device. Surprisingly, no statistically significant differences were found in performance times across trials, although there were trends towards greater and reduced finishing times in the 92 per cent and 107 per cent trials, respectively. Physiological responses (heart rate and blood lactate) and perceived exertion scores (RPE) were also similar between trials. The authors concluded that either a set physiological capacity constrained the performance or that a pacing strategy had been initiated with regard to the muscle activation, which determined the stroke length or some other biomechanical behaviour and marshalled the physiological capacity to allow completion of each trial within the fastest possible time (Thompson et al. 2009).

In another study, breaststroke swimmers completed a 200 m time trial and then swam three additional 200 m trials 48 hours apart and in random order, at 98 per cent, 100 per cent and 102 per cent of the mean time trial speed (Thompson et al. 2004a). The 98 per cent and 100 per cent trials were swum at an even pace, whereas the 102 per cent trial was swum at a positive pace (i.e., the swimmers slowed down significantly in the second 100 m of the trial). The researchers found that physiological responses, which included heart rate, blood lactate and oxygen consumption, were similar for the 98 per cent and 100 per cent trials, indicating a similar metabolic cost. This suggests that pacing a heat swim more slowly (2 per cent slower) to conserve energy may not be effective, perhaps as a result of reduced streamlining and greater drag when swimming just below racing pace. Notably, blood lactate values were greater after the 102 per cent trial, which indicates a greater muscle lactate release and a reduced muscle pH (increased acidity). The RER ratio (volume of oxygen consumed divided by the volume of carbon dioxide expired) was also greater, indicating that a greater anaerobic energy contribution was required towards the end of the 102 per cent trial. Because the profile of the heart rate and oxygen consumption measurements were similar between the 100 per cent (even-paced trial) and the 102 per cent trial, the investigators concluded that a similar aerobic energy contribution was likely. The investigators also suggested that because the finishing time was 0.8 per cent better in the positively paced 102 per cent trial than in the 100 per cent trial, positive pacing could be more effective as a pacing strategy and lead to faster race times. However, this strategy would also require a greater anaerobic energy contribution. Since the anaerobic energy contribution is considered finite, a positive pacing strategy would need to be carefully considered to allow the swimmer to marshal this limited resource to the end of the race. Perhaps as a result of the greater metabolic acidosis arising from positive pacing, the swimmers in this study reported greater perceived exertion in the 102 per cent trial. Therefore, mental toughness appears to come into play to a greater extent with a positive pacing strategy—it hurts more!

In another the study, the same investigators (Thompson et al. 2003) asked breaststroke swimmers to complete 175 m breaststroke trials without a dive start using one of the following strategies:

- An even pace (the same average speed as a maximal 200 m swim)
- A positive pace (2 per cent faster than the average maximal 200 m swim for the first half of the trial and then 2 per cent slower than the average maximal 200 m swim for the second half)
- A negative pace (the reverse of the positive pace trial, swimming 2 per cent slower than the average maximal 200 m swim for the first half of the trial and 2 per cent faster than the average maximal 200 m swim for the second half)

So what happened? The aerobic energy contribution (measured at the end of each trial) was no different among the trials, suggesting a similar aerobic contribution. This is not surprising given that all of the trials were near maximal in terms of effort. Stroke rates were lower during the first half of the even-pace and negative-pace trials; however, they were similar across all trials during the second half of each trial. Stroke length fell in consecutive laps in all the trials, clearly demonstrating increasing fatigue. The even-pace trial appeared to result in a less stressful response, in that blood lactate levels were lower after the trial and the swimmers reported a lower perceived exertion and demonstrated less variability in their turns and pacing precision.

Even-pace swimming, therefore, appears to be less stressful on the swimmer, but is it the preferred strategy for race pacing over the 200 m breaststroke event? As mentioned previously, 200 m events on the whole are swum at an even pace. However, in the 200 m breaststroke, a 6 to 7 per cent decrease in mid-pool swimming velocity has been shown in international swimmers, which is clear evidence that positive pacing is favoured in this event (Thompson and Haljand 2000). It seems that for this particular stroke the increased stress and the risk of incorrectly implementing a positive pacing strategy are offset by the perception (or belief—perhaps gained from race experience) that implementing this strategy correctly will lead to an optimal performance.

In the 400 m freestyle there is a fast first 100 m due to the dive start, then an even pace over the second and third 100 m, followed by a faster final 100 m (an end spurt). This pattern suggests that the swimmers anticipate the end of the race and use feedback from various receptors in the body (both mechanical and metabolic) during the race to guide their efforts and to keep energy in reserve for a prolonged push over the final quarter of the race. Therefore, performance in the 400 m event appears to be more determined by central control mechanisms than are performances in shorter events in which the accumulation of fatiguing metabolites and the depletion of high-energy substrates lead to peripheral (muscle) fatigue.

In the 400 m the brain centres are probably more actively involved in subconscious and conscious decision making. The brain centres have more time to assimilate the feedback from body receptors and to precisely calculate the muscle activation required to maximise performance on an ongoing basis throughout the race. As a consequence, swimmers in this event are likely to pace reasonably well, unless they are inexperienced and do not have the benefit of prior knowledge of the event, or allow strong emotions to dictate their early efforts and set themselves a suicidal early pace. Therefore, a muted or nonexistent end spurt in a 400 m freestyle could be due to a number of factors. For example, the swimmer may have swum sub-maximally throughout perhaps because of a lack of motivation, or may have been operating well above their critical power in the severe exercise intensity domain (85 to 90 per cent of $\dot{V}O_2$max) and as such used much of the anaerobic capacity in the early stages of the race so that it was too depleted to fuel an end spurt.

Role of the Brain

Coaches, athletes and researchers understand that prior experience from training or competition is critical for judging the early pace of a race correctly. Controlling emotion at the start of races is also important to avoid overriding the planned pacing strategy and internal pacing algorithm because of high motivation or arousal levels (e.g., deciding in the moment, 'blow the strategy, I am just going to go for it!'). Furthermore, during the early stages of a race, the brain centres may not be sensitive enough, or may have insufficient signalling from the body receptors at that point, to accurately compute a pacing algorithm. Indeed the brain might not be receiving sufficient information or be able to process information rapidly enough, during the majority of a shorter event, to form a conscious or subconscious decision about the appropriateness of the pacing strategy. This makes it difficult to adjust a poor pacing strategy in time to affect the outcome of a short-distance race. Rather with no warning the muscles might demonstrate sudden fatigue, causing the stroke technique to begin to fail and in turn the swimming velocity to decrease. Muscle fatigue (known as peripheral fatigue) would seem to set in before the brain is even aware that the pace is not appropriate. In contrast, during a longer race there is more time for feedback to reach the brain and be interpreted; the brain can initiate a response to a potential problem, such as fatigue developing too quickly, by slightly reducing the level of muscle activation to produce a slower but more sustainable pace.

The role of the brain in pacing is now being actively researched. What is fascinating is how reliably swimmers can pace themselves, at least when not at maximal racing speeds. Table 6.1 shows a training session for a junior international swimmer who can accurately pace with respect to the target time as speed and heart rate increase during a low-intensity training session.

Table 6.1   Pacing Data for an International Junior Backstroke Swimmer During a Low-Intensity Training Set

Number	Target time	Actual time	Stroke count (str/50 m)	Stroke rate (str/min)	Heart rate (bpm)
1	40	40.4	42	33.30	132
2	39	39.3	42	34.31	147
3	38	37.4	42	36.34	147
4	37	37.7	42	35.34	150
5	36	35.9	42	38.35	155
6	35	35.6	42	38.36	156
7	34	34.4	42	40.38	159
8	33	34.1	42	40.37	164
9	32	32.0	42	42.41	169
10	31	31.5	42	44.43	175
11	30	30.0	42	47.44	179
12	29	29.5	42	47.45	177
Personal best time	28				

When swimming speeds are much higher and the exercise intensity becomes much greater, increasing levels of discomfort occur and emotions can come into play. Figure 6.2 shows the self-reported repetition times and heart rate values of a sprint swimmer attempting to complete 15 × 100 m with approximately a 1:1 work-to-rest ratio. Unfortunately, the swimmer had little experience with this type of speed-endurance set and set off too fast. As a result, on repetition 8 he highlights his discomfort by emphasising the heart rate of 170 beats per minute, but then on repetition 9 he reports that he is angry! On repetition 10, pacing is entirely forgotten and he attacks the swim with an almost all-out effort, using much of the anaerobic capacity remaining and elevating his heart rate to close to maximum. Thereafter, he suffers the consequences of his actions with catastrophic results, and the set is stopped after repetition 13. Following a prolonged rest period, the swimmer, still emotional, chooses to swim another repetition at a maximal effort and produces a slow time (57 seconds for 100 m) as a result of the earlier fatigue from which he had still not recovered.

Repetition	Time(s)	Heart rate (bpm)
1	64.2	158
2	65.37	160
3	65.6	166
4	63.3	168
5	63.2	170
6	64.2	170
7	64.7	170
8	64.4	(170)
9	64.0	182 ANGRY !!
10	62.0	173
11	62.4	178
12	69.0	170
13	68.0	170

Figure 6.2 Self-reported heart rate and swimming times recorded by an international sprint swimmer incorrectly pacing a 15 × 100 m endurance training set.

Swimmers currently learn how to pace during training sessions using the pool-side clock, their own judgement and feedback from the coach who hand-times splits and finishing times with a stopwatch (unfortunately, as noted previously, this is somewhat imprecise). Pacing devices are available for swimmers who wish to go further, although there is not a single widely accepted one at present. Various systems have been tried over the years. For example, pacing lights have been placed either above the water on the pool side, which can lead to unwanted lateral movements, or at the bottom of the pool below the swimmer. In either case the lights are visible only for part of the stroke cycle, and swimmers may struggle to determine where their bodies should be in relation to the lights, causing a significant pacing error (D'Aquisto et al. 1988; Sano et al. 1990). Keskinen (1997a, 1997b) did report that light sequencing could help swimmers pace accurately if correct guidance were provided to the swimmer on body position relative to the lights. Audible sound systems have also been tried, although when placed above the water, they cannot be heard properly during the underwater elements of the stroke and the turn.

The Aquapacer system addresses some of these issues by providing a preprogrammed, coin-size, audible bleeping unit that is placed under the swimming cap, close to the ear so the pacing sound can be heard both above and below water. A number of studies demonstrated the accuracy of the system (Martin & Thompson 1999; Thompson et al. 2002) and concluded that it could more accurately pace the swimmer than a pool-side clock at submaximal speeds and that it allows accurate pacing at near-race speeds and when the swimmer changes pace midway through a high-speed swim. Caution is in order, however, because the error in pacing was reported to be approximately 1 to 3 seconds over 200 m, which is large in terms of the improvements generally possible in the race times of elite swimmers at this distance (1 to 1.5 seconds) over a year or so. Experts have debated whether using a pacing system to guide swimmers' progress against pool markings is accurate enough to train a pacing strategy. However, reputedly, a number of world-class swimmers have used the Aquapacer system to match their stroke rates with the audible bleep signal to train their stroke rate to a particular frequency in training, and this has anecdotally coincided with improved times in competition.

At the elite level of swimming, performance changes are small among competitors and competitions such that a 0.4 per cent change in performance either positively or negatively is a meaningful change. We take care to specify 'meaningful change' because within each day and from day to day, performance times can change slightly in response to factors such as differences in physiology or motor coordination as well as external factors such as the pool environment and the reliability of the measuring equipment (this is why the calibration of measurement instruments is critical). As a result of such factors, New Zealand junior and open national standard swimmers exhibited variability in performance of 1.3 per cent in finishing times in competition performances over a 20-day period (Stewart & Hopkins 2000). However, a controlled pre-race warm-up can negate some of the variation in performance by preparing the swimmer physiologically (Martin & Thompson 2000).

At the elite level at which competition is so strong that a 0.5 to 1.0 per cent improvement in performance can be the difference between glory and failure, meticulous preparation is critical. Taking particular care to set a correct early pace is especially important because the overall pacing pattern appears to be somewhat fixed and inflexible during a race. Therefore, what matters is to achieve a consistent reduction in lap times, which may equate to just over 0.2 second per lap in, say, a men's 200 m freestyle event lasting approximately 107 seconds! Although being able to swim faster accounts for the majority of the improvement in lap times, coaches and swimmers must also pay attention to starts and turns because appreciable time gains can also be made here. Thompson and colleagues (2000) reported that male 100 m breaststroke swimmers complete their start phase to 15 m 0.22 second quicker than 200 m breaststroke swimmers on average. Whether this is because 200 m swimmers, based on prior experience, already have a slower race pace in mind and so start slower or because less emphasis is placed on starting practice by coaches because the start element is less critical in the longer race is debatable. The key point here is that each aspect of performance needs to be evaluated and scrutinised, including the pacing strategy, because each aspect of the race is both marginally and critically important.

chapter 7

Cycling

The relative efficiency of cycling as compared with a sport such as swimming results in the need for a different pacing strategy. For example, sprint swimmers consider a positive pacing strategy, rather than an all-out strategy, in a 100 m event lasting 60 seconds or less, whereas riders in the men's kilo (1000 m) track cycling event, which takes slightly longer than 60 seconds, can use an all-out strategy. Also, because of the high speeds achieved in cycling, atmospheric conditions (air temperature, humidity, barometric pressure) affect this sport more than in many other sports.

Key Factors in Determining a Pacing Strategy for Cycling

Track cycling coaches use sophisticated tables to calculate gearing options depending on the air density resulting from the climatic conditions. Rolling resistance and frictional losses can also account for as much 10 per cent of the rider's total energy expenditure (Kyle 1996). Therefore, the weight of the rider and the bike, as well as the tyre pressures, chain drive and brake systems (where fitted) are all scrutinised to minimise energy costs. The GB Olympic track cycling team famously work with car racing manufacturers such as Lotus and McLaren to produce racing bikes that are extremely light and efficient and yet rigid enough to transfer 2000 W of power effectively onto the track surface.

In road cycling, the wind direction and speed and course topography, as well as the rider's hydration status, energy stores and food intake, all play a part in the race pace strategy. The ability to conserve energy by adopting an aerodynamic position becomes important above 15 km/h (9.3 mph), when the air resistance becomes a major retarding force and squares as a function of cycling velocity (Atkinson et al. 2007). Drafting behind other riders also plays a major part in race pace strategy because it can reduce power output by approximately 30 per cent (Atkinson et al. 2007). Cycling into a headwind of 15 km/h (9.3 mph) means that when you are cycling at 30 km/h (18.6 mph), you are actually expending similar amounts of energy as you would if you were cycling at 45 km/h (28 mph) in conditions of no wind! These factors all affect the pacing strategy adopted, playing a greater or smaller part depending on the event.

Pacing patterns generally observed in cycling are as follows:

- If the cycling event lasts around 1 minute, an all-out pacing strategy is adopted.
- If the event lasts less than 10 minutes, a fast start is observed, which then settles down to an even pace.
- In events lasting beyond 10 minutes under stable conditions (e.g., a velodrome), performance is optimised with an even distribution of work rate (Atkinson et al. 2007).
- In multistage road races, variable pacing is adopted except for the time trial stages, in which even pacing is observed.

Pacing in Events of 1000 Metres or Less

In the track cycling sprint events, the riders accelerate as rapidly as possible to their peak speed and then attempt to maintain that speed until the end of the event. Because sprint cyclists are muscular, they have a large frontal surface area and mass to move (see figure 7.1). In short-duration cycling events (60 seconds or less), athletes can maintain a speed close to their peak despite their power output reducing. In the Olympic Games, the sprint events now comprise the match sprint (4 × 250 m laps, with the last 300 m often flat-out), the team sprint (three riders complete a three-lap race with a rider dropping out each lap) and the keirin. The keirin may not seem like a sprint event because it is ridden over 2 km; however, in essence it is. In this event, the riders ride behind a pacer (usually a small motorcycle known as a derny), which starts at about 25 km/h (15.5 mph). The pacer increases in speed over successive laps until it achieves 50 km/h (31 mph); it then leaves the track approximately 600 to 700 m before the end. At this point the riders race each other, sometimes finishing at 70 km/h (43.5 mph).

The kilo time trial event (1000 m) occurs at the World Championships (the female equivalent is the 500 m time trial). In the kilo track cycling event, the riders' mechanical power output declines significantly; however, their speed falls by only around 10 per cent, because relatively little mechanical power output is required to maintain the terminal speed compared to when accelerating towards it. Shane Sutton, head coach of the hugely successful British cycling team, described it this way: 'With the kilo event (1 km sprint), the riders used to give it full gas for 350 m, then cruised, then brought it home. Now, the riders keep driving all the way through 500 to 750 m and hold on. They get as high as possible (power output) and so have further to fall. Bicarbonate is used to numb the effort'. This quote demonstrates not only that pacing tactics have changed in this event as riders have become fitter and as bikes have become more sophisticated (e.g., thinner profile, less mass and rolling resistance) but also that ergogenic aids are used to stave off fatigue processes.

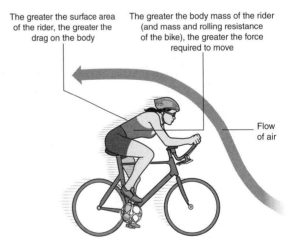

The greater the surface area of the rider, the greater the drag on the body

The greater the body mass of the rider (and mass and rolling resistance of the bike), the greater the force required to move

Flow of air

Figure 7.1   The larger the rider is in terms of surface area and body mass (weight), the greater the drag and rolling resistance will be. Therefore, the force production a large rider requires to achieve a certain speed is greater than that required by a smaller rider. A sprinter's muscular build creates more resistance, but it also provides the strength and power needed to produce great speed.

Strength and power training is a critical component in the sprint events because the riders have to rotate a large fixed gear up to 110 to140 revolutions per minute from a standing start. The fixed gear ratios are extreme; for example, elite riders might use 50/14 or 48/14 (front sprocket teeth/rear sprocket teeth) combinations. Riders' peak torque and power output relate significantly to the performance outcome in track sprint events (Gardner et al. 2007).

The ability to produce high levels of peak torque and power when cycling is highly related to the force-producing capabilities of the hip and knee extensors. For this reason, elite riders commonly undertake strength training exercises to increase the maximal *force-producing capabilities* (strength) *and rate of force production* (power) of the hip and knee extensors, such as squats, vertical jumps and power cleans. Male elite riders with a body weight around 90 kg (198 lb) might squat over 210 kg (463 lb) and power clean 130 kg (287 lb), and female sprinters with a body weight of 60 kg (132 lb) might squat over 100 kg (220 lb) and power clean 70 kg (154 lb). However, peak power values during cycling are most impressive: the very best elite male sprinters demonstrate values of 2,000 to 2,200 W over a 6-second sprint! This level of starting power allows a cyclist to achieve a sub-7-second quarter lap and a sub-10.5-second flying 200 m on a 250 m velodrome track. The ability to start fast is critical, because the first lap time is the primary determinant of the total time in the kilo event (Corbett 2009). The rider with the highest power output is better able to overcome greater air friction and rolling resistance and hence create more kinetic energy and faster motion.

Figure 7.2 demonstrates that, following the start of the men's kilo and women's 500 m events, the race pace is maintained through approximately 50 per cent and 75 per cent of the race distance in the kilo and 500 m events, respectively. Greater fatigue is evident in the men's race because it takes significant longer to complete. If you were to calculate the times taken for the first half of these races and compare them to those of the second half, you might conclude that a negative pacing strategy had occurred because the second half took less time than the first. However, this is simply the result of the time taken to accelerate the bike from rest at the start. The rider's pedal rate, or cadence, is important, because pedalling too quickly or slowly will lead to a loss of efficiency. Pedalling too fast might fatigue the rider prematurely because fast Type IIX muscle fibres are recruited, leading to a rapid accumulation of metabolites associated with fatigue (hydrogen ions, inorganic phosphate and ammonia) (Cherry et al. 1997).

Figure 7.3 demonstrates the high rate of energy production required to accelerate and compete in a kilo race. The figure shows that the initial energy requirement, to get the bike moving, is predicted to be more than 3.5 times the maximal energy production possible from the aerobic energy system! The energy production at this point will of course be primarily provided by the anaerobic energy system, which is rapidly depleted, leading to fatigue. The figure is for illustrative purposes and should not be taken literally because (1) oxygen uptake and hence aerobic metabolism take time to increase at the start of exercise and (2) $\dot{V}O_2$max cannot rise beyond 100 per cent. Therefore, what this graph demonstrates is the reliance on the anaerobic metabolism in the kilo event.

The gear ratio selection is critical to allow the rider to pedal at the optimal rate with the maximum power output. The power output is related to the rider's strength and power characteristics, muscle fibre composition, limb length and pedalling technique. Riders often choose a gear ratio that gives them the most rapid acceleration and hence the fastest start, which is not surprising given that the fastest starter often triumphs in a race. However, this gear ratio may well compromise the final part of the race because the pedal rate will be higher than is optimal at this point, activating the easily fatigued fast-twitch fibres. Peripheral fatigue in the muscles can lead to impaired muscle contraction and prematurely reduced force production, resulting in power output and speed dropping away too much for the rider to win the race. For these reasons, sprint cyclists must identify the best combination of gear ratio to optimise the pedal rate across the race. Riders often have to consider adopting higher gear ratios, which reduces their pedal rate to a less fatiguing range but does not adversely affect their initial acceleration.

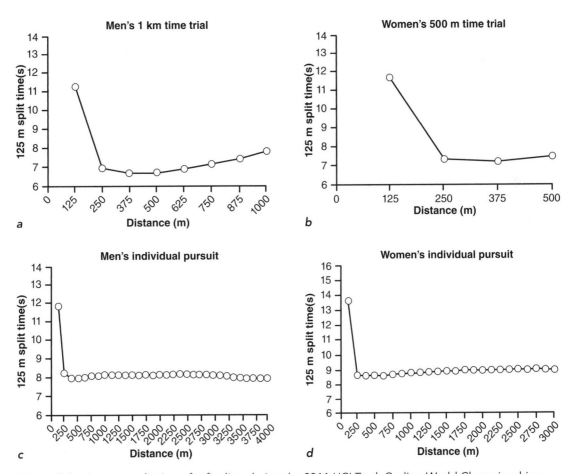

Figure 7.2 Average split times for finalists during the 2011 UCI Track Cycling World Championships.

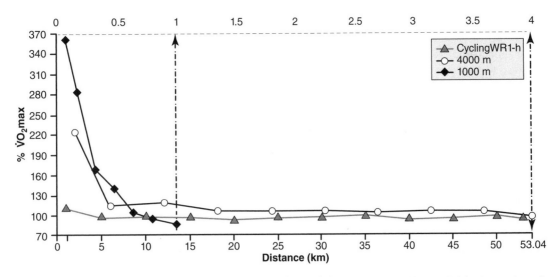

Figure 7.3 Predicted oxygen uptake requirements for the kilo sprint event, 4 km individual pursuit and world record for 1 hour (for distance covered in 1 hour).

Reprinted, by permission, from C. Foster, J.J. de Koning, S. Bischel, et al., 2012, Pacing strategies for endurance performance. In *Endurance training—Science and practice*, edited by I. Mujika (Vitoria-Gasteiz, Basque Country: Iñigo Mujika S.L.U.), 85-98.

Pacing in Individual and Team Pursuit Events

The individual pursuit is completed over 4 km for men and 3 km for women. After the 2008 Olympic Games, it was dropped from the Olympic programme; however, the team pursuit was retained for the London 2012 Olympic Games. In the men's team pursuit event, four riders work as a team and three of them have to finish; in the shorter women's event, three riders compete and all have to finish. A common trend is for road riders to transfer into these events following a relatively short period of training on the track. Bradley Wiggins, for example, won Olympic gold medals in the individual and team pursuit events in the 2008 Olympic Games and gained fourth place in the Tour de France the following year. Male riders in the pursuit events and indeed road races possess a high aerobic capacity ($\dot{V}O_2$max) of 5.0 to 6.4 L/min, or around 75 to 80 ml/kg/min, and can maintain more than 90 per cent of their $\dot{V}O_2$max for up to an hour (i.e., severe intensity exercise) (Atkinson et al 2007).

Figure 7.3 demonstrates how in the 4 km individual pursuit the riders start at an exercise intensity considerably greater than their maximal aerobic capacity (approximately 2.2 times greater than their $\dot{V}O_2$max). However, this is somewhat misleading because the uptake of oxygen actually takes some time to get up to speed at the beginning of high-intensity exercise. As a result, a significant proportion of the energy supplied to the muscles in the first minute of the race is from anaerobic energy metabolism. Once the cyclists reach race speed (after about 250 to 500 m), the race settles down to an even pace. The oxygen uptake reaches a peak after approximately 1000 to 1500 m of the race and then remains at or close to 100 per cent of its maximal capacity (i.e., $\dot{V}O_2$max) until the end of the race. In figure 7.3, you can see that the exercise intensity in the first kilometre of the race is still above the $\dot{V}O_2$max, which means that the anaerobic capacity is still being used to supplement aerobic energy supply. In fact, because it takes around a minute for the rider's oxygen uptake to reach its peak, little of the anaerobic capacity remains. For this reason, following a fast start, riders prefer an even pacing strategy to reduce any further metabolic disturbances, as the anaerobic capacity is depleted and the aerobic capacity is operating at maximum.

A mathematical model of a 4000 m pursuit estimated that the fastest time in a pursuit race is achieved by an all-out start, but after 12 seconds the anaerobic capacity that remains has to be used evenly for the remainder of the race. This confirms the importance of the aerobic energy contribution after the start phase and the need to maintain an even pace (de Koning, Bobbert & Foster 1999). In some races riders may be able to increase their speed in the final lap (an end spurt), although this is possible only if some anaerobic capacity remains.

Corbett (2009) analysed the 2006, 2007 and 2008 World Championships and found that after the first 250 m lap, in which the cyclists were getting up to speed, the second 250 m was the fastest lap. Thereafter, the pace decreased slightly until the end, and the riders demonstrated no end spurt. This probably demonstrates excellent pace judgement in these elite riders because they had fully used their anaerobic capacity and kinetic energy by the end of the race. The analysis, however, also showed that slower riders had been overly ambitious at the start and therefore slowed to a greater extent by the end. The same trends were evident in the men's 4 km individual pursuit.

Broker, Kyle and Burke (1999) reported that elite individual pursuit riders would have to produce an average of over 520 W to break the world record. They also calculated that when the team pursuit world record was set at 4:00.96 (an average speed of 60 km/h, or 37 mph!), the average power output of the riders was calculated to be around 480 W. The German Olympic team pursuit riders in the 2000 Sydney Olympic Games were reported to possess considerable aerobic and anaerobic capacities ($\dot{V}O_2$max of 65 to 73 ml/kg/min and peak blood lactate concentrations of 10 to 21 mmol/L). Their personal best individual pursuit times ranged from 4:18.8 to 4:33.6, and their estimated power outputs were 452 to 551 W. More recently, a world-record holder and Olympic gold

ATHLETE'S PERSPECTIVE:
Pacing for the 4 km Team Pursuit

Paul Manning
Team GB Cycling, national coach

> Manning was a 2008 Olympic gold medallist in the 4 km team pursuit (track). The team set a new world-record time in the final 3 minutes and 53.314 seconds, a world record by nearly 2 seconds! He was also a 2008 World Championship gold medallist in the 4 km team pursuit (track), where the team also set a new world-record time. Manning coached the GB women's 3000 m team pursuit riders, who broke the world record and won a gold medal at the 2012 London Olympic Games.

Pacing is even with little decay—you do not want to drop off any earlier than two (laps) to go. You will not go quickly if the pacing is not right. You need to know where your limits are and make the right decision to change position (within the team), to get off the front and allow the next person to maintain pace. If you get this wrong, you slow the whole team down for another half lap before you get another chance to change.

Over the years, there have been times when somebody (in the team) has not been able to hold pace. The opportunity to change is every half lap. Typically, it is hard to know when you are losing 1K (1 km/h from your speed), and that can quickly add up to 2 or 3 seconds for the team! Also, if you accelerate too early in the race, you can lose a man early (from the team)—this has a 'knock-on' effect as the remaining three riders get half a lap less time off the front as a result and have to do more turns at the front. But this can also sometimes be a strategy—where one rider stays at the front for longer and then drops out. Only three (of the four) need to finish in the men's event. Ideally, you always carry four (men) to the end of the team pursuit; in the women's event there are just three riders, so they all have to finish.

To set the right pace, you break down the time that you want to achieve into segments, you build in some contingency and then in training you refine the strategy and hold optimal speed. We develop the pacing strategy at the Manchester Velodrome, but then when we move to a new venue, we need to relearn it—as track conditions have changed.

In qualification rounds the fastest teams go through, so the heats are time trials, but the final is a race. If you are the last team to ride in the heats, then you can see what the opposition does and can confirm right up to the start point what the pacing will be—but you keep it in the realms of the right speed and cadences so you do not drop too far off the pace.

Over time the Great Britain track team pursuit squad has developed a collective knowledge of what each person is capable of, who would be man 1, man 2. It relies on individuals making the right decision to change before they lose speed. In the final in Beijing (the 2008 Olympic Games 4 km team pursuit final), Geraint (Thomas) could see that we were catching the opposition (teams start the event half a lap apart) and was chasing them down. He saw the opportunity to go faster and was even accelerating at the end of the race! We were not aware how fast we had gone until we finished; you never do when you are going, focusing on the effort in a race.

COACH'S PERSPECTIVE:
Pacing for the 4 km Team Pursuit

Shane Sutton
GB Cycling, head coach

Sutton is the performance adviser and former head coach of Team Sky. At the 2008 and 2012 Olympic Games, GB cyclists won 14 gold, 4 silver and 3 bronze medals. Under Sutton, Team Sky riders finished first and third in the 2012 Tour de France.

Pacing is hitting a certain time for a distance. We know what to add on to get the splits right. For example, for a standing start you need to add 5 to 6 seconds for the first lap; in the team pursuit we might look at 63 for the opening kilo and then 58, 59, 59 for the others.

We pace each lap, not the overall time. 'Walking the line' is where we might take two steps forward or back from a certain mark on the track so the riders know they are two tenths up or down on the split. We get this info to them at the half lap on the back straight after the start (e.g., at 12.3 seconds); then each lap might be a 14.5 pace. We used to walk towards them if they were down on time, but they would end up in the banking eventually!

At the track we measure the barometric pressure and air temperature and have developed charts so we know what gearing to use. We might adjust every 0.1 °C and look for a quicker schedule from the rider if it drops to 990 mbar (99 kPa, atmospheric pressure) and goes up to 26 °C (78.8 °F).

medallist reputedly demonstrated a peak power output of over 570 W in a lab-based test! Riders competing in pursuit races complete over 30,000 km per year in training and during racing (mainly road races), so the demands of the sport are clearly considerable.

Team pursuit riders have to change positions within the group regularly and in a particular order; furthermore, they need to judge when to do so to perfectly optimise overall race performance. Usually, riders change after one lap. A fatigued rider who misses a change or changes too late will have to cycle for half a lap with decreasing speed, which is catastrophic for the team. When riders drop back, they move to last position; as they do, they are unshielded for about half a lap. It is critical that they fit back into position correctly to avoid becoming disengaged from the 'train'.

Figure 7.4 illustrates a power output profile (measured using an SRM power meter system built into the chain set), which describes the power output of each of the four team pursuit riders in the order they began the race. The top line in the figure represents the speed profile of man 1, the first rider in the pace line at the start, and it indicates the changes in speed on the straight, during the turn and during a changeover. This figure demonstrates that power output delivery is not smooth, that clear differences in power output exist among riders and that the output varies when riders are not leading the group. Riders who are farther back in the group benefit from the drafting effect and use it to conserve energy.

Figure 7.5 shows the team pursuit data for the German team at the Sydney Olympic Games in 2000. Figure 7.5*a* clearly shows that rider 4 was not able to maintain pace during the qualification round for the German team. Figure 7.5*b* shows that this rider was replaced for the next round, in which a more homogeneous team performance resulted in a world record. The riders in the final race exchanged places with uncanny precision (2.7 ± 0.3 seconds per changeover) and were estimated to maintain only a 5 to 30 cm (2 to 12 in.) gap between riders' wheels when in position. The graphs in figure 7.5 demonstrate these riders' excellent technical skills, which ensure that the train is reformed quickly and precisely once a change is initiated. This ensures that the maximal

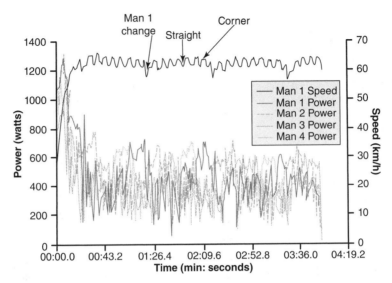

Figure 7.4 Team pursuit power output and profile during training. The initial part of the data line for Man 1 Power is obscured by the data line for Man 2 Power, as they follow almost the same pattern.

Courtesy of the English Institute of Sport.

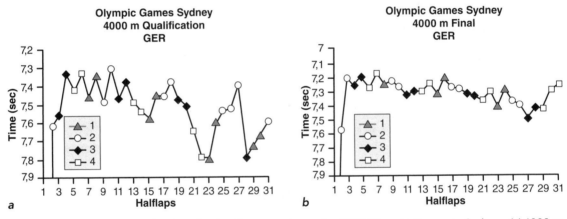

Figure 7.5 Team pursuit split times for the German team at the 2000 Olympic Games in Sydney: (a) 4000 m qualification round and (b) 4000 m final.

Reprinted, by permission, from Y.O. Schumacher and P. Mueller, 2002, "The 4,000-m team pursuit cycling world record: Theoretical and practical aspects," *Medicine & Science in Sports & Exercise* 34(6): 1029-1036.

aerodynamic benefit is recovered in the least amount of time. Finally, it was reported that the riders 1, 2 and 3 rode with a gear of 54 × 14 (achieving 8.3 m per pedal revolution from an average cadence of 120 pedal revolutions per minute; Schumacher & Mueller 2002).

An interesting aspect of pursuit racing is that coaches can provide feedback to the riders as they race in a practice widely known as walking the line (see the Shane Sutton interview). In the pursuit events, the riders start halfway down the straight on opposite sides of the oval track and finish the race at the same point. The coach, who stands to the side of the track at the midpoint of the straight, walks either towards the rider to demonstrate that he is ahead or away from the rider to demonstrate that he is behind, moving a distance in proportion to the gap between the riders. A study by Mauger et al (2011) showed that if incorrect feedback is given by the coach, by adopting the opposite protocol for "walking the line", then the riders seemed to become confused and their finishing times significantly worsened as compared to when correct feedback is given. This study demonstrates that performance feedback is advantageous during exercise, provided it is accurate.

Pacing in Road Races

Road races in cycling can vary enormously in length. Short prologue events might last 6 to 10 km, whereas Olympic time trials might last 40 to 80 km. Multistage races can last many hours on each racing day and may take a few days to a few weeks to complete. The Grand Tours (the Tour de France, Giro d'Italia and Vuelta a Espana) cover vast distances over many days. Long-distance time trials occur in world championships, Olympic Games, and the Tour de France and are specialist events; however, the best Grand Tour road racers in the world are often also among the best at time trials, too. The individual time trials are often where the Tour de France is won and lost because they pit individuals against each other without the protection of teammates for support or to control the pace of a stage. Moreover, drafting is not possible.

The GB Cycling head coach, Shane Sutton, believes that even pacing is the most effective strategy over a 50 km road time trial run over a relatively flat course. He said: 'In the 50 km you work on the rider being at threshold, say, 450 to 460 watts. The rider has to even pace, although he may build into the ride in the first few minutes. Bradley (Wiggins) has ridden two 25 km laps within a second or so of each other when he got his World silver medal in 2011. He will keep an eye on his SRM crank readings, and we will try to have telemetry in the car so we can keep an eye on what he is doing'.

In support of even pacing as the strategy of choice for time trials, Palmer and colleagues (1994) reported that Chris Boardman maintained his heart rate within 5 beats per minute while averaging 178 beats per minute over an elite 80 km time trial. Padilla and colleagues (2000) also observed that the heart rates of 18 elite riders remained remarkably constant (varying by only 5 per cent) during short (less than 40 km) and long (greater than 40 km) time trials, where their heart rates averaged 85 and 80 per cent of maximum, respectively. A fast start also appears to be important even in long time trials before the riders settle down to an even pace (see figure 7.6). A laboratory-based study found that when participants repeatedly completed 40 km cycling time trials over a number of days, they gradually adopted more aggressive starts, which resulted in improved time trial performances (Swart et al. 2009). In another study, Renfree and colleagues (2012) assessed fast- and slow-start strategies over 20 km time trials and found that the riders reported higher levels of positivity with the fast-start strategy, which coincided with better performance times.

Jeukendrup and Martin (2001) developed a model to evaluate road race cycling that incorporated various environmental, training, nutritional and aerodynamic aspects. The model assumed that the rider was cycling over a 40 km course that had varying wind conditions (2 metres per second headwind or tailwind) and gradients (flat to ± 1 per cent). It predicted that improvements in riders' aerodynamic characteristics and training could

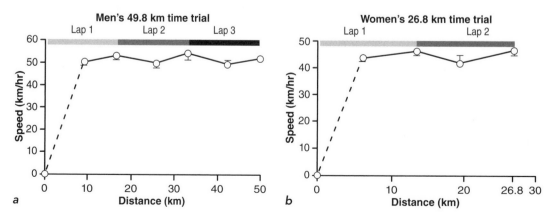

Figure 7.6 Typical pacing profiles for (a) men's 49.8 km and (b) women's 26.8 km road time trials at the 2009 UCI Road World Championships. Values shown are averaged data from the top two finishers. The dotted lines represent the transition from the starting position to the first recorded split time. Error bars represent the deviation from the average speed attained across the time trial.

improve performance by minutes, whereas altitude training, carbohydrate drinks and caffeine ingestion would shed a few seconds to a minute or so. Other research suggests that riders must vary their power output when the course has changeable hill gradients and wind conditions. More specifically, it suggests that the power output should be increased when riding into a headwind or on uphill sections and decreased when riding with a tailwind or on downhill sections. These strategies can lead to many seconds being saved on hour-long time trials, and even small variations in power output (± 5 per cent) in response to slight changes in gradient or wind speed appear effective as compared to maintaining a constant power output (Atkinson, Peacock & Passfield 2007; Swaine 1997).

Ebert and colleagues (2006) examined 207 road races over six years and concluded that despite a relatively low average power output, men's road races were characterised by frequent high-intensity surges above $\dot{V}O_2max$. Depending on whether riders were racing in a criterium, hilly or flat race, they demonstrated higher or lower levels of exertion. For example, in a criterium race, riders exhibited a higher average power output (262 vs. 188 W) and undertook more 6- to 10-second sprints (70 vs. 20) compared to a flat race. Vogt and colleagues (2006) found that six professional riders on a six-day cycle race produced an average power output of 332 to 452 W during an uphill stage. An analysis of 27 top-20 finishers in women's World Cup road races showed that flat courses were raced at an average pedal rate (69 to 83 revolutions per minute) that was similar to that used on hilly courses, but that the riders demonstrated higher average speed (38 vs. 34 km/h, or 23.6 vs. 21 mph) and power output (192 vs. 169 W) during flat races. They also spent more time at a power output of over 500 W.

Clearly, each style of racing has its own demands and associated pacing strategy. However, the sporadic nature of cycle racing means that any rider has to think carefully before embarking on an intense effort to try to break away from the peloton. A misjudged attack will be unsuccessful and result in fatigue, and the consequences are often compounded when other riders choose that moment to attack as the peloton slows, believing the danger is over. Riders commonly launch a strategic attack on hilly sections or after the lead riders have just finished hard efforts at the front and are tired.

Earnest and colleagues (2009) analysed 26 riders who were considered contenders and non-contenders for race victory in the Tour de France and Vuelta a Espana from 1997 to 2003. They found that contenders spent a significantly greater time exercising in the severe exercise intensity domain, even in team time trial stages in which they had the opportunity to draft. This demonstrates that they adopt a more aggressive pacing style than non-contenders do.

Attacks in road races are also more likely to be effective when a number of riders work together. This gives them a drafting effect similar to that of being in the peloton, when they are in a 'pace line'. That said, a peloton is always likely to chase down a breakaway because the riders in the peloton can draft more easily, take fewer turns working at the front and drop back to recover with greater regularity than can the riders in a small breakaway group. There used to be a certain advantage in breaking away from the peloton early in a race, because the peloton would not be motivated to chase with such a long way to go. The breakaway group would then work hard to build up a lead of many minutes; also, because they would no longer be visible they were 'out of sight and out of mind'. Historically, this was a good tactic because the peloton might not react quickly enough to catch them by the end of the stage. However, nowadays radio transmissions and GPS systems report a breakaway group's exact position and time gap to the riders in the chasing peloton, who can pace their chase precisely and decisively.

Pacing in the Grand Tours

The most famous Grand Tour is the Tour de France, which is composed of flat, high-mountain and time trial stages. The length of this race was originally 2,428 km (1,509 miles), but it rose to 5,745 km (3,570 miles) in 1927 before falling to around 3,650 km

(2,268 miles) from 1990 to 2011 (Santalla et al. 2012). From 1985 to 2011, the average age of Tour winners has been 29 ± 3 years which suggests that significant experience is needed to pace a winning Tour (Santalla et al. 2012). The winner's speed has been increasing from below 30 km/h (18.6 mph) in the 1920s to a peak of 41.7 km/h (25.9 mph) in 2005, demonstrating that modern riders compete at high exercise intensities for prolonged periods. In the high-mountain stages, high-intensity efforts of 45 minutes or more are required to reach the top of a mountain pass in stages set over 200 km (124 miles), which take 5 to 6 hours to complete (Lucia, Earnest & Arribas 2003).

Tour riders possess characteristics that lend themselves to certain types of stages and not others. Climbing specialists tend to range from 175 to 180 cm tall (5 ft 9 in. to 5 ft 11 in.) and weigh only 60 to 66 kg (132 to 146 lb; BMI 19-20 kg/m^2); time trial specialists are larger athletes, with heights of 180 to 185 cm (5 ft 9 in. to 6 ft) and weights of 70 to 75 kg (154 to 165 lb; BMI approximately 22 kg/m^2) (Lucia, Hoyos & Chicharro 2000; Padilla et al. 1999). These physical differences allow the climbers to produce greater relative power outputs for success in climbing (more than 6 W/kg of body mass), whereas the time trial specialists produce greater absolute power outputs, which is critical for time trials (e.g., averaging 400 W during long time trials over 40 km [25 miles]; Lucia, Hoyos & Chicharro 2001).

Tour riders also possess particularly high levels of aerobic fitness, with minimal $\dot{V}O_2$max values suggested to be around 80 ml/kg/min for race winners (Santalla et al. 2012). Laboratory-based measurements reveal that riders seem to be able to ride for many hours at 75 to 80 per cent of their $\dot{V}O_2$max while producing around 330 W of power! They do not reach severe exercise intensities (i.e., above their critical speed) until the power output is around 390 W, at which point their aerobic energy production is around 85 per cent of their $\dot{V}O_2$max and their heart rate is over 90 per cent of their maximum (Earnest et al. 2009; Fernandez-Garcia et al. 2000; Lucia et al 1999; Mujika & Padilla 2001; Padilla et al. 2000). Five-time Tour winner Miguel Indurain was reported to be able to achieve 505 W (6.2 W/kg of body mass) when beginning to experience the onset of severe exercise (Padilla et al. 2000).

It is perhaps not surprising that Tour riders demonstrate a high gross mechanical efficiency that can be as much as 25 per cent at about 500 W in Tour winners (Padilla et al. 2000). Top-level Tour cyclists appear to adopt high pedalling cadences to remain efficient, a practice that may improve blood return to the heart and, by lowering the force production required by the contracting quadriceps muscles, mitigate against the interference to blood flow that can occur during powerful muscle contractions (Gotshall, Bauer & Fahrner 1996; Takaishi et al. 2002).

Grand Tours consist of many individual races on successive days, and each day presents different opportunities to different riders. For example, the overall leader is concerned with maintaining a winning margin in terms of the overall race time, whereas other riders are concerned with winning the King of the Mountains, Points Winner or Best Young Rider (less than 25 years old) competition. As a result, pacing a race stage on any particular day is complex. A unique characteristic of Grand Tours is that, because the riders race on long stages over many days, the race in effect becomes an ultra-distance event. Recovering from the exertions of the previous day becomes increasingly difficult as a tour progresses, forcing some riders to decide not to compete on some stages so they can recover and compete successively on another day. Riders stay in the midst of the peloton to shield themselves so they can pedal at a significantly lower intensity than they could if they were at the front. In some cases riders simply do not recover and are forced to retire from the event, exhausted or injured. It has been suggested that there might be a physical limit that tour riders can experience during the hardest of a tour's stages, which affects the amount of exercise that is possible the next day. This would mean that the body is regulated by a central controller to prevent riders from reaching dangerous physiological disturbances, such as hormonal exhaustion (Santalla et al. 2012).

A major issue facing Grand Tour riders is eating sufficient amounts of food to maintain their energy levels. Suboptimal food intake can lead to low blood sugar (glucose) levels, a condition known as hypoglycaemia. Cyclists in the Tour de France might expend around 6,000 kilocalories of energy per day, and so they try to take in more than 13 grams of carbohydrate per kilogram of body weight per day to ensure that their muscle and liver glycogen stores are intact prior to each day's racing (Santalla et al. 2012). Because riders tend to under eat during race stages, their post-stage nutrition has to be well designed to maximise the restoration of their carbohydrate (glycogen) stores in the muscles and liver in the 18 hours or so before the next day's stage.

An additional issue is that tour riders cover stages (particularly time trial stages) at high velocities that require them to push high gears for 4 or more hours. This can result in muscle damage that can affect carbohydrate store restoration and force production capacity. Cumulative muscle damage from high-speed, flat stages can compromise riders' performances on subsequent stages such as mountainous stages and time trials. Therefore, Grand Tour riders not only have to pace their efforts on any given day to maximise their race position, but they also have to consider the Grand Tour as a whole and have a pacing strategy for the overall event.

Finally, a significant factor in Grand Tour races is the environmental temperature, particularly during long climbs in mountainous stages in which the wind speed, which cools riders down, may be minimal. Abbiss and colleagues (2010) found that trained, but not elite, riders who rode on a cycle ergometer for 100 km (62 miles) in an environmental chamber at 34 °C (93 °F) or 10 °C (50 °F) demonstrated very different responses. The researchers noted a lower power output and muscle activation in the cyclists exercising in the hot condition, but perhaps more important, this trend began *before* any difference was detected in the internal body temperature compared with the cold condition. The authors suggested that the brain had made an anticipatory decision based on the rate of the rising body temperature, metabolic conditions and knowledge of the distance remaining, which restrained the riders' pace. In short, the brain reduced activation to the leg muscles, thus reducing their power output and their requirement for metabolic energy production, which then reduced the related internal heat production.

This adaptive response is possibly a protective effect to circumvent attaining critical body temperatures before the end of a race. That said, when a *maillot jaune* (or yellow jersey) is at stake in the Tour De France, riders can be so motivated that they exercise beyond this protective internal setting and risk thermal injury and collapse. Furthermore, because mountain stages often finish at moderate altitude (greater than 2,000 m, or 6,562 ft), riders may suffer some gas exchange impairments resulting from a reduced pressure of oxygen in the surrounding air, which affects diffusion processes in the lungs and blood. As a consequence, muscle activation decreases, and riders reduce their pedal rates (to below 80 rpm). However, riders with lower body weights coupled with a high $\dot{V}O_2$max (approximately 80 ml/kg/min) can maintain higher pedal rates (Lucia, Hoyos & Chicharro 2001).

chapter 8

Speed Skating

Competitive speed skating takes place on oval ice tracks. In long-track speed skating, the standard track length is 400 m, but tracks of 200, 250 and 333.3 m are also used. In short-track speed skating, races often take place in an indoor ice hockey rink on a 111 m oval track. The main difference between short-track and long-track speed skating, aside from the track size, is that in short-track speed skating the competitors race out of lanes following a mass start of four to six skaters, whereas in long-track two competitors race in their own designated lanes and are timed over a set distance (Bullock, Martin & Zhang 2008; Foster et al. 2000).

The relevance of pacing to each of these versions of the sport is rather different. Pacing strategies in long-track speed skating are somewhat similar to those of swimming, in that competitors might almost view a race as a time trial (albeit with a fellow competitor alongside) and set their own paces throughout. In short-track speed skating, race tactics and group dynamics affect the pacing strategy in real time, as the race progresses, making it difficult to adopt a particular pacing strategy over a whole race. In short-track speed skating, rather like middle-distance running in track and field, race tactics play a significant role (e.g., competitors are often impeded by others when they are not in the optimal race position). Also, short-track skaters often draft behind others for a period to conserve energy before trying to dictate the pace of the race later on.

Key Factors in Determining a Pacing Strategy for Speed Skating

As in cycling, air resistance is a significant consideration in speed skating as a result of the high speeds skaters achieve during competition. In long-track, speed skaters attain maximum speeds of 64 to 69 km/h (40 to 43 mph); even in short-track, speeds of over 40 km/h (25 mph) are achieved during races (Rundell 1996b). To minimise air resistance, speed skaters wear tight-fitting Lycra and coated fabric skin suits with hoods. The power produced from the skater's muscle contractions are used to overcome air and ice friction. The magnitude of the resisting forces from air and ice friction depend on the skater's speed, posture and upper-body length and weight, as well as the ice friction coefficient (a measure of the resistance to the sliding of ice across another surface—the skate). Using computer simulations, researchers have tried to produce pacing models that can determine how skaters should regulate their power output—and subsequently their race pace—to achieve an optimal performance (de Groot et al. 2007; van Ingen Schenau 1982). This will be discussed in more detail later in this chapter.

Speed skating is a complex skill requiring high levels of power while remaining well balanced and in an optimal aerodynamic position to achieve high speeds. It involves cyclic movement patterns that include a single leg push-off completed approximately once per second (de Groot el al. 2007). While racing, skaters crouch, keeping their upper bodies as horizontal as possible to attain a balance between maximising their force production and minimising their air resistance. A more pronounced crouch allows for a greater extension of the leg (out to the side) when pushing, which lengthens the time spent in contact with the ice. This in turn, extends the time over which force can be applied. At push-off, the propelling leg produces force of around 130 per cent of the skater's body weight, with an instantaneous power output greater than 2,000 W (de Boer et al. 1986; de Groot, de Boer & van Ingen Schenau 1985).

Speed skating is characterised by cycles of high levels of force production and high muscle contraction velocities (Kandou et al. 1987). During short periods of fast skating, as at the start of a race, the skater's fast-twitch muscle fibres are extensively recruited, rapidly depleting anaerobic capacity. Therefore, pacing is critical to success, particularly in the 1000 m and 1500 m events in long-track speed skating, in which high speeds must be maintained for 60 to 100 seconds.

Pacing in Long-Track Speed Skating

The power output produced by elite females while skating over 500 m has been calculated to be 5.4 W/kg of body weight, from combined right- and left-leg push-offs taking 2.1 seconds to complete. Over 5000 m this changed to 3.6 W/kg of body weight, from combined right- and left-leg push-offs taking 1.3 seconds (van Ingen Schenau, de Groot & de Boer 1985). In speed skating, maintaining good technique and coordination and an effective frequency of push-offs becomes increasingly difficult as fatigue develops. Deleterious changes to technique, balance and posture that accompany fatigue have a significant impact on the muscular and frictional forces affecting the skater's speed. For example, when skaters become fatigued, they are less able to control the natural activation of their calf muscles, which occurs as the knee extends at the end of the push-off phase. This can lead to unwanted plantar flexion (downward pointing of the foot), which increases ice friction (de Groot el al. 2007). Therefore, regulating exercise intensity—or pace—during skating to maintain an efficient technique is an important consideration.

Elite-level skaters have been observed to consume 5 to 10 per cent less oxygen when skating maximally than when cycling maximally and 10 to 20 per cent less oxygen than when running maximally (Seiler 1997). This reduced oxygen consumption has been suggested to be due to the aerodynamic crouch position, which might reduce blood flow and hence the delivery of oxygen to the muscles when they are contracting powerfully (Rundell 1996a). An alternative theory is that skaters do not use as much oxygen in their leg muscles during propulsion, because the muscle activity of their legs is limited by the skating technique. Traditionally, skaters have been coached to push from their heels and not extend their ankles, which is what normally takes place during running, for example (Seiler 1997). The purpose of this technique is to reduce plantar flexion and prevent the skate from creating too much friction and digging into the ice, disturbing balance and power production. The reduced requirement for plantar flexion at push-off and the associated muscle activity might be a cause of the lowered oxygen uptake observed in skating compared to cycling and running during severe-intensity exercise.

A recent technological innovation in long track speed skating has been the introduction of the clap skate, which allows the heel to detach from the blade and features a spring-loaded hinge at the front of the skate that snaps the blade back into position when the skate is lifted (see figure 8.1). The development of this skate has been attributed to Gerrit Jan van Ingen Schenau and co-workers in the Faculty of Human Movement Sciences of the Vrije Universiteit (Free University) in Amsterdam beginning in 1978. Since the 1990s, an increasing number of skaters have adopted the clap skate in place of the fixed-blade skate because it allows them to push with their toes and more efficiently activate their calf muscles. The clap skate system aids the application of force during push-off by allowing the blade to stay in contact with the ice longer, because the ankle can be extended at the end of the stroke. In addition, by allowing a greater ankle extension, the clap skate may better use the knee extensor muscles.

Interestingly, a similar rate of energy breakdown has been observed in sprint runners, cyclists and speed skaters both while accelerating during the first 4 to 5 seconds of races and after the start phase when a power output of more than 10 W/kg of body weight is generated to maintain their speed. Computer simulations have calculated that an all-out pacing strategy might best suit sprint-type events taking up to 100 seconds to complete for these sports, whereas an even pacing strategy might be more effective for events of longer duration (van Ingen Schenau, de Koning & de Groot 1994). To put this into context, the winning time in elite women's 1000 m World Cup races during the 2013 long-track speed skating season was typically around 72.5 to 74.5 seconds. Because the 1000 m event is on the cusp of being 80 seconds long, an all-out pacing strategy may not be the optimal strategy. However, a pacing strategy involving a very fast start is certainly required, with the aim being to try to finish with as little kinetic energy remaining as possible.

Notably, even in 1500 m races, speed skaters start with a velocity similar to what they can achieve over only 300 m! However, there is a significant risk of miscalculation in pacing in speed skating because technique is so critical, perhaps more so than in cycling. For this reason a fast start that leads to a rapid development of fatigue challenges the ability of the skater to maintain good technique and balance during the complex and highly dynamic propulsion phase. Even a small miscalculation of pacing can be catastrophic and lead to a marked reduction in overall performance. Pacing optimally in speed skating clearly involves walking a fine line between success and failure. To manage the risk, elite skaters devise precise pacing strategies with their coaches, which are developed through trial and error in competition and training practices.

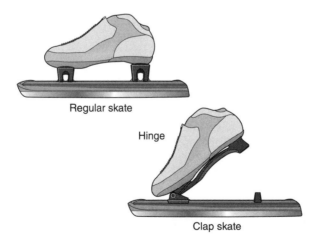

Figure 8.1   The clap skate allows skaters to maintain maximal contact with the ice while pushing.

The Olympic events in long-track are as follows:

- 500 m
- 1000 m
- 1500 m
- 3000 m (women's)
- 5000 m
- 10,000 m (men's)
- Team pursuit (four-person)

Pacing in the 1000-Metre Event

Modelling studies suggest that in sprint events (i.e., those lasting less than 80 seconds), skaters achieve optimal performance with a fast start, or all-out pacing strategy (Muehlbauer, Schindler & Panzer 2010c). It is believed that the fast start develops kinetic energy, and provided the sprinter paces effectively and maintains good technique, speed will deteriorate optimally, leaving little kinetic energy at the end (i.e., little energy will be wasted). For elite skaters, speed and external power output depend on their movement frequency (Farfel 1977). Technique is critical because small changes in push-off mechanics (work per stroke) determine skaters' success or failure (de Groot et al. 2007).

Muehlbauer, Schindler and Panzer (2010c) undertook a study of 34 elite female and 31 elite male skaters who competed in either four or five indoor World Cup speed skating competitions in the 2007/2008 season. They found that, irrespective of rank or gender, elite speed skaters demonstrate a similar pacing pattern during 1000 m races: an acceleration section during the 0 to 200 m start phase, followed by a fast second race section from 200 to 600 m before reducing speed in the final race section (600 to 1000 m). This pacing pattern is common in the sprint disciplines (de Koning et al. 2005; Foster et al. 1994; Kuhlow 1974). Higher-ranked (upper-ranked) skaters exhibited greater speed from 200 to 1000 m, showing that they were better able to maintain their speed than lower-ranked competitors were (see figure 8.2).

Muehlbauer, Schindler and Panzer (2010c) also observed that in races undertaken at a higher altitude, such as in Salt Lake City and Calgary, skaters exhibited shorter times in sectors 2 and 3, of around 2 to 3 per cent and 3 to 4 per cent, respectively, which led to shorter race times. This was presumably due to lower air resistance at altitude because

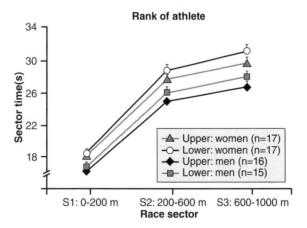

Figure 8.2 Comparison of upper- and lower-ranked elite male and female 1000 m speed skaters.

Reprinted, by permission, from T. Muehlbauer, C. Schindler, and S. Panzer, 2010, "Pacing and sprint performance in speed skating during a competitive season," *International Journal of Sport Physiology and Performance* 5(2): 165-176.

of the reduced air pressure, and it suggests that skaters can and should adopt a more aggressive pacing strategy when racing at altitude (Foster et al. 1994).

Muehlbauer, Schindler and Panzer (2010c) also compared skaters who started races from the inner lane and those who started from the outer lane. International rules require skaters to change lanes (cross over) every lap to equalise the distance covered. Although the skater in the outside lane has the right of way, these rules effectively give all skaters a fair chance regardless of the lanes they are racing in. Muehlbauer, Schindler and Panzer (2010c) found no significant differences in finishing times between skaters who started in the inner lane and those who started in the outer lane. In support of this finding, a similar pacing profile was evident in these races.

Muehlbauer, Schindler and Panzer (2010c) also investigated trends in race profiles to determine whether increasing speed in sectors 1 and 2 would improve race times, as one might expect. They calculated that this would in fact result in an increased overall race time, because it would lead to a disproportionate increase in fatigue and a poor final sector time. A similar finding was observed in a study of 1500 m national skaters in which the pacing strategy was manipulated to induce a faster start than normal (Hettinga, de Koning & Foster 2009). However, Muehlbauer, Schindler and Panzer (2010c) did find a strong association between increasing speed in sector 3 and an improvement in overall race time. This probably relates to skaters being able to maintain good technique in the final sector.

Because speed skating is a highly technical event, a loss of balance, posture or technique leads to a marked deterioration in speed across the ice (Akahane et al. 2006; de Groot et al. 2007). This might suggest that an all-out pacing strategy in 1000 m speed skating would be unlikely to result in an optimal performance. Indeed, it would seem that an optimal race performance would require that skaters regulate their energy resources across the race. Therefore, in the 1000 m, it is likely that skaters need to aggressively positively pace the race, as opposed to adopting an all-out pacing strategy. They would also need to anticipate their developing fatigue during the race and adjust their pace accordingly to avoid fatiguing too quickly.

Finally, Muehlbauer, Schindler and Panzer (2010c) reported that the upper-ranked skaters in their study were more consistent in their pacing profiles. More specifically, higher-ranked male competitors were more consistent in their performances at the start of races (up to 200 m) and during the final stages (600 to 1000 m) than were lower-ranked competitors, and this finding was similar for female skaters.

Pacing in the 1500-Metre Event

Muehlbauer, Schindler and Panzer (2010a) analysed the pacing profiles of 53 female and 61 male skaters in the 1500 m event held on an indoor 400 m oval track during the Essent World Cup event in Calgary in 2007. As in the 1000 m event, the skaters showed a rapid increase in velocity up until 300 m, but thereafter demonstrated a progressive slowing down. Faster skaters demonstrated a similar pacing profile to slower skaters except that they were faster through each sector of the race and by a similar margin each time. The researchers found that improvements in sector 3 (700 to 1100 m) conferred the highest probability of an improved race time. This agrees with a comment by Diane Holum, coach of Olympic gold medallist Eric A. Heiden, who argued that the skater needs to accelerate at the 700 m point and then try to maintain velocity in the last 400 m (Holum 1984). However, Muehlbauer, Schindler and Panzer (2010a) also warned against starting too fast, because they observed that skaters with relatively faster starts were relatively slower later in the race. In fact, producing maximal velocities in sector 1 risked a catastrophic slowing down late in the race (de Koning & van Ingen Schenau 2000; Foster & de Koning 1999).

In the 1500 m it is important to finish as fast as possible late in the race. Skaters need to control their early pace so they are not quite as fast in the first part of the race. This allows them to minimise the decline in velocity towards the end of the race and aligns somewhat with the assertion that a more uniform velocity is optimal for middle-distance events (Foster & de Koning 1999; van Ingen Schenau et al. 1990).

A fast start rapidly depletes the skater's anaerobic capacity, because anaerobic energy metabolism is heavily used, which leads to a significant blood lactate accumulation. Kindermann and Kuel (1980) reported speed skaters finishing 1000 m races with arterial blood lactate concentrations of 14 to 15 mmol/L, which would indicate the development of peripheral fatigue in the closing stages of races. This would lower the force production of the muscle fibres, affecting skaters' technique and reducing speed.

Van Ingen Schenau and colleagues (van Ingen Schenau, de Groot & Hollander 1983; van Ingen Schenau et al. 1989) detected that elite skaters used a high stroke frequency and better skating position, which would presumably help them maintain their technique in the latter stages of races. They also found that elite/highly trained skaters had a higher $\dot{V}O_2$max than well-trained skaters, a finding also reported by Foster and Thompson (1990). If better skaters possess a higher $\dot{V}O_2$max, their oxygen uptake kinetics would also likely be faster. This would allow them to produce more energy in the early stages of races from aerobic energy metabolism, which would spare the anaerobic capacity so that it could be husbanded across the race to better maintain speed. De Koning and colleagues (2005) looked at how skaters distribute their energy across a 1500 m race and concluded that they retain an appreciable energetic reserve to either increase velocity or prevent deceleration during the closing stages of the race.

Hettinga, de Koning and Foster (2009) attempted to impose an optimal pacing strategy on seven national-level speed skaters over a 1500 m trial, which they then compared with a self-paced trial. In the imposed-pace trial, the skaters were asked to start at a faster pace than normal, which was outside of their normal pacing range but, based on results from studies by de Koning, Bobbert and Foster (1999), would theoretically produce an optimal pacing strategy. The skaters practised this faster start by undertaking 3×300 m and 2×700 m sets at maximal velocity over two training sessions. The researchers believed this was necessary because national-level skaters, when self-pacing, actually begin 1500 m races at a velocity close to their maximal velocity for a one-off 300 m repetition. Given that the theoretical optimal pacing strategy would require an even faster start than the normal self-paced start, the skaters had to get used to the idea of an almost all-out approach when beginning the imposed-pace 1500 m trial.

So what happened? In the self-paced trial, the skaters managed a 1500 m time around 2 seconds faster than they did for the imposed-pace trial. In the imposed-pace trial, the skaters did produce more power over the first 300 m, which led to a relatively faster pace at this point compared to the self-paced trial. However, over the final 400 m, the pace was significantly lower in the imposed-pace trial. Therefore, despite the overall power output being the same as in the self-paced trial, the finishing time was worse in the imposed-pace trial. Skaters were more able to maintain their velocity in the latter half of the self-paced trial than they were in the imposed-pace trial. This was attributed in part to more favourable external conditions (barometric pressure and ice conditions) during the self-paced trial; however, the major reason for the difference in performance was attributed to changes in the skater's technique in the imposed-pace trial.

The researchers concluded that the effort of the increased early pace in the imposed-pace trial led to an increased air friction coefficient potentially due to a postural change that increased skaters' frontal surface area and subsequent drag, which in turn reduced their speed. This unfavourable technical change outweighed the benefit of the faster start in the imposed-pace trial and led to a slower finishing time. The researchers highlighted how national-level skaters, through experience gained in training practices and competitions, can accurately anticipate the correct pace to optimise performance when self-pacing. (Chapter 1 provides an excellent account of how practising different pacing strategies in the 1500 m event led to an improved performance by American skater Pat Seltsam because he better understood the pacing requirement of the event.)

Pacing in the 3000-, 5000- and 10,000-Metre Events

Muehlbauer, Schindler and Panzer (2010b) studied speed skaters' performances in long-distance events during a complete World Cup series in the 2008/2009 season. They observed that regardless of performance level (i.e., among the world's top 10 or outside of it), gender or the location of the rink (low or high altitude), all of the skaters adopted a positive pacing strategy in the 3000 and 5000 m events. All the skaters also demonstrated a similarly shaped velocity (pacing) profile over races. As in the other long-track events, faster skaters demonstrated a similar pacing profile to slower skaters except that they were faster through each sector of the race and by a similar margin each time. In the 3000 and 5000 m races, a fast start was followed by a progressive slowing down (see figure 8.3). Males had faster velocities than females for each lap, but demonstrated a similar pacing profile. When competing at high altitude, the skaters demonstrated slower race times (by 4.5 per cent for women, 6 per cent for men) in the 3000 and 5000 m events compared to when they raced at low altitude. This meant that the lap time profile shifted upward, although the overall shape of the pacing profile remained similar. However, in the men's 10,000 m event a different pacing strategy was evident. Here the skaters tended to demonstrate a slow opening lap, which was then followed by relatively evenly paced laps. Notably, during the period of the study, a new world-record time was set in the 10,000 m, which was achieved by the skater slightly increasing his pace over the final five laps. He presumably finished the race close to, or at, his $\dot{V}O_2$ max, with little of his anaerobic capacity remaining.

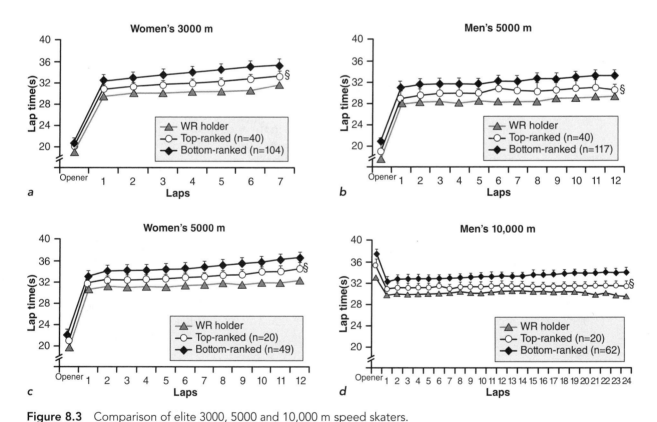

Figure 8.3 Comparison of elite 3000, 5000 and 10,000 m speed skaters.

Reprinted, by permission, from T. Muehlbauer, S. Panzer, and C. Schindler, 2010, "Pacing pattern and speed skating performance in competitive long-distance events," *Journal of Strength and Conditioning Research* 24(1): 114-119.

Pacing in Short-Track Speed Skating

Having appeared as a demonstration sport in the 1988 Calgary Games, short-track speed skating was first contested as a fully recognised Winter Olympic Games sport at the Albertville Games, held in France in 1992. A short track competition involves a series of elimination rounds requiring the skaters to use various tactics to be first to the finish line. Finishing position rather than finishing time is the deciding factor. In individual competitions, 32 skaters begin the competition and participate usually in groups of 4 at a time. Only the first, 2 finishers progress to the next round with the last four remaining competitors competing for the medals in the final. The relay involves 8 teams of four skaters. Only the first, 2 teams from each semi-final progress to the final. It is up to each team as to how many laps each skater completes however the last 2 laps must be completed by the same skater.

The following race distances were included in the Winter Olympic Games in Vancouver (2010) and Sochi (2014):

- 500 m
- 1000 m
- 1500 m
- 3000 m relay (women's)
- 5000 m relay (men's)

Bullock, Martin and Zhang(2008) examined race tactics during six World Cup and one World Championship speed skating final (2003/2004) in the 500 m (4.5 laps), 1000 m (9 laps) and 1500 m (13.5 laps) events (see figure 8.4). They observed that to have a good chance of winning, male and female skaters, respectively, had to be capable of lapping in a time of 8.6 and 9.2 seconds in the 500 m event, 9.1 and 9.5 seconds in the 1000 m event and 9.3 and 9.7 seconds in the 1500 m event. In the 1000 m, skaters had to maintain a near-optimal pace from lap 2, ideally drafting behind others to conserve energy; in the 1500 m, this pacing strategy was required from around lap 6.

In all three events, being in the top three positions in the final three laps significantly increased the likelihood of success. Being at the front at this stage in the race and so not needing to overtake other competitors could be argued to outweigh the benefits of drafting behind a number of skaters because it mitigates against the risk of falling, particularly in the 500 m (Rundell 1996b). In the 500 m, a fast start was crucial to either gain the lead or be at least in second place on the penultimate lap to have a chance of winning (Bullock, Martin & Zhang 2008; Maw et al. 2003).

Muehlbauer and Schindler (2011) studied three short-track European and World Championships incorporating 321 female and 386 male skaters' races. They observed a shift in the pacing strategy with increasing race distance: Skaters reduced their efforts to get to the front of the race as the distance of the race increased. In 1500 m races, it would seem that skaters initially conserve their energy for an end spurt in the last few laps by drafting initially behind others (van Ingen Schenau 1982). However, in the 500 m event, competitors adopt an all-out approach, because of the need to be in front as soon as possible to have any chance of success. Finally, starting position and finishing position correlate more strongly in the finals than in the preliminary rounds, indicating that skaters need to force the pace more in the later rounds of a short-track competition (Muehlbauer & Schindler 2011).

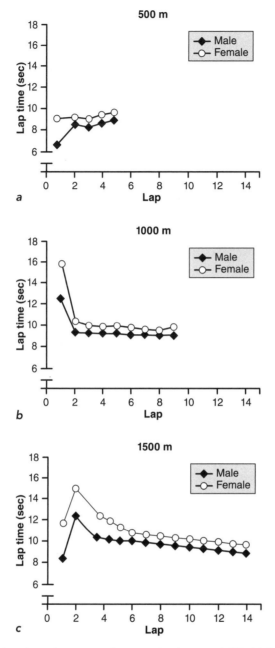

Figure 8.4 Mean lap times for men and women in short-track World Cup races.

Adapted from N. Bullock, D.T. Martin, and A. Zhang, 2008, "Performance analysis of world class short track speed skating: What does it take to win?" *International Journal of Performance Analysis in Sport* 8(1): 9-18.

chapter 9

Running

Athletics is a collection of running, walking, jumping and throwing events. With regard to the running events, athletics competitions might feature either track running, road running or cross-country running. However the focus of this chapter on pacing in running will be limited to the pacing strategies in the track running and marathon events. In major championships, the track running program is comprised of nine individual events (100 m, 110 or 100 m hurdles, 200 m, 400 m, 800 m, 1500 m, 3000 m steeplechase, 5000 m and 10,000 m) and two relay events (4 × 100 m and 4 × 400 m). In addition, a marathon race is held over 42.2 km (26 miles 385 yds) on a road course; although the final 400 m to 600 m of the race can often take place in the athletics stadium where the track running events are being held. Given the large number of events and the particular challenges each presents, the pacing strategies used in these running events are complex and varied.

Key Factors in Determining a Pacing Strategy for Running

Many factors can affect the pacing strategies adopted in running events. One is the different performance goals for the various events. For example, sprint runners are interested in achieving the shortest possible time over the race, whereas middle- and long-distance runners might race tactically to simply win the race; the finishing time is less relevant. Distance runners also produce distinct surges in speed (variable or parabolic pacing) during races to tire opponents so they cannot sprint at the end of the race.

Other factors that affect pacing strategies are environmental and track conditions. In events that require runners to complete a certain number of laps, they can be exposed to headwinds, tailwinds and crosswinds all on the same lap. High temperatures and high altitude can adversely affect the race performances of endurance runners, but can benefit sprinters. Notably, in the 1968 Mexico Olympic Games (altitude 2,300 m, or 7,546 ft), world records were achieved in men's running events of 400 m or less as a result of the reduced air friction. However, as a result of hypoxia, prominent long-distance runners such as 5000 m and 10,000 m world-record holder Ron Clarke produced notably slower-than-expected race times. Course topography is a pacing strategy consideration in marathon running given that some races are held on relatively flat courses and others expose the runners to long hills and downhill sections such as the Athens Marathon at the 2004 Olympic Games.

The pacing strategies of elite sprint runners and long-distance runners are also related to body size and composition and vary markedly depending on the events they specialise in. For example, sprint runners are larger, more muscular and often taller than long-distance runners. Their additional muscle mass affords them the ability to produce powerful strides and starts from the blocks. Sprint runners possess a greater relative complement of fast-twitch muscle fibres than long-distance runners, who in turn possess relatively more slow-twitch muscle fibres. A greater complement of fast-twitch muscle fibres gives sprint runners the ability to produce more force more rapidly, which is critical in an all-out 100 m race. However, a greater reliance on anaerobic energy metabolism means that sprinters fatigue rapidly during races. Therefore, pace judgement, particularly in the longer sprints such as the 400 m, is almost an art form!

In contrast, long-distance runners train to maximise their running economy at racing speeds, rather than to develop rapid force production as sprint runners do. Long-distance races require a more even-paced strategy to achieve fast times, although race tactics can regularly interfere with this strategy. Possessing a highly economical running action becomes vitally important in longer-distance events in which aerobic energy production predominates. This is because reducing the amount of oxygen required for aerobic energy production at a given racing speed delays the attainment of maximal oxygen uptake ($\dot{V}O_2$ max) and the fatigue that follows a few minutes later.

Possessing a large aerobic capacity (i.e., $\dot{V}O_2$ max) is also important for endurance runners because it then takes longer to attain it during a race, especially if their running economy is good. Sport scientists often measure not only the $\dot{V}O_2$ max of endurance runners but also the speed at which they achieve it, using laboratory-based treadmill protocols with a number of incremental speed increases. This provides a more complete view of runners' aerobic capacity and running economy.

Endurance runners must have a high $\dot{V}O_2$ max relative to their body weight to be able to run at a high speed for prolonged periods. Therefore, endurance runners, and even their racing shoes, need to be relatively light. Carrying excess weight (non-functional muscle mass or body fat) therefore affects the pacing strategy. Finally, possessing a superior running economy can also mean that the finite anaerobic capacity can be spared and eked out for longer during the race. This can allow the athlete to produce a faster surge or sprint finish during the final stages of the race.

Pacing in middle- to long-distance events can also depend on the purpose of the race for the main contenders. A world-record attempt often involves one or more pacemakers who set the correct pace to allow runners to draft behind them for long periods of the race before making the run for home. However, championship races are often tactical in that athletes choose to sit in the pack while watching for a breakaway attempt. In this style of race, the speed often builds in the final laps to its conclusion. The runners may have a pacing strategy in mind, but it might not be executed until the final stage of the race; the early part of the race is run at a comfortable pace.

Following are the pacing patterns generally observed in running events:

- All-out pacing in the 100 m event
- Positive pacing (at least after the start phase) in the 200 m to 800 m events
- Parabolic pacing in the 1500 m event
- Even pacing (generally) in the 3000 m to 10,000 m events
- Positive pacing in the marathon, which is completed on a road course (although more successful athletes can demonstrate even pacing)

Sprint Events (400 Metres or Less)

The acceleration phase is particularly prominent in the 100 m event; it can take 45 to 55 per cent of the race distance to reach peak speed. Following the start and transition to top speed, the sprinter tries to maintain that speed as the energy stores, specifically the phosphocreatine store, in the fast-twitch fibres rapidly decrease. For example, at half-distance only 50 per cent of the phosphocreatine store might remain with less than 30 per cent left by the end of the race. (Chapter 5 provides a more detailed discussion of this process.) Research also suggests that athletes cannot maintain maximal nerve-firing frequencies for the full duration of a 100 m sprint (Ross, Leveritt & Riek 2001). Despite these limitations, elite sprinters can largely maintain their running speed in the second 50 m of a 100 m race. As a result, the race will appear to have a negative pacing strategy because the second half is faster than the first; however, in essence, the runner is actually using an all-out pacing strategy.

Research investigating the physical attributes sprinters must have to perform at the highest levels of the sport suggest that they might possess relatively high percentages of fast-twitch fibres as well as an enhanced ability to conduct electrical signals down their nerves to activate their muscles more quickly, which might be further enhanced through training (Ross, Leveritt & Riek 2001). Sprinters also possess a large muscle cross-sectional area. However, this is not the greatest determinant of performance in elite sprinters; indeed, muscle bulk adds to the weight that needs to be accelerated and, perhaps more important, can restrict range of movement.

Aside from being powerful, the sprinter has to master all the elements of a sprint race, which includes (1) leaving the blocks and achieving peak speed in the shortest possible time, (2) being able to run with correct technique despite becoming fatigued and (3) not false starting or running without relaxation while experiencing the psychological stress of competitors in close attendance. Figure 9.1 shows how sprinters in the 100 m hurdles race lose speed after the final hurdle, as they transition from hurdling to sprinting. This may be the result of fatigue and also technical adjustments; athletes commonly clip hurdles during the race and may be slightly off balance as they leave the final hurdle.

The 200 m race is sometimes run at a higher average speed than the 100 m because the acceleration phase is not so significant and the athletes can run at very close to maximal speed for a greater portion of the event. For example, in 2007 the average running speed for the world record for the men's 100 m was 37 km/h (22.9 mph), whereas the speed in the 200 m was 37.3 km/h (23.2 mph). However, this trend was reversed in the women's events.

Figure 9.1 shows the significant fatigue elite 200 m sprinters experience as the energy production from their anaerobic energy systems falls. This is likely due to a depletion of the active muscles' phosphocreatine stores accompanied by a reduction in the rate of glycogen (carbohydrate) breakdown in the muscle. This latter event is the result of a drop in anaerobic glycolysis activity to around 50 per cent of maximum after 20 or so seconds of exercise. These physiological events are important because they mean that the fast-twitch muscle fibres cannot continue to contract with the same frequency, and so the athlete slows down. For these reasons, the 200 m event is positively paced, after the acceleration phase, because the speed of the athlete diminishes particularly in the last 50 m.

Spencer and Gastin (2001) calculated that the anaerobic energy contribution for 200 m and 400 m events for males and females is about 70 per cent and 55 to 59 per cent, respectively. The aerobic energy system provides an energy contribution of 30 per cent and 41 to 45 per cent, respectively. In addition, male and female sprinters finish 200 m and 400 m races at 71 per cent and 89 to 83 per cent, respectively, of their $\dot{V}O_2$max (Duffield, Dawson & Goodman 2005a; James et al. 2007; Spencer & Gastin 2001). Therefore, it would appear that even 200 m and 400 m sprinters require a developed aerobic system to compete successfully.

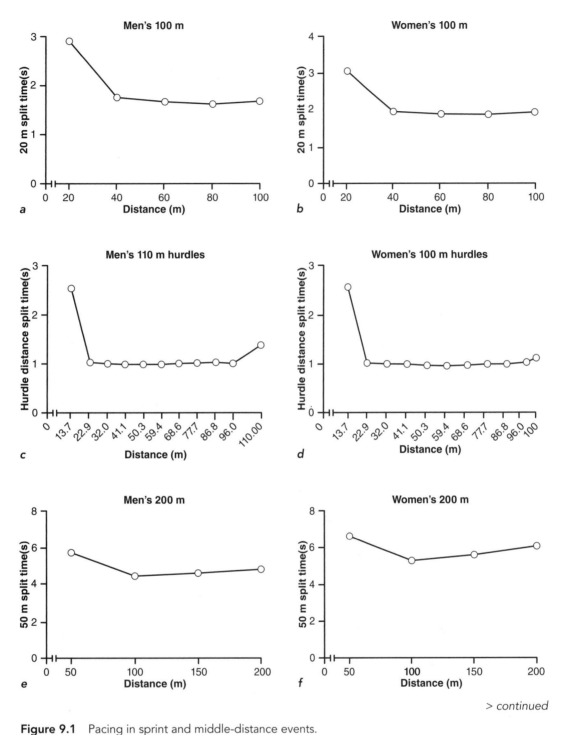

> continued

Figure 9.1 Pacing in sprint and middle-distance events.

Data from International Association of Athletics Associations, 2009, Biomechanics project - Berlin 2009. [Online]. Available: http://berlin.iaaf.org/records/biomechanics/index.html [March 28, 2014].

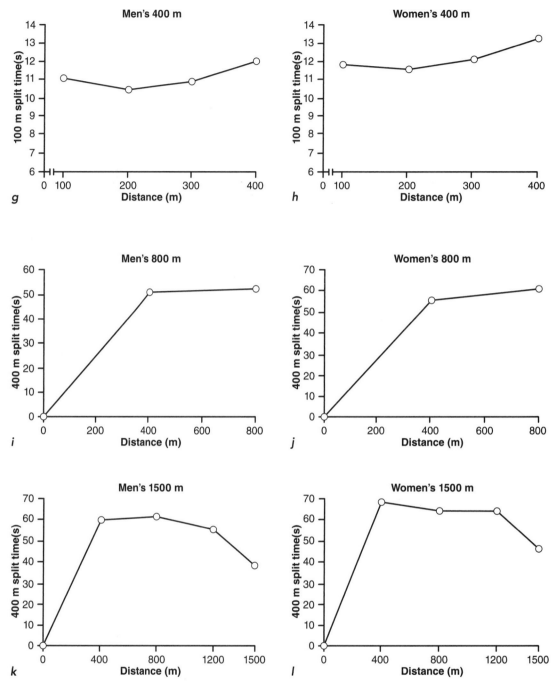

Figure 9.1 *(continued)*

Pacing a 400 m is difficult because the race requires the full use of the available anaerobic capacity and substantially stresses the aerobic system, making it very easy to catastrophically misjudge the race. The 400 m involves accelerating rapidly during the first 100 m to near maximal speed, but not up to it (which would lead to premature fatigue) and not too far below it (which would require having to continue to accelerate in the second 200 m). Because the second and third 100 m require a consistent speed, runners avoid wasteful fluctuations in speed. Finally, athletes attempt to maintain good form and run as efficiently as possible, while having to work physically harder, as fatigue develops causing them to slow down.

Figure 9.1 shows that from 200 m on, runners in the 400 m event slow down, demonstrating a positive pacing profile as their anaerobic energy production rates decline. In the final 100 m of a 400 m race, a measurement of the electrical activity of the leg muscles would reveal an increased signal, despite the athlete's slowing down. This suggests that as the exercising muscle fibres are becoming fatigued, the brain is trying to activate more of them to compensate. However, if the aerobic energy production rate could be improved in the early stages of the race, a 400 m sprinter may be able to maintain more speed in the latter stages of the race, because the anaerobic capacity could be spread over more of the race. In support of this idea, although 400 m sprinters have been shown to have lower aerobic capacities than middle-distance runners ($\dot{V}O_2$ max of 63.7 vs. 68.8 to 71.9 ml/kg/min, respectively; Svedenhag & Sjödin 1984), they have been reported to be able to reach a greater percentage or their $\dot{V}O_2$max during a 400 m time trial compared to 800 m runners (James et al. 2007). This supports the notion that developing a high rate of aerobic energy production is critical in the 400 m event. Studies have shown that high-speed interval training can improve athletes' aerobic capacity ($\dot{V}O_2$max; Dawson et al. 1998), and their oxygen uptake at the start of sprinting exercise would also likely improve (see chapter 5), which could spare their anaerobic capacity.

Evidence also suggests that sprint training might increase the number of anaerobic and aerobic energy pathway enzymes, which would improve the rate of energy production for muscle contractions. However, the buffering capacity of the muscles, which counters the disturbance of the acid–base balance during prolonged sprinting, might not be improved by sprint training (Linderman & Gosselink 1994). Consequently, some athletes take a sodium bicarbonate (or sodium citrate) supplement prior to a 400 m or 800 m race to boost the buffering capacity of their muscles and reduce the build-up of acidity that might affect contractions in their active muscles (Carr, Gore & Dawson 2011; Carr, Hopkins & Gore 2011; McNaughton, Siegler & Midgley 2008).

Middle-Distance Events

The aerobic energy contribution has been reported to be around 60 to 63 per cent and 70 to 71 per cent for males and females, respectively in 800 m events. Additionally, during 800 m races the aerobic energy system provides more energy than the anaerobic energy systems does from around 200 to 400 m into the race (Duffield, Dawson & Goodman 2005a). However, a recent study by Thomas and colleagues (2005) also suggested that the oxygen uptake of runners can dip prior to the end of an 800 m race and reduce the aerobic energy production, possibly as a result of either a fall in the heart's stroke volume or metabolic acidosis. This would mean that conserving some of the anaerobic capacity until the end of the race would be critical for maintaining race speed. Therefore, despite the dominance of the aerobic energy supply in the 800 m event, the eking out of the limited anaerobic capacity still constrains the pacing strategy.

When 800 m races are run fast (e.g., within 2 per cent of the world record), a positive pacing strategy is generally observed (Abbiss & Laursen 2008). Tucker, Lambert and Noakes (2006) analysed 26 world-record performances from 1912 to 1997 and concluded that the optimal pacing strategy in an 800 m race is to attempt greater running speeds during the first lap. In accordance with this strategy, the 1983 world record for the 800 m set by Pamela Jelimo at 1 minute 54 seconds was run with lap times of 27.5, 28.5, 28.5 and 29.5 seconds. In fact, elite 800 m runners typically run the first 200 m, middle 400 m and last 200 m at 107.4 per cent, 98.3 per cent and 97.5 per cent of the average speed for the race (Sandals et al. 2006).

Scientific evidence also suggests that a fast-start, or positive pacing, strategy is physiologically advantageous. Sandals and colleagues (2006) found that positive pacing increased the aerobic energy contribution by the end of an 800 m treadmill trial, compared to even pacing. This suggests that the fast start increased the aerobic contribution, which in turn allowed the runners to eke out the anaerobic capacity for longer to support a higher race speed. However, with this strategy the potential to increase speed during the second lap is limited because the anaerobic capacity is substantially used up by that stage and the aerobic system is also operating at close to maximum during the second lap (Thomas et al. 2005). Therefore, during a 'fast' 800 m race, athletes have difficulty raising a sprint finish; rather, the athlete who slows down the least is often the one who prevails. This also explains the tactic in 800 m races of athletes with excellent speed endurance starting fast to run the sprint finish out of those who are known to be able to 'kick at the end of the race'.

In the 1500 m event a race with a slow pace early on is invariably won by an 800 m specialist because that runner will have the faster finish. Meanwhile, a fast race is run much more evenly and often won by a 1500 m specialist. Peter Elliott won a silver medal in the 1988 Olympic 1500 m event in Seoul, despite being known more as an 800 m runner. He knew where his strengths lay as a competitor.

ATHLETE'S PERSPECTIVE: Pacing in the 800 Metre

Peter Elliott
800 m silver medallist, World Championship, Rome, 1987; 800 m personal best: 1:42.9

After the initial fast start in the 800 m, my strategy was to race at an even pace. I would alert pacemakers to take me out in 50.5 seconds. This took away some of the fear element and made it a more honest race, spreading the field out so there was less chance of being brought down. When an 800 m specialist front-runs, it makes it difficult for someone stepping up from 400 m to outkick you. I preferred to be near the front with a lap to go, because it may be that the last lap is run around 52 seconds, and so if you are at the back, you will need to run 50 or 51 seconds!

My coach and I also worked on accelerating over 80 m to stop other athletes from passing me when they suddenly accelerated. If someone gets a jump on you, then you will lose a second, which you then have to catch up. Someone like Joaquim Cruz would front-run so you could follow; others get to the front and slow the pace down, so you have to get past.

In an 800 m race in Sweden, I asked the pacemaker to go out in 50 to 50.5 seconds, but the problem is that you never know where you are on the first bend. In addition, a friend of the pacemaker asked for the pace to be 49 seconds for the first lap! I went out too fast and knew this in my mind at 200 m (I was 26 years old and so experienced), but I questioned myself as to whether I was just tired as the pace should have been only 50.5 seconds. I also had adrenaline rushing around and a big crowd in the stadium, which made me keep going. At 750 m, I felt like I was crawling to the line. I got passed, and the winner ran more even splits, having come through from the back of the field.

In another race, I battled for position with Joaquim Cruz for 700 m, and we both were overtaken as we wasted energy fighting each other!

ATHLETE'S PERSPECTIVE: Pacing in the 1500 Metre

Peter Elliott
1500 m silver medallist, Olympic Games, Seoul, 1988; 1500 m gold medallist, Commonwealth Games, Auckland, New Zealand, 1990

In the 1500 m you see what happens when the gun goes; you settle into the race and keep looking around. On the third lap, athletes can fall asleep. In Grand Prix events, you know the splits and so you can commit with approximately 600 m to go (sometimes less). If you are in a slow race, you know there is going to be a burn-up!

I developed up to 1500 m races at around 25 years old. In the 800 m I always tried to lead all the way, whereas in the 1500 m I would feel that I had good speed and so would be happy to cover gaps and push on with 400 to 500 m to go. Or if I felt really confident, I would wait until the finishing straight to accelerate hard.

The first and final laps of mile races, when run at world-record pace, are invariably faster than the second or third laps (Leger & Ferguson, 1974; Tucker, Lambert & Noakes 2006). Figure 9.1 shows that the 1500 m event in the IAAF Athletics World Championships in Beijing in 2009 was characterised by a fast final 300 m. The pacing in the 1500 m and mile races is therefore even in the middle portions, but overall is more parabolic. Runners in these events possess high aerobic capacities (65 to 75 ml/kg/min or higher) and can rapidly increase their oxygen uptake at the start of the race allowing then to run fast for a prolonged period and still spare some of their anaerobic and aerobic capacity to increase pace over the final lap (Spencer & Gastin 2001). A recent study suggested that better 1500 m runners have more of their anaerobic capacity remaining with 30 per cent or so of the race remaining, which allows them to increase their pace on the final lap (Billat et al. 2009; also see figure 9.1).

Researchers have also reported that male and female 1500 m runners rely on their anaerobic energy systems for approximately 24 and 19 per cent of their energy, respectively, and produce post-race peak blood lactate concentrations of 15.6 and 13.2 mmol/L. These data demonstrate the high degree of use of the anaerobic energy system during a 1500 m race, particularly in the last lap (Duffield, Dawson & Goodman 2005b; Hill 1999).

Finally, during 3000 m races the aerobic energy contribution for males and females has been estimated to be 86 to 93 per cent and 92 to 94 per cent, respectively. Figure 9.2 demonstrates how an even pace is adopted during the 3000 m steeplechase, which is likely due to the event being run so close to the athletes' $\dot{V}O_2$max, as well as to their need to maintain a rhythm of running between and over the barriers. During fast races athletes' anaerobic capacity is spread thinly across the race, which does not allow them to vary their pace greatly (Duffield, Dawson & Goodman 2005b).

Pacing in Longer-Distance Events

Figure 9.2 shows how the 5 km and 10 km races are evenly paced for much of the race, although an end spurt is evident over the last kilometre. In the men's 5 km, there is also a trend for the pace to increase slightly throughout (a negative pace strategy). Tucker and colleagues (2006) reported that in 32 world-record performances for the 5 km event, the first and final kilometres were generally faster than the second, third and fourth kilometres. However, in 34 world-record 10 km races the times for each kilometre increased for the first 3 kilometres and then stabilised before dropping significantly in the last kilometre, which was also the fastest in the race.

Some experimental evidence supports a strategy of beginning the first mile of a 5 km race with a fast start. Gosztyla and colleagues (2006) had runners complete a 5 km trial at an even pace or with the first 1.6 km completed either 3 per cent or 6 per cent faster.

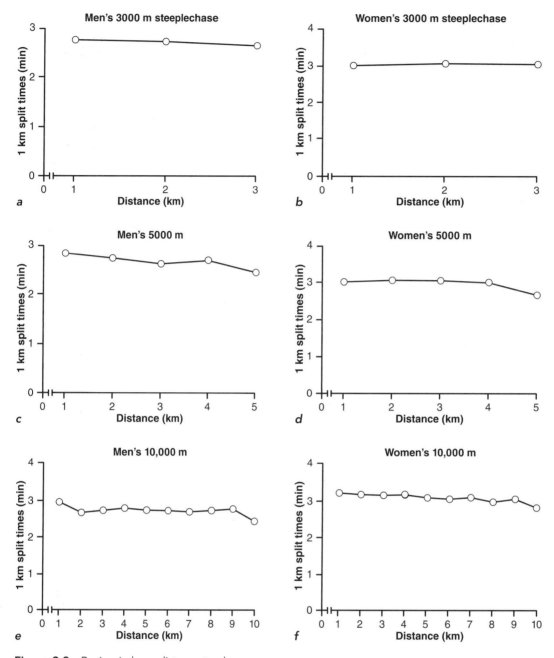

Figure 9.2 Pacing in long-distance track races.

IAAF World Athletic Championships, Daegu, Korea (2011). Source: http://daegu2011.iaaf.org/ResultsByDate.aspx.

They observed no increase in overall energy cost among the three trials, but there was a trend for the runners' performances to improve in the faster-start trials compared to when adopting an even pace throughout. A study by Lima-Silva and colleagues (2009) also demonstrated that better 10 km runners adopt a faster-start strategy than less capable runners.

As noted in chapter 5, exercising above critical power depletes the anaerobic capacity, causing athletes to approach their maximal oxygen uptake ($\dot{V}O_2$ max)—and the more athletes exercise above their critical power, the faster these physiological events occur and the more rapidly fatigue develops. Athletes who misjudge the pace and run too fast achieve their $\dot{V}O_2$ max before the end of the race and fatigue within a few minutes, forcing them to slow down. They also rapidly deplete their anaerobic capacity, which makes it impossible for them to increase their pace in the latter stages of the race.

Distance runners produce surges in speed to tire the opposition so they cannot sprint at the end of the race. This is a common pacing tactic in major championship races. Finally, it is important that distance runners avoid running out of lane 1 when possible during races to minimise the distance covered. Running an extra few metres has been shown to result in defeat as a result of the small winning margins apparent even in longer-distance track races (Jones & Whipp 2002).

Figure 9.3 highlights that runners in 5 km and 10 km races run for the majority of the race below their $\dot{V}O_2$max but above their critical power, which means that their oxygen uptake and aerobic energy production are increasing over the race towards their maximum (Basset & Howley 2000; Jones & Whipp 2002). Although the percentage of the $\dot{V}O_2$max at which the critical power occurs varies among runners, for the purposes of the figure, an indicative value for reaching the critical power might be around 85 to 90 per cent of $\dot{V}O_2$ max. Note that marathon runners run close to their critical power for over 2 hours! It is not possible for humans to take in and use more oxygen than 100 per cent of their $\dot{V}O_2$ max; hence, where this is indicated in figure 9.3, the assumption is that the anaerobic energy metabolism (and capacity) is being rapidly used at this point.

Much of the marathon event is run at an exercise intensity of around 75 to 85 per cent of $\dot{V}O_2$max. Because this is below athletes' critical power, oxygen uptake does not rise to its maximum ($\dot{V}O_2$max) during a race (see chapter 5 for a discussion of the critical power concept). Elite athletes demonstrate incredible running economy in this event and may run at around 85 to 90 per cent of their maximal heart rate for much of the race. A key consideration in marathon races is the ability to husband the muscle and liver glycogen (carbohydrate) stores across the race by also using the fat stores for aerobic energy production. Marathon runners undertake long, slow runs to adapt their bodies so they can metabolise more fat when running at marathon pace to spare their glycogen stores. Chapter 5 provides an in-depth discussion of how these energy demands and other factors (e.g., environmental temperature, wind conditions, variable pacing) affect pacing in the marathon event.

To date, only a few studies have investigated pacing in marathon races. Renfree and St Clair Gibson (2013) studied competitors in the 2009 IAAF Women's Marathon Championship and found that runners in the top 25 per cent were faster in every 5 km segment of the race and demonstrated less variability in their speed during the race (see figure 9.4). The lower the athlete finished in the race order, the greater the variability of speed was,

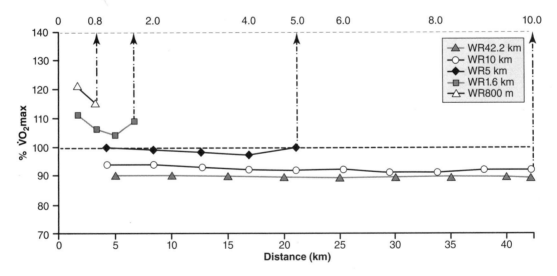

Figure 9.3 Aerobic and anaerobic energy requirements of middle- and long-distance running races.

Reprinted, by permission, from C. Foster, J.J. de Koning, S. Bischel, et al., 2012, Pacing strategies for endurance performance. In *Endurance training—Science and practice*, edited by I. Mujika (Vitoria-Gasteiz, Basque Country: Iñigo Mujika S.L.U.), 85-98.

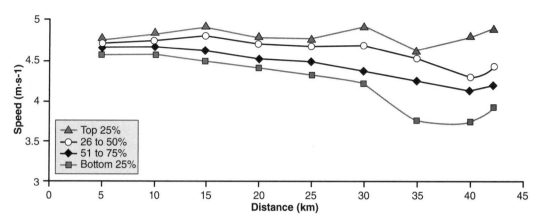

Figure 9.4 Change in the speed of runners in the 2009 IAAF Women's Marathon Championship.

Adapted, by permission, from A. Renfree and A. St. Clair Gibson, 2013, "Influence of different performance levels on pacing strategy during the women's World Championship marathon race," *International Journal of Sports Physiology and Performance* 8(3): 279-285.

suggesting that she had slowed down and speeded up to a greater extent compared to the better runners, which might indicate a reduced ability to pace effectively. One reason for this was that the less able runners followed the pace of the top runners in the early stages of the race, which was clearly too fast for them to maintain. Subsequently, the runners finishing outside of the top 25 per cent demonstrated a positive-pace strategy because they started too fast and then slowed down across the race, whereas runners in the top 25 per cent ran a relatively more even-paced race. Compared to the other runners, those in the top 25 per cent ran the first and second 5 km segments of the marathon at a lower percentage of the average speed for their personal best marathon time. This relatively conservative pace during the early stages of the race allowed them to run at a higher percentage of their personal best average marathon speed from 35 km onward, compared to the other runners.

A statistical analysis of two men's world-record performances (Run 1, 2:03:59, 28 September 2008, and Run 2, 2:03:38, 25 September 2011) demonstrated that, even accounting for environmental conditions (road gradient and weather conditions such as headwinds), during each kilometre of the race, the two world record–breaking athletes demonstrated an oscillatory (variable) pacing strategy rather than an evenly-paced profile (Angus 2013). The author of the study concluded that the runners' pacing strategies were likely suboptimal and probably due, at least in part, to tactical interplay within the race.

Finally, a study of Japanese women's championship marathons observed that warm weather affects the finishing times and pacing strategies of slower and faster marathon runners differently (Ely 2008). In warm conditions (15 to 21 °C, or 59 to 70 °F), slower runners tended to reduce their pace from the outset of the race compared to when racing in cooler conditions (5-10 °C, or 41-50 °F). As a consequence, they demonstrated a proportionately greater increase in their finishing times than did the faster marathon runners. In contrast, the faster marathon runners tended to start closer to the pace they might choose for a race in cooler conditions, but they subsequently slowed to a greater extent than the slower runners did, which was determined based on a comparison of their first and final 5 km times (i.e., the faster runners adopted more of a positive-pace race strategy). These findings suggest that better marathon runners possess a superior ability to regulate their pace in warm races, presumably because they have a better understanding of the feedback from their bodies, more experience racing in such conditions and more accurate knowledge of the pace they can manage over the distance remaining.

chapter 10

Olympic and Ironman Triathlon

Triathlon involves swimming, cycling and running, and consequently there is a carry-over from one event to another in terms of energy expenditure and developing fatigue. Athletes are often stronger in one (or two) of these sports and relatively weaker than their competitors in another. This is often due to their training backgrounds and, particularly, the sports they began competing in as junior athletes (most people transfer to triathlon from another sport). This chapter addresses how pacing in each of the sports affects the next and also how athletes attempt to conserve energy during the swimming and cycling legs to maximise their overall race speed. Drafting, for example, is now a key part of the sport of Olympic triathlon having been deemed a legal tactic by the sport's governing body; this greatly affects pacing strategy.

This chapter addresses pacing in the Olympic distance triathlon first, followed by a discussion of pacing for the Ironman triathlon. However, pacing elements common to both events feature primarily in the Olympic distance triathlon section. Finally, the chapters on general pacing strategies and on pacing in swimming (chapter 6), cycling (chapter 7) and running (chapter 9) that precede this chapter also provide detailed discussions relevant to the sport of triathlon.

Key Factors in Determining a Pacing Strategy for Triathlon

Triathlon is a complex and time-consuming sport to train and prepare for. Triathletes need a keen sense and understanding of their physical and technical capacities to position themselves correctly in races to optimise their performances. They also require special equipment to cope with variable environmental and course conditions (wetsuit, bicycle, gear ratios, wheels). These factors all feed into the pacing strategy. Mastering each of the three exercise modalities requires many hours of training as well as enormous commitment and discipline.

Olympic triathletes have to strike a balance between exercising at a severe intensity (i.e., above critical power; see chapter 5), perhaps to make a break in the race, and settling into an even pace (i.e., below critical power) to conserve aerobic and anaerobic capacity. Rather like marathon running, the event is too long (1.5 to 2 hours) for triathletes to exercise beyond their critical power for the whole race; doing so would lead to premature fatigue because they would reach their $\dot{V}O_2max$ and deplete their anaerobic capacity well before the end of the race. When deciding when to exercise at a severe intensity, triathletes need to take into account issues such as their relative efficiency in each of the exercise modalities, whether a prolonged surge could catch them up to the leading bunch and then allow a reduction in intensity by drafting behind others, or whether they can gain a time advantage from the course conditions ahead (e.g., heading into a transition zone or climbing a hill).

In longer triathlon races lasting more than 3 hours, carbohydrate (glycogen) depletion, hyperthermia (when racing in hot conditions), muscle damage and a loss of central drive and motivation are the most likely causes of fatigue, which might derail the pacing strategy (Burnley & Jones 2007). The mental aspects of enduring hours of training and then competing for many hours in an Ironman triathlon are particularly daunting. For the much shorter Olympic distance triathlon, these factors are still a significant concern in training but perhaps less so in competition. Nevertheless, common to both forms of triathlon is the fact that successful competitors require considerable mental toughness to persevere with their pacing strategies while suffering worsening levels of fatigue and discomfort as the race progresses.

Physically, triathletes face a number of challenges that affect their race preparation and pacing strategies. The cumulative fatigue that results from training in three exercise modalities can easily lead to overuse injuries and high degrees of muscle soreness. In addition, maintaining the correct energy and fluid balance is also a challenge; a deficit can lead to ill health and poor training. To be able to train and compete at the appropriate exercise intensities, triathletes must maintain optimal muscle glycogen (carbohydrate) levels so they can execute their pacing strategies. A reduced rate of carbohydrate metabolism towards the end of a race will adversely affect exercise intensity and subsequently the race pace. In Ironman triathlon, sufficiently lowered carbohydrate levels can even lead to hypoglycaemia (abnormally low blood glucose) and ketosis (excessive accumulation of ketones) and a resultant loss of coordination or collapse (St Clair Gibson et al. 2013).

Elite triathletes train two or three times daily and therefore need to consume a high-carbohydrate diet to replenish muscle and liver carbohydrate (glycogen) stores. They also need to diligently replace water and salt losses from sweating during exercise. To maximise carbohydrate stores in the 24 hours prior to a sprint or Olympic distance triathlon, the triathlete might take in around 7 to 8 grams of carbohydrate per kilogram of body weight. In the 48 to 72 hours prior to an Ironman triathlon, a carbohydrate intake of around 10 to 12 grams of carbohydrate per kilogram of body weight per day is recommended (Australian Institute of Sport 2014).

Triathletes tailor their nutrition intake to the duration of the race and the environmental conditions. The longer and hotter the race is, the greater is the risk of severely depleting their glycogen stores and also dehydration. General recommendations as to the amount of carbohydrate a triathlete needs to take in during a race vary. However, for short races lasting around 2 or 3 hours a carbohydrate intake of between 30 and 60 grams (1 and 2 oz) per hour is recommended, whereas in a race lasting beyond 3 hours an intake in excess 90 grams (3 oz) per hour is recommended (Gatorade.co.uk 2014). Ironman triathletes are advised to take in 1 to 1.5 grams of carbohydrate per kilogram of body weight per hour—for example, 70 to 105 grams (2.5 to 3.7 oz) each hour for a 70 kg (154 lb) competitor (Australian Institute of Sport 2014).

Triathlons often take place in hot and humid conditions and so competitors need to acclimatise by training and practising their pacing in similar environments. This ensures that they adapt physiologically and psychologically to the conditions. A well-considered hydration strategy, taking into account the triathlete's personal rate of sweating, can mitigate against exercise-induced dehydration. Avoiding dehydration during a triathlon is important because it affects the body's ability to maintain sufficient blood volume to adequately support heat loss and to maximise oxygen delivery to maintain the desired race pace (see the section "Considerations for Longer-Term Endurance Events" in chapter 5).

Triathlon races occur under various changeable environmental conditions (e.g., weather, course topography, road surface, water temperature, tides). Thus, 'laboratory' studies simulating triathlon races are, of course, limited by the environmental conditions imposed. Power outputs, or speeds, vary greatly and frequently during competitive races, whereas in the laboratory, triathletes often demonstrate more constant power outputs. Nonetheless, findings from research studies do inform our understanding of the pacing strategies of triathletes.

Olympic Distance Triathlon

The Olympic distance triathlon takes approximately 2 hours to complete and consists of a 1500 m swim followed by a 40 km cycling leg and a 10 km run. Recent studies suggest that the most common ways pacing is manipulated during the Olympic triathlon is through drafting and adjustments in power output and cycling cadence (Hausswirth & Brisswalter 2008). In addition, triathlon performance has been found to be related to the maximal oxygen uptake ($\dot{V}O_2$max) athletes can reach during swimming, cycling and running, but not to swimming economy. This is possibly because triathletes are not skilled swimmers and because the nature of racing results in pacing surges throughout a race. What is perhaps critical to triathlon performance is a high aerobic capacity, which allows athletes to adjust their pace significantly at times while still predominantly using their aerobic energy stores rather than anaerobic metabolism for muscle contractions.

Swimming

The start and first 500 m of the swimming leg appears to be a major determinant of triathlon success because of how it relates to the position after the swimming stage (Vleck, Bentley & Bürgi 2006). Completing the swimming leg in a leading position is important because the leading triathletes will set an aggressive early pace during the cycling leg to gain an early lead. This tactic requires the slower swimmers to cycle significantly faster over the first half of the cycling leg to catch up. In contrast, the faster swimmers do not have to chase and can draft in a bunch of riders conserving their energy.

Chapter 6 describes a trend in which better swimmers set a faster initial pace than their competitors and then maintain that gap throughout the race. This can occur in the triathlon when strong swimmers build up a significant lead during the swimming leg. A swimming background can be a significant advantage in triathlon because, on average, elite triathletes are not as efficient at swimming as specialist swimmers. Millet, Chollet and Chatard (2000) observed that elite female triathletes produced shorter propulsive phases and longer recovery phases at high swimming speeds compared with elite swimmers. These technical deficiencies led to reduced stroke lengths and swimming speeds in the triathletes studied.

A number of factors determine the less efficient propulsion of triathletes compared to specialist swimmers. First, triathletes might not have an extensive swimming background when they begin the sport and so are less technically efficient, and in addition they do not spend as much time in swim training as full-time swimmers do. Second, the swimming leg of triathlon is swum in open water and bodysuits are worn, and both of these factors affect technique. Finally, triathletes can draft behind or to the side of their competitors, which can have a marked effect on energy expenditure.

Using the front crawl, triathletes attempt to reduce their hydrodynamic drag by swimming in the depression made in the water by the swimmer just ahead of them (Chatard & Wilson 2003). This is thought to decrease the pressure gradient, facilitating their forward movement and reducing their energy expenditure. Various studies have suggested that swimmers should draft within 0 to 50 cm (0 to 20 in.) for the greatest effect, but a positive effect can occur up to 150 cm (60 in.). Intuitively, high-level athletes stay within

60 cm (24 in.) of their immediate competitors (Chatard & Wilson 2003; Hausswirth & Brisswalter 2008; Millet, Chollet & Chatard 2000). Drafting behind a swimmer demonstrating either a two-beat or six-beat kick makes no difference, despite there being a lower passive drag when swimming behind a two-beat-kick swimmer (Millet et al. 2000). Swimming behind another person over a distance of 400 m has been demonstrated to increase swimming speed by 3.2 to 3.7 per cent, and so is a highly significant tactic (Chatard, Chollet & Millet 1998; Chollet et al. 2000).

The bodysuit worn by triathletes might also result in a higher swimming speed or a reduced metabolic cost when swimming at a certain speed compared to when not wearing a suit (Mollendorf et al. 2004). Delextrat and colleagues (2003) reported a 7 per cent reduction in heart rate when swimmers donned a wetsuit over a 750 m race, suggesting that their oxygen uptake might have been reduced and subsequently their rate of energy expenditure.

It has been demonstrated that following the 750 m swim in a sprint triathlon event, the cycling efficiency of competitors fell by 17.5 per cent when compared to cycling during a pre-race trial without having swum beforehand (Delextrat et al. 2003). Also, the early stages of the cycling leg have been found to be predictive of overall race performance, and so the physiological state that the triathlete is in when leaving the water is important. Drafting effectively during swimming can reduce the immediate oxygen uptake and hence aerobic energy requirement during the start of the cycling leg and improve cycling efficiency by 4.8 per cent (Delextrat et al. 2003). Bentley and colleagues (2007) found that cycling power output was enhanced over a 20-minute trial when subjects drafted during a 400 m swim compared to when they did not draft.

Cycling

Positive pacing has been observed during the cycling legs of elite-level Olympic distance triathlon races in a number of studies. A reduction in speed, power output and heart rate were observed in 10 triathletes (5 male, 5 female) during the cycling leg of the Beijing Olympic test event in 2006. Riders spent less time above their critical power and at higher exercise intensities over consecutive laps of the course (Bernard et al. 2009). In addition, the athletes demonstrated increased variability in these responses, suggesting that they were suffering worsening fatigue and losses of efficiency during each lap of the cycling leg, which resulted in positive pacing.

It is no wonder that drafting is also a major tactic of triathletes during the cycling leg, as they attempt to conserve energy and also keep up with the pace of the race. Research revealed that cyclists drafting during a stage of the Tour de France reduced their average power output to only 98 W, which is 152 W below the estimate required for a lone rider (Jeukendrup, Craig & Hawley 2000; Jeukendrup, Jentjens & Moseley 2005). Cycling behind a pack of eight riders has also been found to be more beneficial than drafting behind one, two or four riders (McCole et al. 1990). Hausswirth and colleagues (1999) reported that drafting at a distance of 0.2 to 0.5 m (8 to 20 in.) during a triathlon cycling leg significantly reduces energy expenditure and cardiorespiratory strain. Hausswirth and colleagues (2001) also showed that drafting continuously is better than drafting intermittently because it reduces oxygen uptake (16.5 per cent) and heart rate (11 per cent) significantly, which was also found to coincide with improved performance (4.2 per cent) during a subsequent 5 km run.

Another advantage of drafting is that it can reduce cyclists' cadence (pedal rate) significantly (Hausswirth et al. 2001). Triathletes have been reported to adopt a freely chosen cycling cadence of 80 rpm during constant cycling for 30 minutes, although this might be less during longer bouts of cycling (over 1 hour; Hausswirth & Brisswalter 2008). However, some evidence suggests that using a lower cadence (e.g., 70 to 75 rpm) might reduce energy cost over 30 minutes of cycling and during a subsequent 15-minute running trial when exercising at a severe intensity (Vercruyssen et al. 2002). Bernard and colleagues (2003) have also suggested that cycling with a high cadence (close to 100 rpm) before running is a poor strategy; they found that subjects ran closer to their $\dot{V}O_2$max over a 3000 m run when they had cycled with a low cadence (60 rpm) beforehand than when they had cycled at higher cadences (80 to 100 rpm). The subjects after the 60 rpm cycling leg also achieved running times 4.3 and 12 seconds faster on average than when running after the 80 or 100 rpm cycle legs, respectively. However, this was not found to be statistically significant because of a high variability in running times among subjects.

In practice, it is debatable whether triathletes would attempt a reduced cadence during the cycling leg for a number of reasons. They might prefer higher cadences for neuromuscular reasons because they feel as though they are not pushing such a high gear. Also, a slow cadence can reduce speed early in the cycling leg, which might result in the rider missing out on getting into a pack and then losing out on the opportunity to draft. An alternative pacing strategy might therefore be to change cadence to a lower rate only towards the end of the cycling leg. But would there be any metabolic benefit from doing that? Vercruyssen and colleagues (2002) asked subjects to decrease their cadence to 75 rpm during the last 10 minutes of a cycling leg and found that they subsequently demonstrated an increased running time to exhaustion (894 vs. 624 seconds) compared to when they increased their cadence as they approached the end of the cycling leg. However, increasing cadence just prior to the end of the cycling leg is common practice among triathletes, and so again they would need convincing that this rather contradictory strategy, identified under laboratory conditions, could be applied successfully to race conditions.

Research studies have demonstrated that varying cadence by around 5 per cent while cycling uphill or downhill or in windy conditions can help riders maintain an even pace, particularly if they react quickly to the changing conditions (Atkinson, Peacock & Passfield 2007). However, although adopting variable pacing is useful when course topography or wind conditions demand it, variable pacing on a flat course is not a good tactic. Also, another study had subjects frequently varying their power output (variable pacing) using large variations of 5 to 15 per cent of the average power during a 20 km triathlon cycling leg. This led to a reduction in performance during a 5 km run, when compared with a constant cycling power output strategy (Lepers et al. 2007). Therefore, small variations in power output are beneficial to performance, but larger variations might not be.

Running

Running well following the cycling leg is difficult. During a 30-minute triathlon run, competitors were unable to maintain their stride length or running speed (which fell from 14.5 to 13.6 km/h, or 9 to 8.5 mph), which indicates positive pacing (Hausswirth, Bernard & Vallier 2002). The stride length of triathletes appears to be shortened when they begin their running leg, compared to when they run without having cycled beforehand; this may be due to the fact that the knee extension during the flight phase of running is affected by the previous bout of cycling (Heiden & Burnett 2003). An analysis of the running leg of 107 finishers in the 2009 European Triathlon Championships (42 females, 65 males) demonstrated that they positively paced, although the better athletes adopted a more evenly paced strategy (Le Meur et al. 2011). Perhaps because of this more measured pacing strategy, the better runners reduced speed to a lesser degree on the hill sections, where substantial time can be gained on opponents. Running faster during the hill sections would also explain the more even-paced strategy observed.

An aggressive start to the running leg is a common tactic in triathlon to position oneself to draft effectively and also to maintain contact with the athletes one is racing. Nevertheless, some researchers have argued that triathletes should adopt a less aggressive pace and control their high levels of emotion and motivation as they transition from the bike, to resist the temptation to run too fast too soon. Male and female triathletes have been observed to run 3 to 4 per cent faster on the first lap than over the remaining laps, where their paces settled down and fluctuated by only 0.2 km/h (0.12 mph; Le Meur et al. 2011).

Hausswirth, Bernard and Vallier (2002) suggested that a lower running cadence and speed over the first kilometre of an Olympic triathlon might be beneficial. They found that following the cycling leg it was better to run the first kilometre of the 10 km run 5 per cent slower (rather than 5 per cent faster) than the usual running speed observed for a stand-alone 10 km running time trial (when no cycling was undertaken beforehand). The study demonstrated a 40-second difference, or greater, over a 32- to 33-minute 10 km run time. They believed that the strategy of a slow start was important to keep the energy cost constant during the run. By starting too fast, athletes would exercise well above their critical power and so achieve or exercise close to their $\dot{V}O_2$max soon after and rapidly deplete their anaerobic capacity, leading to premature fatigue.

Pugh (1971) observed that drafting during running reduced the oxygen cost of overcoming air resistance by 80 per cent when running at 6 m per second (21.6 km/h, or 13.4 mph) and could lead to a 6.5 per cent reduction in overall oxygen uptake when running at 16 km/h (10 mph). Given that triathletes often run at speeds above 16 km/h (10 mph), drafting during races is beneficial, particularly in windy conditions. Being able to draft, or at least conserve, energy during the running leg can be critical because it might conserve sufficient energy to allow for an end spurt. Le Meur and colleagues (2011) reported that 38 per cent of finishers at the 2009 European Championships demonstrated an end spurt on the last lap. Therefore, the running leg pacing profile for these athletes was more reverse-J-shaped than positively split (refer to figure 2.6). Clearly, not all triathletes positively pace (although the majority do), and in fact, a proportion of competitors do attempt to speed up at the end to gain places.

Gender Differences

The pacing strategies of 12 elite triathletes (6 male, 6 female) were analysed during an International Triathlon Union (ITU) World Cup event (Le Meur et al. 2009). The researchers observed that men and women adopted similar positive pacing strategies during the swimming and running legs. However, the men pushed harder when transitioning from swimming to cycling, and the women had to work relatively harder on hilly cycling sections. Heart rate values for both men and women averaged 92 per cent of maximal heart rate during the overall race, demonstrating high levels of aerobic fitness.

A study that examined 68 male and 35 female triathletes over an ITU course revealed gender differences and similarities in race strategy. In both sexes, the initial swim position over the first, 222 m of the swim leg was associated with both the finish position and the time difference from the leader at the end of the swim leg. This demonstrates that the leaders at the end of the swim leg were in leading positions after only 222 m of the swim leg. The study also found that the difference from the leader at the end of the swim leg determined which bike pack the triathlete was able to join on lap 1 of the cycle leg which in turn affected their finish position at the end of the cycle leg and the overall race position in both sexes. Therefore, the ability to produce a strong swim in the early stages of the race seemed to affect many aspects of the race. However, bike speed and pack number on laps 1 and 2 as well as average bike speed appeared to affect the finish position in males less than it did in females, whereas average running speed was more predictive of the overall finish position in men. The researchers found that females did not tend to bridge gaps in the cycling section and also concluded that female triathletes need to develop their bike performances to increase their chances of success. Both sexes demonstrated positive pacing in the 10 km running leg (Vleck et al. 2008).

COACH'S PERSPECTIVE: Pacing in Triathlon

Ben Bright

Men's coach, 2012 GB triathlon team

2000 Sydney Olympian for New Zealand

Founder and head coach at Triathlon Performance Solutions

The pacing strategy depends on how the race develops. If a large pack comes off the bike together, then athletes are forced into a faster start, similar to a cross country running race in which a selection is made and the race is normally decided among the athletes still together at the 3 or 4 km mark. If there is a smaller break-away group with a substantial lead, then athletes can pace the beginning of the run much better and try to employ a more even-paced strategy.

With endurance sports, one of the keys to best performance is the measuring out of your reserves over the race duration. By using too much energy early, you will suffer late, but you also don't want to have too much in the tank at the finish. Drafting in triathlon makes this difficult because you also have the tactical element of swimming, biking and running in packs, where there is great advantage. So in an individual time trial you may aim for an even pace, but in a competitive drafting event you also have to react to the race, so there are a lot of calculations going on in an athlete's mind during an event.

In the London World Triathlon Series in 2010, Alistair Brownlee had a poor second transition and then ran extremely hard in the first kilometre to get back on terms with the leaders. He managed to do this, but late in the race that early effort—combined with a stomach problem and hot, humid conditions—meant he overheated in the final kilometre and was in a lot of trouble at the finish. If he had eased into the run rather than sprinting up to the leaders, I believe he would still have managed to win or at least place in the top three.

With such a large field at the end of the bike in many races, the pressure is on to get to the front early on the run to establish position and cover the other favourites. I think there is a lack of confidence with many athletes about whether they can run at a more controlled pace and then move through when other athletes begin to fade and they maintain their speed.

The perfect pacing strategy for an Olympic distance triathlon would involve a fast start on the swim, allowing the athlete to fall into a position between third and fifth at the first turning buoy, where he would remain for the rest of the swim, swimming at a strong but controlled pace. The run into transition 1 should be fast to make sure those in front do not get away but to also ensure that those behind have to chase hard. The initial few kilometres on the bike should be hard, to see if a breakaway opportunity is possible and to again ensure that those behind have to work hard to catch up. After the first lap of the bike (between 5 and 8 km), the athlete can assess whether to continue riding hard in a small group. If a larger group has caught the athlete, he should fall into the top 10 per cent of the group because this position is the safest and most energy efficient, especially on a technical course. At the end of the bike, the athlete should be in the top three coming into transition 2. This may cost a bit more energy at the end of the bike, but it makes transition 2 much easier, smoother and faster.

The athlete should then run the first kilometre just above threshold before settling into threshold pace. The competition would move past at around 1 to 1.5 km and extend the pull-away until around the 3 km mark, where they would be between 5

> continued

> *continued*

and 10 seconds ahead. At around the 5 to 6 km mark the athlete would rejoin the lead of the race and be able to maintain his threshold until the final 2 km, where he could accelerate to above threshold.

This strategy for the swim and bike is often applied, but on the run the most successful athletes tend to run very quickly. It is common for the first kilometre off the bike in the men's event to be around the 2 mins 45 s per km mark, then 2 mins 50 s per km, then 2 mins 55 s per km before settling into a 3 mins to 3 mins 5 s per km pace from kilometre 4 to 7 before accelerating again to just below 3 mins per km pace for the last 3 km. The initial fast pace is used by the best athletes to create an immediate selection, but I believe a slightly slower pace in the first 3 km would result in a faster overall pace—but this requires a great deal of patience and confidence.

Each athlete has specific strengths and weaknesses. A strong swim-biker will aim to start quickly to build a lead and then hold on during the run, whereas a fast runner will look to conserve energy during the swim and bike whilst staying in contention before aiming to run down the competition. All of this is discussed between the coach and athlete prior to each event. Some events are used to experiment with strategies and refine tactics for the major championships.

The more important the event, the more planning. For a major race, strategy would be decided upon years out, to allow athletes to train specifically. But a key part of being an elite triathlete is the ability to adjust or change tactics during the event depending on circumstances.

As athletes get older and gain experience, they learn what is possible and what is not. They learn to differentiate between a calculated risk and a risk. Pacing at the elite level is about very fine lines. One second too fast for 400 m during the swim, or 1 km during the run, can be the difference between winning and losing. Athletes also learn that there is real cause and effect during a race. Too much energy expended during the swim or bike will have an effect during the run. Athletes with more experience tend to have a better feel for where their energy gauge is and when to use that energy to best effect.

Ironman Triathlon

The Ironman triathlon involves a 3.8 km swim, 180 km bike and 42.2 km marathon run and can take between 8 and 17 hours to complete depending on ability (Bentley et al. 2008). For this reason, the energy demands and exercise intensities are very different from those of the Olympic distance triathlon event. Exercise intensities are much lower in the Ironman; well-trained triathletes have been reported to perform the cycling leg at a moderate exercise intensity (55 per cent of $\dot{V}O_2$max, a heart rate of 80 to 83 per cent of maximum and a cycling power output of 55 per cent of maximum) (Abbiss et al. 2006; Laursen et al. 2002, 2005; O'Toole, Douglas & Hiller 1998). The Ironman is generally performed with a positive pacing strategy; that is, the exercise intensity decreases over the course of the race (see figure 10.1).

It is thought that an even-paced strategy would be most effective during an Ironman race given that athletes exercise at moderate to heavy exercise intensities, around their first ventilatory threshold or lactate threshold. However, in practice this is very difficult to achieve. During the cycling leg of the Ironman race, athletes' average heart rates were similar to those observed at the ventilatory threshold (150 beats per minute, or bpm) measured during an incremental laboratory cycling test, but cycling power output was lower (Laursen et al. 2002). Another study investigating the 180 km cycling leg measured the responses of six triathletes who placed in the top 10 per cent of finishers and

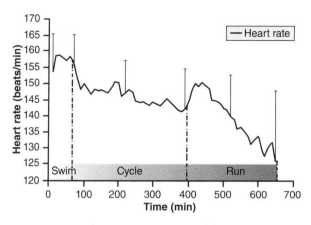

Figure 10.1 Heart rate response during an Ironman triathlon.

Data averaged from 27 athletes.

revealed an average power output of 221 W, a speed of 34.8 km/h (21.6 mph), a cadence of 85 rpm and a heart rate of 146 bpm. However, all these parameters fell during the ride, confirming that even pacing might not be possible during an Ironman, although these findings were partly attributed to an increase in wind speed over the duration of the ride (Abbiss et al. 2006). There is some evidence that if triathletes can exercise below their first ventilatory threshold during the cycling phase, they might be able to run faster marathon legs and produce lower overall Ironman finishing times (Laursen et al. 2005).

It is vital to get to the marathon run in good order because during this leg the overall race placing can change markedly. The heart rate will generally fall in the marathon after 90 to 120 minutes as a result of fatigue. Key considerations are to retain sufficient muscle glycogen stores and to limit the effects of eccentric muscle damage, dehydration and hyperthermia to minimise a reduction in speed. By exercising at a moderate exercise intensity during the cycling leg, athletes can use their bodies' fat stores for aerobic energy production and spare the muscle glycogen stores for the running leg, which results in a higher running speed. Perhaps more important, blood glucose levels can be maintained to protect brain function and movement coordination. Therefore, Ironman triathletes need to plan their pre-race diets carefully to boost carbohydrate (glycogen) stores using a carbohydrate intake regimen of around 10 to 12 grams of carbohydrate per kilogram of body weight. Kimber and colleagues (2002) found that 18 triathletes in the 1997 New Zealand Triathlon took in 1.2 to 1.5 grams of carbohydrate per kilogram of body weight per hour during the cycling leg and 0.6 to 0.8 grams per hour during the marathon run. The female participants in the study demonstrated a positive relationship between their total carbohydrate intake and cycling leg carbohydrate intake and their finishing times. These findings demonstrate that a more evenly paced race strategy can only be possible with correct nutritional practices.

Because drafting during the cycling leg is not allowed in the Ironman, athletes have to sustain a more constant power output than do those in the Olympic distance event, although the power output will of course still need to vary with course conditions. Ironman triathletes wear wetsuits to counter the thermoregulatory effects of the prolonged swimming leg. However, these suits are also thought to aid swimming speed by providing positive buoyancy and hydrodynamic lift, which raises swimmers in the water and reduces their drag as a result (Bentley et al. 2008). Evidence suggests that the lower-intensity swimming observed in Ironman events lessens the detrimental effect the swimming leg has on cycling performance in comparison with the Olympic distance event.

chapter 11

Rowing

Rowing is one of the oldest of the Olympic sports. It requires a blend of power, speed, endurance and technique. Olympic rowing events use both the anaerobic and aerobic energy systems, because they generally last between 5 and 7.5 minutes. The rower sits facing the stern of the boat, away from the direction of travel. In the sculls rowing events, each rower uses two oars; in the other Olympic events, each rower uses just one oar. In some of the events, a coxswain (cox) is also part of the crew. The cox's roles include steering the boat; observing the course conditions, the distance remaining and the opposition's position; and calling out to the crew to coordinate their power and rhythm (pacing). In coxless crews the rowers have complete responsibility for their pacing strategies during races.

The Olympic rowing programme includes the following 14 events, all of which take place over a 2000 m course:

Men's single sculls	Women's single sculls
Men's double sculls	Women's double sculls
Men's lightweight double sculls	Women's lightweight double sculls
Men's quadruple sculls	Women's quadruple sculls
Men's coxless pair	Women's coxless pair
Men's eight	Women's eight
Men's coxless four	Men's lightweight four

The lightweight events feature males weighing less than 72.5 kg (160 lb) with an average crew weight of no more than 70 kg (154 lb), and females weighing less than 59 kg (130 lb), with an average crew weight of no more than 57 kg (126 lb). Standard, non-lightweight (or heavyweight) crews might be 15 to 20 kg (33 to 44 lb) heavier and 10 cm (4 in.) taller than their lightweight counterparts.

Competition rowing can take place on rivers, lakes and the ocean as well as indoors on portable rowing ergometers. This chapter focuses primarily on the Olympic rowing events, which typically take place on lakes—sometimes those specifically created for rowing. However, a section on indoor rowing is included because rowing ergometers have become widely used as a training tool. Their popularity has increased to the point that indoor rowing has now become popular as a sport in its own right. In addition, it is interesting to compare and contrast the pacing strategies adopted during on-water (open-water) and indoor rowing because rowers undertake both forms as part of their competition preparations.

Technique is critical for success in rowing. The rowing stroke itself is a closed skill made up of three main elements: the catch, the drive and the extraction. The catch occurs when the rower quickly places the oar in the water. At this point the drive phase begins and the rower applies force, first by extending the legs, which pushes the seat forward towards the bow of the boat, and then by pulling the arms towards the chest. The extraction (also called the finish, release or recovery) phase of the stroke occurs immediately following the drive phase, as the oar is removed from the water. Once the oar leaves the water, it is rapidly rotated so the blade is parallel to the water (known as feathering the blade), and moved back to the catch position by the action of pushing the oar handle away from the chest. At the same time, the rower flexes the knees, moving the seat back into position in preparation for the next catch phase. The blade is rotated (squared) back into a perpendicular position to re-enter the water, and the cycle begins again. The boat's maximum speed occurs after the drive phase—that is, during the recovery phase (Baudouin & Hawkins 2002).

The rowing technique is highly complex and the coordination and synchrony of each of the rower's oars during each stroke is critical because it affects the boat's overall velocity (Baudouin & Hawkins 2002). Maintaining coordination and synchrony becomes increasingly difficult during a race because the rowers in the crew fatigue at different rates based on their individual levels of fitness. Therefore, the overall pacing strategy adopted by the crew is a significant issue because it affects each crew member differently.

The drag force of a rowing boat shell is proportional to the square of the speed of the boat. An increase in the boat's speed in turn exponentially increases the rower's energy expenditure (Hagerman et al. 1978; Secher 1990). The blade force of the oar acts as the propulsive force that counters the drag force (Baudouin & Hawkins 2002). Perhaps unsurprisingly, sport biomechanics experts are currently researching both boat and oar design to try to improve propulsive efficiency. The mechanical efficiency of the sport has been estimated to be around 20.9 per cent under normal conditions (Hagerman 1984) and approximately 17.5 to 27.5 per cent while rowing a boat in a rowing tank (Fukunaga et al. 1986). Rowing is therefore less mechanically efficient than cycling but more efficient than swimming. Rowing has also been shown to require a high rate of energy expenditure—estimated to be at 36 kilocalories per minute based on a review of rowing physiology studies (Hagerman 1984).

Key Factors in Determining a Pacing Strategy for Rowing

Environmental conditions can adversely affect course conditions and subsequently the pacing strategy. In a strong tailwind, rowers may choose not to feather their oar blades but rather to use them as sails by facing them into the wind. Tailwinds can significantly increase the pace of the boat, whereas headwinds can have the opposite effect. Moreover, smaller boats are the most greatly affected by changes in wind speed and direction. Water temperature can also affect boat speed (e.g., colder water slows the boat); however, changes in water temperature have much less of an impact on boat speed than do changes in wind speed. River races can be significantly affected by pre-race heavy rain, which can lead to choppy water conditions and increased water speeds, which in turn can undermine the stability of a rowing boat and might even cause the cancellation of a race due to safety concerns. How well a rowing crew reacts psychologically to poor or markedly changing race conditions certainly affects the execution of the pacing strategy and the chances of a successful performance.

Through training practices, rowing crews attempt to identify the stroke rate that will optimise their power production and efficiency for the various stages of a race. The pacing profile decided on for the race determines the boat speed, which in turn affects the stroke rate, stroke mechanics and energy cost at each stage of the race. One of the key aims in rowing is to attain as high a stroke rate as possible during the race while maintaining stroke efficiency and propulsion. Higher stroke rates lead to smaller changes in boat speed during strokes and so the boat achieves a more constant velocity, which is helpful. However, realising a higher stroke rate requires that rowers significantly increase their force production, which places substantial additional physiological demands on them (Baudouin & Hawkins 2002). To manage an increase in their stroke rate, rowers have to regulate their exercise intensity and stroke rate sufficiently during races to keep fatigue from developing too early in the event.

At the start of a rowing race, between 1,000 and 1,500 Newtons (N) of force are generated on the oars to accelerate the boat. Thereafter, speed is maintained at a lower level (i.e., 500 to 700 N of force produced for 210 to 230 strokes); hence, rowers must have a high degree of muscle mass and large physiological capacities (Steinacker 1993). Rowers are generally tall with long arms that provide extra leverage. Rowers can afford to be heavy because body weight is supported by the water, although they tend to be lean. This is helpful because the forward movement of the boat is significantly affected by the weight of the vessel and its crew; therefore, carrying excess body fat, which has no functional benefit, is disadvantageous (Shephard 1998). One study suggested that rowers are increasing in height and weight by 2 cm (0.8 in.) and 5 kg (11 lb), respectively, per decade (Carter 1982a, 1982b). Another study of lightweight rowers revealed that the more successful rowers in the 2003 Australian Rowing Championships had relatively less body fat and more muscle and were subsequently heavier than their less successful counterparts (Slater et al. 2005).

Because of the cyclical movement of rowing, which involves both arms and legs, a large proportion of muscle mass is used in a rather unusual way: High force and power are required at low contraction speeds dictated by the slow rate of stroking. To achieve this motion, rowers have been reported to possess high complements of slow-twitch fibres (70 to 75 per cent) in their skeletal muscles, which allow them to produce large forces at low contraction speeds (Secher 1990). Perhaps surprisingly, then, elite rowers undertake regular heavy strength training sessions, which typically recruit their fast-twitch muscle fibres, alongside rowing training to develop their physical capacities. This type of training might be undertaken primarily to improve their ability to get the boat moving at the start of the race.

Interestingly, there is evidence that competitive rowers can complete a typical heavy strength training session up to 24 hours prior to a 2000 m time trial undertaken on a rowing ergometer, with no detrimental effect on their performance. However, evidence of muscle soreness and a reduction in leg power was detected in jump tests (Gee et al. 2011). This finding probably relates to the fact that fast-twitch muscle fibres, rather than slow-twitch muscle fibres, were recruited and subsequently fatigued during the heavy strength training session. The rowers' 2000 m time trial performance the following day was unaffected because the contractile properties of the slow-twitch muscle fibres are most critical to 2000 m rowing performance. Elite rowers typically train for 1,000 hours and cover 5,000 to 7,000 km (3,106 to 4,350 miles) in training per year. Most international teams undertake large amounts of low-intensity training to cultivate economical rowing techniques and well-developed aerobic energy systems.

During races, rowers take a breath with each rowing stroke. This synchronisation would seem to impinge on their ventilatory capacity by restricting opportunities to breathe. However, despite this limitation, rowers have demonstrated very high ventilatory volumes: Male and female competitive rowers breathe more than 200 litres and 170 litres of air per minute on average, during 6 minutes and 3 minutes of rowing, respectively (Hagerman 1984). One review noted that male rowers demonstrated ventilation volumes of 243 litres of air per minute (Secher 1990)! Another characteristic of rowing is that the static component of the rowing stroke—at the catch—significantly elevates the rower's blood pressure to values around 200 mmHg (Secher 1990). To succeed in races, elite rowers certainly have to possess excellent cardiorespiratory efficiency and capacity.

The aerobic nature of the sport is demonstrated by the fact that successful rowers have high proportions of slow-twitch (oxygen-dependent) muscle fibres and a large capacity to take in oxygen and use it for energy production. Male rowers have been found to possess large maximal oxygen uptakes ($\dot{V}O_2$max) of between 6.0 and 6.6 litres per minute (or 65 to 70 ml/kg/min) and an anaerobic threshold at 80 to 85 per cent of this level of oxygen uptake, which demonstrates a high level of aerobic fitness (Ingham et al. 2002; Secher 1993; Steinacker 1993). Female rowers have demonstrated $\dot{V}O_2$max values of 4 litres per minute (Hagerman 1984). By developing their aerobic fitness, rowers can reduce their blood lactate levels at low to high training intensities and by the end of 6- to 7-minute maximal rowing efforts, indicating that aerobic training reduces the need for anaerobic energy production or improves the ability to use lactate more effectively as a fuel for energy production, or both. As a result, it has been estimated that around 65 to 79 per cent of the energy used for rowing in races comes from aerobic energy metabolism (Hagerman 1984; Secher 1990; Shephard 1998; Steinacker 1993).

There is good evidence that rowing performance can be predicted by four factors:

- Well-developed aerobic capacity
- Ability to produce a high power output at maximal oxygen uptake and anaerobic threshold
- Ability to maintain a high percentage of maximal oxygen uptake ($\dot{V}O_2$max) and maximal power output at the anaerobic or lactate threshold
- Ability to produce a high power output and force over five maximal rowing strokes (Bourdin et al. 2004; Cosgrove et al. 1999; Ingham et al. 2002; Steinacker 1993)

The former components (points 1-3) benefit the rowers in maintaining speed endurance during the final 1000 m of the race, whereas the latter component (point 4) allows the rower to produce high levels of force and power, which is critical to the pacing strategy at the beginning of the race. It must not, however, be assumed that all rowers on a boat crew demonstrate the same power profiles, even though they might exhibit similar physiological profiles. Renfree and colleagues (2013) found that the power profiles of rowers in a men's coxless four boat (stroke to stroke), measured during 2 km and 4 km maximal-effort on-water time trials, demonstrated a wide variation. This suggests that they were pacing their efforts quite differently over the time trial.

Common Pacing Strategies in Rowing

Aside from researching the physical, kinematic and drag characteristics of rowing, sport scientists have also investigated the influence of a number of other factors on pacing in rowing races. This section addresses the influence of race positioning, boat type, class, event and gender on pacing strategy during on-water rowing races.

In general, Olympic event rowing races demonstrate a significant acceleration phase to get the boat up to racing speed in the first 100 to 200 m of the race. Thereafter, a parabolic pacing profile is observed as the boat speed initially slows somewhat by 500 m to a pace that is then maintained to 1500 m, at which point an end spurt occurs in most events, but not all (Brown, Delau & Desgorces 2010; Garland 2005; Hagerman 1984; Kleshnev 2001; Muehlbauer, Schindler & Widmer 2010). This parabolic pacing strategy has been termed a reverse-J-shaped pacing strategy. The graph of the force being produced by a rower on the handlebar of a rowing ergometer during a 2000 m test shows a similar pattern: a high force at the start of the test followed by a reduction over the middle portion and an increase at the end as the rower attempts an end spurt (Simoes, Velosa & Armada-da-Silva 2006).

A common tactic in rowing is to lead the field following the start phase (100 to 200 m); this not only provides a psychological advantage but also allows the members of the leading crew to observe the opposition trailing them, so they can adjust their pace to counter any attacks. The pacing strategies for a number of rowing events are depicted in figure 11.1. In this figure, the variability in the 50 m split times evident across races suggests that changes in pace are frequent during rowing races and that boat speeds fluctuate with the sporadic bursts of speed among the crews. Another advantage of leading is that you can avoid the wake of other boats.

The importance of heading a race, or being in close contention, was demonstrated in a study of Olympic, World, and French national championship crews. The researchers found that 78 per cent of the winners were in first position in the middle of the race and 100 per cent of the winners were in the first three places at the halfway point. This clearly supports a fast-start strategy (Brown, Delau & Desgorces 2010).

Interestingly, pacing strategies have been found to be similar irrespective of the boat's finishing position, boat type, event or gender (Brown, Delau & Desgorces 2010; Garland et al. 2005; Kleshnev 2001; Muehlbauer, Schindler & Widmer 2010). Garland (2005) analysed the 500 m split times of 918 heavyweight crews during Olympic and World Championships between 2000 and 2002 who took on average around 381 seconds (males) and 417 seconds (females) to complete the course. This analysis deliberately left out boats finishing last or trailing a long way behind, whose crews may have reduced their efforts prior to the end of the race. In fact, 664 boats were discounted from the findings on this basis! Typically, the crews in this study completed the first 500 m with a time 5.1 seconds faster than subsequent 500 m sectors. In the remaining sectors, split times varied by much less, around 1.3 seconds per 500 m, which suggests that crews were almost evenly pacing the last three-quarters of the race.

The power production required to accelerate the boat and complete the first 500 m of a race significantly faster (1 to 5 per cent) than in the following sectors is substantial, and so it is perhaps not surprising that rowers reduce their pace during the middle portion of a race. The anaerobic energy system is highly used in the first 500 m of the race, and because this system has a finite capacity, rowers need to conserve it in the middle portion of the race so they can use any remaining capacity for an end spurt. In the latter stages of the race, rowers are operating at their maximal aerobic energy production capacity, and so an end spurt largely depends on the remaining anaerobic capacity.

Muehlbauer, Schindler and Widmer (2010) analysed 500 m split times for all boats in heavyweight heats and finals during the 2008 Olympic rowing regatta and had similar results to those of Garland's 2005 study. However, they noted that the pacing strategies during heats and finals were different in the boats that qualified for the finals. In general, it seems as though the crews who qualified for finals adopted a more conservative start (i.e., slower pace) over the first half of the final race compared to the heat race, but were relatively faster in the last quarter of the final race. This subtle change in pacing strategy in the final would presumably be designed to conserve some of the finite anaerobic capacity for the closing stages of the race in order to deliver a decisive end spurt. Alternatively, the faster start in the heat races might be indicative of a strategy to try to dominate the opposition by gaining the lead position early to control the race. This would presumably increase the leading crew's chances of qualification for the final and potentially allow that crew to conserve energy in the latter stages of the heat, if the lead were long enough to permit a reduction in pace. This strategy could allow the leading crew(s) to complete the final stages of the heat in a more even-paced manner, because by controlling the race, they might be able to avoid the need for an end spurt.

Although pacing strategies have been shown to be similar across various events, a study of pacing strategies in seven World Championships reported that the single sculls event often lacked an end spurt. This is certainly the case for the men's single sculls event depicted in figure 11.1. The researchers suggested that having multiple rowers in a boat increases the likelihood of a sprint finish because, even if one rower is too fatigued to accelerate near the end of the race, one or more of the others might be fresh enough to do so. However, in a single sculls race this would not be possible (Muehlbauer & Melges 2011). The comments from Paul Thompson (British and former Australian

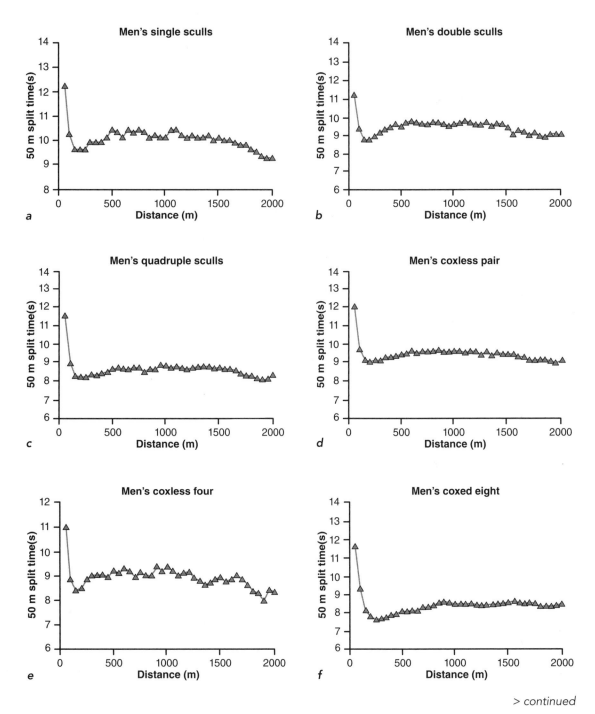

> continued

Figure 11.1 Pacing in the 2011 Rowing World Championships.

Data was publicly available for the 2011 World Rowing Championships, Slovenia, from www.worldrowing.com

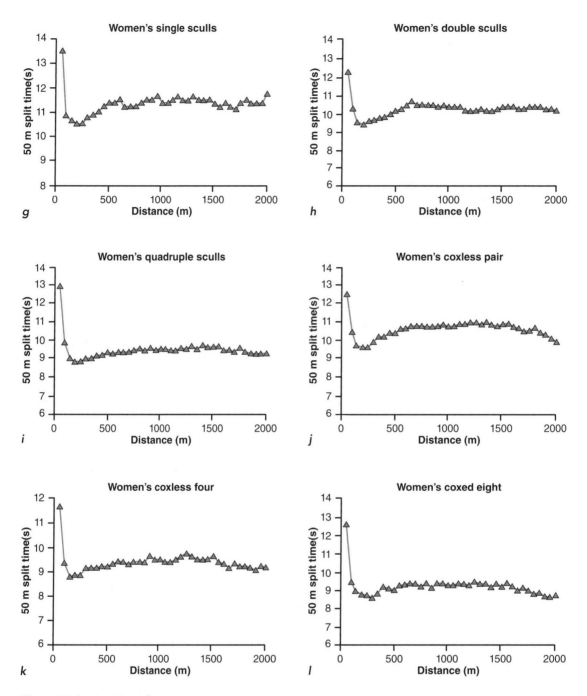

Figure 11.1 *(continued)*

Data was publicly available for the 2011 World Rowing Championships, Slovenia, from www.worldrowing.com

Olympic team rowing coach) in this chapter might suggest another reason for the lack of an end spurt in the single sculls class. If the rowers in this small boat class tend to change pace often during races, this might deplete their anaerobic stores. And as they would be exercising close to or at their $\dot{V}O_2$max towards the end of the race as well, an end spurt would not be possible.

Current British Rowing coach and former Australian Rowing coach Paul Thompson had this to say on the subject:

> Generally speaking, the smaller boat classes have a greater ability to change pace and so tend to be the races that are the most volatile. The bigger boats, especially the eights, tend to have the most powerful people, requiring them to get the heaviest boat up to speed and maintain it. These boats don't tend to have such large variations in the race speed and race volatility. So while the shape of their race profile might be similar, generally the profile is not as pronounced in the heavier boats. In addition, boat and athlete gearing and rigging have an effect on how the crew's power is distributed over the course of the race, which therefore impacts upon rowers' ability to pace their race.

A study of 580 on-water 2000 m races featuring elite, national and sub-elite rowers revealed that the elite rowers were more able to sustain a relatively even pace (i.e., less exaggerated parabolic curve) than lower-level rowers were (see figure 11.2). The investigators attributed this difference to the higher physiological effort and technical competence of elite rowers (Brown, Delau & Desgorces 2010). Therefore, it would appear that better rowers are better able to regulate their efforts during races than lesser rowers are. A further interesting finding of this study was that race winners were in front at the halfway point to a greater extent in elite-level races (78 per cent) than in national (56 per cent) or sub-elite races (60 per cent). This demonstrates that a fast start is more critical in elite-level races.

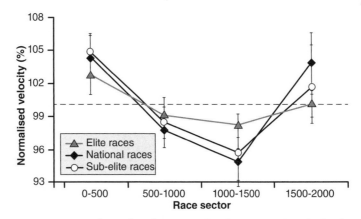

Figure 11.2 Comparative analysis of performances by elite, national and sub-elite rowers. Rowing times have been normalized as a percentage of the average velocity over the race and this is represented by the dashed line on the figure.

Reprinted from *Journal of Science and Medicine in Sport*, 13(6), M.R. Bown, S. Delau, and F.D. Desgorces, "Effort regulation in rowing races depends on performance level and exercise mode," pp. 613-617, 2010, with permission from Elsevier.

COACH'S PERSPECTIVE: Pacing in Rowing

Paul Thompson
Chief coach for women and lightweights for British Rowing

Thompson has coached world and Olympic champions for both his native Australia and his adopted Great Britain. In Beijing the GB women and lightweights squad delivered a gold, a silver and a bronze medal; in London his squad won three gold and two silver medals. Thompson has personally coached medal-winning boats at the last five Olympics (including the double scull of Katherine Grainger and Anna Watkins) to a winning streak of 23 races that included three World Cup series wins, two World Championship titles and the Olympic crown in London. In 2007 he was World Rowing's coach of the year. Thompson shares his thoughts on leading the race, the importance of training and the differences between pacing on water and on the ergometer.

By virtue of facing backwards, rowers face a challenging situation to judge what the pace of the race will be, and indeed their own race pace. They need to either be leading or be close to the lead to set the pace of the race, and often they will only find out how well they have paced the race at the end of it, if they are challenged by another boat and have to sprint. By having the advantage of being in the lead, you can counter your opposition and control the race. The interesting races are when you have two or more crews doing the same thing here. I would suggest that psychological factors reinforcing confidence and race delivery would be a great advantage to the leading crews.

Generally speaking, crews do only what they need to do to qualify in what they feel is the best position for themselves. The fastest crews will do as little as possible to qualify first. To really understand racing strategy and pacing, at the top level, it is important to differentiate between the standard of competition at regattas. The racing is thicker and more volatile at the Olympics than at the World Championships, which is a big step up from the World Cups.

A crew's pacing is developed in training; it is determined in the long miles on the water during the preparation phase and then practised and honed specifically during the race practice phase. Pacing has physiological, technical and mental components, which is why it has to be rehearsed time and time again in training. The efficiency and rhythm of the crew developed during training lay the foundation for racing.

Pacing through rhythm needs to become part of the crew's racing DNA; experienced rowers need to know how to pace over the whole 2000 m. They never know which stroke will win the race—it could be the first or the last. Therefore, the crew or sculler has to learn how to pace for a front-loaded race in which they gain the ascendency and cover their opposition and at the same time be prepared to battle it out gladiatorial style, stroke by stroke, all the way down the course. Pacing this latter sort of race relies on the crew's not being too greedy to take too much of a lead that is too expensive physiologically, but rather to work with the boat and be relaxed and then decisive with their move. There is a physiological cost, and the crew needs to be psychologically and technically prepared to (1) deliver a rhythm with the crews around them and (2) maintain the faster boat speed until an advantage is gained and the race is won.

I have seen some good ergo (rowing ergometer) performances, and I would always say that even pacing, being more physiologically efficient, is the best way to achieve this. The ergo provides stroke-by-stroke feedback that you don't get in the boat and allows rowers to be very structured in their performance and apply a more physiologically efficient profile. It is also a battle with themselves as they don't have to respond tactically to others, even in the ergo competitions. I would suggest that this, and being better able to monitor their work output, is why that first 500 m split variation is different between the water and ergo, producing a more even profile.

2000-Metre Indoor Rowing Competitions

Garland (2005) analysed data from 200 m indoor rowing trials (170 of them) at the British Indoor Rowing Championships in 2000 and 2001. As with on-water (open-water) rowing, he found that pacing strategies were similar, irrespective of finishing position during indoor rowing. However, the pacing strategy of on-water and indoor rowing differed significantly over the first 500 m and also from 500 to 1000 m and from 1000 m to 1500 m. Both on-water and indoor rowing races demonstrated a parabolic pacing strategy with a fast start over 500 m, a gradually slowing pace from 500 m to 1500 m and an end spurt. However, the difference in split times between the first 500 m and subsequent 500 m sectors was more marked in the on-water event (5.1 seconds) than in the indoor rowing event (1.7 seconds). In addition, on-water rowers slowed more in the 500 to 1000 m and 1000 to 1500 m sectors than indoor rowers did. These differences might represent a physiological and biomechanical preference for a relatively faster start on water, perhaps because of the need to overcome greater resistance from the water at the start of the race.

One study suggested that a 2000 m on-water race would be more similar in terms of physical stress to a 2500 m indoor rowing race than a 2000 m indoor rowing race. The researchers suggested that on-water and indoor rowing have different technical and energy requirements (De Campos et al. 2004). On-water rowing may be less efficient than indoor rowing because drag increases to a greater extent with speed on the water and because there is a need to accelerate and balance the boat to overcome currents and waves. This would also explain a requirement for a greater reduction in speed in the middle portion of on-water rowing races: Rowers would have a greater need to conserve energy to allow for an end spurt. A further explanation for these differences in pacing is that, during on-water rowing, a fast start gains placement at the front of the race, where the boat can stay out of the waves generated by other boats and the crew can monitor the opposition.

Finally, although the reverse-J-shaped pacing strategy illustrated in figure 11.1 appears well established during on-water rowing, there is some debate as to whether indoor rowing performance might be better served by a positive pacing strategy. This may depend on the level of the athlete, however. National-level rowers and high school rowers have been shown to positively pace races, whereas both elite and well-trained indoor rowers exhibit a reverse-J-shaped strategy (Brown, Delau & Desgorces 2010; Schabort et al. 1999; Soper & Hume 2004). A couple of studies have revealed that when rowers repeatedly complete maximal effort 2000 m indoor rowing ergometer tests, their pacing profiles can change from a positive to a more even-paced or J-shaped strategy. In one study this coincided with a 3 per cent improvement in performance (Gee et al. 2013; Schabort et al. 1999). This is an example of the concept of teleoanticipation, in which the person amends the pacing strategy based on experience gained from previous bouts of exercise and consciously or subconsciously adjusts the pacing strategy based on this additional knowledge, which results in an improved performance.

chapter 12

Football

This chapter examines the potential role of pacing in the football codes of Association football (soccer), Australian Rules football (AFL), rugby union and rugby league. These sports are characterised by their frequent, multiple bursts of sprint activity and by abundant changes in movement and exercise intensity during matches. The energy expenditure of players in these sports is rarely held constant for more than a brief period of time. Rather, it fluctuates repeatedly as players react to the game around them, which can be unpredictable. Therefore, any attempt players might make to regulate their energy supply would have to occur in a somewhat reactive fashion as well. Sport scientists have only recently begun to investigate whether pacing is, or could be, used by football players and what its effect on match play might be. This chapter looks at the evidence published to date related to pacing in football and attempts to draw some tentative conclusions.

Research specifically addressing the role pacing might play in the various football codes is limited. However, a number of performance analysis studies of soccer and AFL have described the movement characteristics of these sports in detail. Researchers have capitalised on advances in video-based player tracking and global positioning systems (GPS units worn by players) to capture large amounts of data (during match play when allowed by the rules of the sport, and in simulated, or 'friendly', competitive matches when not allowed). Developments in miniature accelerometers and radio frequency identification (RFID) technology have resulted in ever-more sophisticated and precise data being captured in team sports. Real-time software packages are being developed to analyse the data during matches to allow coaches and their support teams to make tactical decisions based on rather subjective data, including the work rate of players. Unfortunately, the majority of football performance analysis studies have been of professional male players and so might not reflect the match play characteristics of female players. However, as the cost of performance analysis technologies falls and their use becomes more widespread, this shortcoming should be addressed in the near future.

Key Factors in Determining a Pacing Strategy for Football

Many factors affect whether pacing is evident in the various football codes and to what extent. These factors include the requirements of the game (e.g., playing time, pitch size, substitutions, recovery time between consecutive matches); the team's playing style and match tactics; the players' physical attributes, capacities, injury management plans and nutrition; and the prevailing environmental conditions.

Data provided in published studies indicate that pacing is likely to play a significant role in soccer and a much less significant role in AFL. Part of the reason for this difference is rules based. Soccer regulations limit how many player substitutions the coach can make during matches. As a result, the majority of the team is required to stay on the pitch and adapt their playing styles by pacing their efforts as they fatigue over the course of a match. In contrast, substitutions are used extensively in AFL; teams are allowed to rotate their players on and off the field in an unrestricted fashion during matches. In addition, stoppages in play are more common in AFL than in soccer, which provides more recovery time for AFL players. Therefore, although AFL players might fatigue rapidly because of the high-speed nature of the game and the large pitches they play on, they have less of a need to pace themselves than soccer players do. More frequent stoppages give AFL players time to recover while on the pitch, and those who are tired can simply be rotated off until they are ready to return to play.

Playing position is another factor that determines the need for a pacing strategy. Work-to-recovery ratios and the frequency and duration of high-intensity efforts vary from sport to sport, player to player and match to match. However, players in certain positions are more likely to fatigue during matches than others are because their positions require a greater overall level of speed endurance. The players most likely to consider pacing during soccer and rugby union matches are the full backs or midfield players and forward players, respectively, because of the greater volume of moderate- to high-speed exercise required in these positions.

Coaches typically attempt to develop in their players the fitness conditioning and 'game intelligence' they need to minimise the risk of the opposition taking advantage of their fatigue and maximise their chances of capitalising on the opposing players' fatigue. Today, many elite football teams employ performance analysts to analyse the opposition's tactics and playing styles as well as their own strengths and weaknesses. This informs the match strategy and pace, provided the strategy can be executed successfully.

Teams often try to identify and 'play-on' tired opposing players, giving them little respite in the hope that a mistake or poor tactical decision from them will lead to a scoring opportunity. Knowing when to raise the tempo (pace) of the match as the opposing players are becoming fatigued is important for increasing scoring opportunities. In support of this tactic, a number of team sports show increased scoring opportunities towards the end of playing halves when players are most fatigued (Mohr et al. 2005).

Team tactics clearly play a significant part in the pace of a match. A coach may instruct the team to attack aggressively during a certain period of the match or to adopt a defensive posture after building up a significant lead. As their skill levels decrease with fatigue, some players deliberately conserve their energy towards the end of football matches to maintain their technical abilities, perhaps to make the most of scoring chances that may transpire or to ensure that they defend effectively. (See the perspectives from former Australian international rugby union player Joe Roff and 2007 World Cup–winning rugby union coach Jake White for some interesting insights on the use of tactics and pacing in match play.)

Environmental conditions such as climate and topography vary considerably during football matches, and their impact on strategy and energy management is now being investigated. In modern sport, elite football players regularly travel to compete in international competitions for their clubs or national teams, so they are frequently exposed to significant variations in climate. A common pacing tactic when playing in hot conditions, or at moderate to high altitude, is to build up play slowly. This gives players significant recovery periods between attacks.

Playing any form of football in extremely high temperatures most certainly affects the pacing and performance capacities of players, and coaches consider this in their team selections and substitution strategies. Not surprisingly, then, there has been a great deal of speculation about the 2022 World Cup for soccer being held in Qatar in June or July. This time of year typically coincides with the warm European summer; however, in Qatar air temperatures are typically much higher! Indeed, temperatures in Qatar can easily reach 40 °C (104 °F), although 53 °C (127 °F) is possible, and humidity levels may also be high. Many are concerned that these extreme conditions will adversely affect player performance and health. The tournament organisers and the international football federation, FIFA, have looked into various solutions, including whether covered, air-conditioned stadiums would provide controllable environmental conditions and even whether holding the tournament between November and January, when temperatures can fall to 25 °C (77 °F), would be more desirable.

Playing soccer at altitude also affects performance. An analysis of approximately 100 years of home and away South American World Cup matches found that competition at moderate to high altitude (>2000 m) favours the home team (Gore et al. 2008). This is likely due to a reduction in the aerobic capacity and running economy of sea level–based teams at altitude, which affects their ability to play at the same pace as teams that reside at altitude.

Finally, in rugby union, when wet weather makes passing and catching the ball difficult, teams often favour a 'kicking game', in which the ball is regularly kicked downfield to rapidly gain territory with minimal risk of error.

Pacing in Association Football

Association football, also known as soccer, is probably the sport with the largest participation and fan base in the world. The FIFA World Cup finals in 1998 attracted an estimated audience of 40,000 million television viewers (Reilly, Bangsbo & Franks 2000). ESPN Soccer (2011) reported that an estimated 1 billion people witnessed the 2010 World Cup final, and FIFA research reported that 3.2 billion people (46.4 per cent of the world's population at that time) watched live coverage for at least 1 minute. However, despite this popularity, few studies have investigated whether players actually pace their activity during matches. A number of studies have compared activity levels during matches to try to understand fatigue and its relationship to tactics. However, few studies specifically mention pacing.

A soccer match consists of two 45-minute periods (halves) with a 15-minute half-time recovery period between them. Time does not stop during play for restarts, injuries or other interruptions; however, the referee tallies this 'stoppage' time and tacks it on to the end of the match. Association football pitch sizes do vary, but the stadiums of professional teams are generally around 105 m long and 70 m wide. In Association football, a goal is scored when the entire ball passes the opposition's goal line between the goalposts and under the crossbar, usually from kicking the ball. A goal cannot be scored if there has been an infringement of the rules prior to it. The team with the most goals at the end of the match wins. Compared to other football codes, the frequency of scoring is low.

At any one time 11 players from each side play in a match, unless a player has been sent off by the referee for a disciplinary offence, in which case the team loses a player for the rest of the match. The number of substitutes allowed during a match varies depending on the football league of the country. For example, in the English leagues each team is allowed to have 5 substitute players in addition to the 11 players in the starting line-up, but only 3 of the substitutes can play a part in the match. In Association football, the team can make only a few substitutions during the match, and so most of the team's players complete the full 90 minutes of the match—longer if there is added stoppage time (usually only a few minutes).

Evidence suggests that when substitutes come on during the second half of a match, they sprint and compete at a higher intensity than the players who complete all 90 minutes of the match (Mohr, Krustrup & Bangsbo 2003). This finding demonstrates that coaches must carefully consider when to make player substitutions. For example, replacing a defensive player who is showing signs of fatigue with another more attacking style of player could inject more pace into the attacking formation and take advantage of an opposition's tiring defenders if done at the right time.

Energy Requirements and Activity Levels of Association Football Players

Outfield soccer players (players other than the goalkeeper) typically cover 8 to 13 km (5 to 8 miles) during a match. They change activity every 5 seconds or so (e.g., from walking to dribbling to tackling to running to jogging to sprinting), leading to well over a thousand changes of activity per match (Di Salvo et al. 2009; Mohr, Krustrup & Bangsbo 2005). Energy is predominantly supplied by the aerobic energy system, and players exercise at around 70 to 75 per cent of their maximal oxygen uptake (75 to 85 per cent of maximal heart rate) over the course of a match.

Midfield players tend to cover the greatest distances and have been observed to possess the highest oxygen uptakes—60 ml/kg/min or more (Reilly, Bangsbo & Franks 2000; Sporis et al. 2009). Full backs and midfield players cover the greatest distance at high-intensity or very high-intensity running speeds (Rampinini et al. 2007). The anaerobic energy system is used intermittently during more intense play, which is typically under-taken every 30 seconds or so. Blood lactate values of 3 to 6 mmol/L are common, and individual players produce 12 mmol/L at times during very intense playing periods (Di Salvo et al. 2007; Dupont et al. 2010; Mohr et al. 2004; Rampinini et al. 2007; Reilly, Bangsbo & Franks 2000; Stolen et al. 2005). These findings demonstrate that players, particularly full backs and midfield players, exercise within the heavy to severe exercise intensity domains for prolonged periods during matches, for which they need a well-developed endurance capability. The attackers, or strikers, often demonstrate greater sprint ability than the other outfield players over distances of 5 to 15 m, but less endurance performance capability (Sporis et al. 2009).

Producing a maximal effort over 10 seconds of match play can deplete the creatine phosphate store in the muscle. This 'fast-energy' store can only be regenerated if the player's activity level falls to a moderate intensity; however, this pacing of effort is not always possible. For example, if the opposing team attacks suddenly during what would otherwise be a regenerating period, then fatigued players might have to sprint again and further deplete their anaerobic stores. If this pattern of play persists, at some stage players will no longer be able to sprint at full speed and chase down opposing players. Hence, players need to judge (or pace) their activity cleverly when deciding when to get involved in play and when not to.

Television commentators often take note when a defensive player undertakes a long attacking run down the outside portion of the field, because they know that this tactic is risky. The defender is out of position in the defensive formation, and should the opposition attack, the defender may not be able to run back quickly enough to defend because of temporary fatigue. Because outfield players can become fatigued during a match, elite players likely pace themselves by choosing to work at moderate intensity levels at certain times and occasionally choosing not to be involved in a developing attack or defensive situation (Orendurff et al. 2010). Consider a situation in which an attacking player appears to be isolated with the ball in the final quarter of the pitch. The television commentator might say, 'There is nobody [from the attacking player's team] supporting the player'. In this scenario one or more players might have chosen to hold their positions and not attack with their teammate because they were pacing themselves.

Anecdotally, English Premiership League forward players have been known to wait until the last quarter or so to become more involved in the match in order to conserve energy, particularly their anaerobic capacity, so they can use it when defending players might be tiring. In support of this tactic, one study found that 3 per cent of players produced their most intense period of activity in the last 15 minutes of a match, while 40 per cent of players were producing their lowest activity levels of the match (Mohr, Krustrup & Bangsbo 2005).

Evidence of Pacing in Association Football

Players undoubtedly pace themselves according to their fitness levels, the importance of the match, their playing positions, team success and tactical considerations such as the match score (Di Salvo et al. 2009; Edwards & Noakes 2009). For example, the better the opposition is, the greater the total distance covered and the amount of high-intensity running required by players (Rampanini et al. 2007). However, fatigue may also play a part in the activity levels of players. Time-and-motion analyses during football matches have determined that players' performances are generally reduced

- following short-term, intense efforts,
- during the early stages of the second half and
- in the final period of the match (Mohr, Krustrup & Bangsbo 2005).

Fatigue following short, intense efforts might be caused by a number of factors that affect the anaerobic capacity, such as creatine phosphate depletion, the build-up of metabolites associated with fatigue (inorganic phosphate, a change in acidity from hydrogen ion accumulation, ammonia, potassium) and the related effects on the nerves and how they stimulate the muscles. In the latter stages of matches, the reduction of muscles' carbohydrate (glycogen) stores is another factor thought to reduce players' sprint activity. In addition, heat and humidity may affect physical performance because players feel increasingly uncomfortable as they become hot and dehydrated, and this might affect brain function.

Evidence shows that following a short, intense effort over a 5-minute period, football players are less active during the next 5 minutes of play. A study found that the distance covered by players at a high intensity (greater than 15 km/h, or 9.3 mph) dropped significantly in the following 5-minute period, and that this reduced activity was less than the average 5-minute activity value for the whole match (Mohr, Krustrup & Bangsbo 2003). In another study in which players performed a repeated sprint test following a short, intense period of match play during the first half of a competitive match, their ability to repeatedly sprint was reduced (Krustrup et al. 2003). Taken together, these studies demonstrate that a reduction in high-intensity activity following an intense 5 minutes of play might not be due simply to a natural variation in match play; rather, physical fatigue is likely to have contributed.

As illustrated in figure 12.1, a number of studies investigating both male and female elite football players have reported that the amount of sprinting and high-speed running as well as distances covered are less during the second half of matches (Bangsbo 1994; Di Salvo et al. 2009; Mohr et al. 2008; Mohr, Krustrup

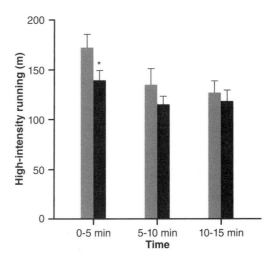

Figure 12.1 Changes in the amount of high-intensity activity of elite soccer players between the first half (lightly-shaded bars) and the second half (darkly-shaded bars) of competition.

*Significant difference between the two halves.

From M. Mohr, P. Krustrup, and J. Bagsbo, 2005, "Fatigue in soccer: A brief review," *Journal of Sports Sciences* 23(6): 593-599. Data from J. Bangsbo, P. Krustrup, and M. Mohr, 2003, "Match performance of high-standard soccer players with special reference to development of fatigue," *Journal of Sports Sciences* 21(7): 519-528. Reprinted with permission of Taylor & Francis Ltd.

& Bangsbo 2003, 2005; Reilly & Thomas 1976). This might be partly explained by a reduced amount of carbohydrate available in the muscles for aerobic and anaerobic energy production towards the end of matches. There are some scientific reports of players having low levels of carbohydrate in their muscles towards the end of matches, and more specifically, that their fast-twitch (Type IIA) muscle fibres and slow-twitch muscle fibres can be low in muscle glycogen (carbohydrate) at the end of matches, although this is not always the case. Thankfully, scientific studies do not report critical levels of blood glucose, which might affect a player's health, during football matches (Jacobs et al. 1982; Krustrup et al. 2003; Smaros 1980).

A criticism of time-and-motion studies to date is that they tend to measure only the time a player spends in certain speed zones (e.g., walking, jogging, running, high-speed running, sprinting) rather than the ability to accelerate. The ability of a player to accelerate might be more important than the actual average speed or even the maximal running speed attained, because being able to accelerate past an opposing player is critical when attacking or defending. Osgnach and colleagues (2010) also argued that a greater energy cost is associated with a change of speed (i.e., acceleration or deceleration). In addition, acceleration is of course a prerequisite to high-speed running and has been shown to be different from maximal speed in that it requires greater nerve activation to the working muscles (Little & Williams 2005; Mero & Komi 1986, 1987).

Akenhead and colleagues (2013) demonstrated that the accelerations and decelerations of players are affected by fatigue over the course of matches, suggesting that pacing must play a part in soccer. These researchers analysed 36 English Premier League club players over six 15-minute periods and observed that distances covered using a low, moderate and high acceleration and deceleration fell by 8.0 to 13 per cent from the first 15-minute period to the third 15-minute period of the first half and by 9 to 16 per cent for the same 15-minute periods in the second half. A reduction of between 15 and 21 per cent in the distance covered while accelerating and decelerating was also observed in the final 15-minute period in the second half, compared to the first 15-minute period in the first half. In addition, when players exhibited their greatest distance covered at high rates of acceleration over a 5-minute period, they were then found to suffer a drop of 10 per cent during the next 5 minutes of play.

There is evidence that exercising (e.g., on a stationary bike) at a low to moderate intensity for 7 to 8 minutes at half-time helps maintain body and muscle temperature, which can fall by 2 °C otherwise. In addition it may also increase the muscles' ability to take up oxygen (i.e., improve the so-called oxygen uptake kinetics) and enhance aerobic energy production when the second half begins. This would allow players to operate more aerobically in the initial period after half-time, sparing their anaerobic capacity and allowing for a greater overall playing intensity (i.e., a higher pace), which might provide a competitive advantage (Mohr, Krustrup & Bangsbo 2005).

Dehydration and high internal body temperatures have also been suggested as possible causes of fatigue in soccer. Studies have detected players losing 3 litres of fluid (3 kg, or 6.6 lb, in weight) primarily through sweating during matches in normal temperatures and 4 to 5 litres in hot and humid match environments (Mohr et al. 2004; Mustafa & Mahmoud 1979). The average internal body temperatures of football players after matches have been between 39 and 39.5 °C (102 and 103 °F); however, some players have been found to have temperatures beyond 40 °C (104 °F). An internal body temperature over 40 °C (104 °F) has been associated with what is known as central fatigue, because at this temperature it is thought that the brain might reduce a person's activity levels to protect against developing a heat-related illness. However, high internal temperatures are not a feature of most football matches. In fact, in one study no differences were found in the body temperatures of players following the first and second halves of a match, which demonstrated that they had suffered no net gain in heat over the match (Eckblom 1986; Mohr et al. 2004).

The relatively small levels of dehydration (1 to 2 per cent of body weight) and rises in body temperature detected in players during soccer matches have been argued to be evidence of their pacing their activity to avoid large changes in these parameters (Edwards & Noakes 2009). Edwards and Noakes (2009) argued that a part of the brain (termed the central governer) ensures that no single physiological system is maximally used during a match. Rather, the brain modifies the player's behaviour subconsciously as the match progresses to prevent exhaustion or a heat illness. They also suggested that the thirst players develop over a match may alert the brain to reduce high levels of activity and hence the match pace.

To conclude, some sport science researchers suspect that feedback from various physiological systems (e.g., thirst, metabolite levels, body temperature, carbohydrate levels), players' knowledge of how much time is left to play and their previous match experiences might result in their subconsciously and consciously modifying their activity levels to reach the end of the match in a competitive physical state. This degree of pacing might also maintain skill levels. A recent study revealed that French League 1 players were generally able to maintain their skill-related performance as they reduced their high-intensity activity during the final period of matches (Carling & Dupont 2011). Therefore, pacing determined by central regulation from the brain is a possible explanation for the reduction in distances observed for high-intensity running, sprinting, accelerations and decelerations during the latter stages of football matches. This reduced activity might be a strategy for maintaining competitive physical capacity and skill level towards the ends of matches.

Pacing in Australian Rules Football

Australian Rules football, the most popular football code in Australia, is also played in over 30 countries worldwide (Gray & Jenkins 2010). The game consists of two teams playing four 20-minute periods, with 18 of each team's 22 players on the field at any time. However, stoppage time can be significant and can increase total playing time to over 120 minutes (10 or so extra minutes each quarter). The main way to score points is by kicking the ball between the two major inner goalposts, which earns 6 points, although 1 point can be earned by kicking the ball between one of the two smaller outer posts and one of the larger inner posts. The winning team is the one who scores the most points through goal kicking.

Eighteen teams representing all seven Australian states compete in the Australian Football League (AFL). Australian football is an invasion game involving less contact than in rugby; however, tackling (between the shoulders and knees) and collisions are common. Players can also shepherd opposing players by pushing them with their bodies or arms when they are within 5 m of the ball. The pitch is oval in shape and generally 135 to 185 m long and 110 to 155 m wide. There are six forward, six midfield and six back players who have different roles and responsibilities. Forward and back player groupings tend to contain at least two taller players along with four smaller and more mobile players. Midfielders (centre, wings and followers) link play to both the forwards and backs and play the game with a more nomadic style as a result. Midfield players and ruckmen, who are often the tallest players (over 2 m, or 6 ft 6 in., tall) and the major ball winners when the ball is in the air, have long been established as playing with more frequent bouts of high-intensity exercise and with greater overall physical loads (Wisbey, Montgomery & Pyne 2008).

The game has recently become increasingly professionalised, resulting in an increasingly faster pace and necessitating the need for players to be regularly substituted in and out of matches as they fatigue (Gray & Jenkins 2010; Wisbey, Pyne & Rattray 2010). Rule changes have also contributed to the speed at which the game is played, requiring the fitness levels of players to change commensurately. For example, the playing period length has fallen from 25 minutes to 20 minutes (1994); deliberate kicks out of bounds are disallowed (1968); player interchanges have become unlimited (1978); four substitute players are available to interchange with on-field players (1998); and modern umpires are required to take less time to restart play. Consequently, modern players require a greater ability to sprint repeatedly and higher levels of upper- and lower-body strength than their earlier counterparts did, as well as high levels of endurance fitness. Between the 2005 and 2008 seasons, the average running velocity during matches rose by 8.4 per cent; and exercise intensity, by 14 per cent (Wisbey et al. 2010).

Players tend to be around 1.85 to1.92 m (6 ft 1 in. to 6 ft 3 in.) tall, to weigh between 80 and 95 kg (176 and 209 lb) and to have low levels of body fat. The modern game of Australian Rules football consists of shorter periods of play at high intensities interspersed with more frequent and longer stoppages (Gray & Jenkins 2010). Coaches have also moved away from the tactic of players kicking over long distances to one another and moved towards shorter kicks and a more possession-focused style of playing in which the players move in groups. The modern game also features players kicking the ball to teammates who are in positions back towards their own goal to maintain possession, although this can also be used to slow the pace of the match down briefly. Another trend is for fewer players to remain on the field throughout matches—only 20 per cent in 2005 (Norton 2007). Play is also more intermittent; bounce-downs (to restart play) have increased from 11 in 1961 to 60 in 2003, despite stoppage time falling overall (Anderson 2005; Gray & Jenkins 2010; Norton, Craig & Olds 1999).

Energy Requirements and Activity Levels of Australian Rules Football Players

Players tend to cover between 12 and 12.5 km (7.5 and 7.8 miles) per match, with nomadic players often covering around 0.5 km (0.3 miles) more than forwards and backs. More in-depth analyses that split the total distance covered into high, moderate and low speeds demonstrated that for approximately 70 per cent of the time players are operating at low speeds (covering less than 7.9 km/h or 4.9 miles/h); however, this might be less in nomadic midfield players (65 per cent) who complete more activity at moderate speeds than do those in other positions (Wisbey, Montgomery & Pyne 2008). Midfield players also tend to spend the most time sprinting (5.6 per cent) and take part in more high-intensity bouts (208 vs. 158) than forwards or backs. Fast running and sprinting has been found to account for around 4.4 to 6.3 per cent of match activity for the various playing positions (Dawson et al. 2004).

In the 2008 AFL season, most sprint efforts lasted less than 3 seconds, and all sprints lasted less than 6 seconds; however, longer fast-running efforts averaged between 11 and 13 seconds for all positions (Wisbey, Rattray & Pyne 2008). Because of the short durations of sprinting, players rarely reach maximal speed in matches. As a result, the ability to accelerate up to, say, more than 80 per cent of maximal speed within a couple of seconds is perhaps more important than outright speed, unless a longer effort can be undertaken in which outright speed will give an advantage. Players who can sprint and recover more quickly to sprint again (i.e., those with repeat sprint ability) have been judged to also be the better players in one study of elite Australian Football players (Young et al. 2005).

Players spend approximately 21 minutes (forwards and backs) to 24 minutes (midfielders) undertaking steady running (below their critical power threshold). However, this represents a minor part of matches, which can regularly take over 100 minutes with stoppages (Wisbey, Rattray & Pyne 2008). Players do have recovery periods during play (moving at less than 5.0 km/h or 3.1 miles/h) for periods of around 90 to 120 seconds and regularly spend twice as much time at relatively low exercise intensities compared to moderate or high exercise intensities. This suggests that they pace themselves or that the match is sufficiently spread out that they are not engaged with play for long periods at a time. Nonetheless, the regularity of substitution suggests that players do become significantly fatigued on a regular basis.

Researchers reported that individual playing time fell by 9 per cent from the 2005 to the 2008 season, which suggests that less playing time is necessary to allow for the higher playing intensity of the modern game (Dawson et al. 2004; Wisbey, Montgomery & Pyne 2008; Wisbey et al. 2010). For example, Aughey (2010) reported that players commonly undertake two periods of play during each quarter and that teams might have up to 100 substitutions per match.

Australian Rules football players possess similar maximal oxygen uptake ($\dot{V}O_2$max) scores as soccer players (around 55 to 65 ml/kg/min), which suggests that they need to recover quickly between sprints and be able to spare their anaerobic capacity where possible as well. A high $\dot{V}O_2$max has also been found to distinguish successful AFL club draftees, which suggests that the ability to produce energy aerobically is important. Most likely, this ability furnishes the majority of the muscle's energy requirement for low to moderate running and also ensures that the anaerobic capacity (and specifically the creatine phosphate store of muscles) is replenished between sprints during recovery periods (Pyne et al. 2005). This would help to maintain the anaerobic capacity for fast runs, jumps, tackling, wrestling and shepherding activities, which require high levels of upper- and lower-body strength and power. Thus, it seems clear that pacing is something Australian Rules football players have to consider during matches, although because they can be easily substituted throughout a match, they can also recover on the bench when significantly fatigued.

Evidence of Pacing in Australian Rules Football

AFL players' mean speeds are greater in the early stages of each quarter, and those who interchange more frequently can also undertake more high-intensity efforts (Gray & Jenkins 2010). Clearly, then, players are not being required to pace themselves as much as they would have, say, 20 years ago, because they are now covering ground at higher speeds and can rest with unrestricted frequency when the coaching staff perceives they are tiring.

Coutts and colleagues (2009) studied 16 elite-level AFL players over one to nine matches (a total of 65 matches) between 2005 and 2007, using global positioning systems (GPS), and found that players covered 12 to 14 km (7.5 to 8.7 miles) per match. Approximately 3.2 to 4.5 km (2 to 2.8 miles) of that distance was covered at a high intensity (i.e., running speeds above 14.4 km/h, or 8.9 mph). Total distance covered decreased by 7.3 per cent, 5.5 per cent and 10.7 per cent in the second, third and fourth quarters compared to the first quarter, and high-intensity running also decreased after the first quarter. Players who covered large total distances or large distances at high intensity during the first half of a quarter or in the whole quarter subsequently reduced the distance they covered in the next half or quarter, respectively, demonstrating a reduction in effort that might indicate pacing, or at least positive pacing. In an analysis of the 2010 AFL season, Wisbey, Pyne and Rattray (2010) reported moderate decreases (7 to 12 per cent) in average speed, exertion index per minute and total distance covered.

Aughey (2010) took a slightly different approach and attempted to account for the fact that players rotate on and off the field by analysing distances covered according to the actual time players were on the pitch. He found that when the total distance covered and the distance covered while undertaking low-intensity activity were expressed in terms of metres covered every minute, these parameters did not change significantly during a match in 18 elite AFL players. However, bouts of high-intensity running at speeds ranging between 15 and 36 km/h (9.3 and 22.4 mph) decreased as the match progressed, which indicates fatigue. In addition, the ability to accelerate also decreased over the course of the match. Aughey concluded that these findings did not support the belief that team sport players pace their efforts because the players had not reduced their low-intensity running or total distance covered to maintain their high-intensity running or frequency of maximal accelerations. The researcher also made the point that players do not know the duration of quarters because stoppage time can be significant. Therefore, the classic premise of pacing—that an athlete paces by anticipating the end point of the event because it is known in advance (teleoanticipation)—is not fully met in Australian Rules football.

However, a study in which changes in the internal body temperature of AFL players were monitored during two pre-season matches in hot conditions (>29 °C, or 84 °F) did reveal evidence that players reduced their low-intensity activity, but not their high-intensity efforts, during matches. This suggests that players were attempting to control the rise in their internal body temperatures during the matches. The researchers concluded that pacing strategies might have been employed to control the internal heat load (Duffield, Coutts & Quinn 2009).

In summary, the reduction in high-intensity exercise during match play suggests that fatigue develops during the course of a match and is consistent with the notion that some degree of pacing takes place during Australian Rules football matches. In addition, players are regularly rotated (i.e., substituted), which clearly suggests that they demonstrate significant fatigue. However, because players can leave the field at any time, they presumably pace themselves accordingly and no doubt undertake an exhausting period of exercise just prior to leaving the field. Most players no longer complete a match, or even a quarter, without rotating, which is clearly a very different strategy to that observed in soccer, in which players generally play the full match without interruption except for the half-time break. Indeed, in contrast to soccer players, Australian Rules football players might deliberately positively pace and produce a number of nearly all-out efforts in quick succession because they know that a rotation is imminent and they will have time to recover before rejoining the match.

Pacing in Rugby

Rugby is a full-contact invasion game based on running with an oval-shaped ball in hand. It involves repeated high-intensity sprints and a high frequency of physical contact. The sport is generally played on a pitch that is 100 m long and 70 m wide with H-shaped posts on either goal line. Rugby matches consist of two 40-minute periods, with a 10-minute half-time break between them.

Two codes of rugby are played worldwide: rugby union and rugby league. In rugby union, each side has 15 players on the pitch at one time and seven reserve players on the sideline, whereas in rugby league there are 13 players on the pitch and four reserve players. Scoring is also different between codes. In rugby union, 5 points are awarded for a 'try' (when the ball is grounded after the goal line) and a further 2 points are awarded for the conversion kick (kicked goal) that follows. Three points can also be scored by a kicked drop goal or a penalty goal. In rugby league, 4 points are awarded for a try, and a conversion is worth a further 2 points. Two points can also be scored by performing a kicked penalty goal but only 1 point for a kicked drop goal.

The style of play differs between the codes in a number of ways. First, the scrum in rugby league is largely uncontested. There are no line-outs, but rather a 'put-in' to a scrum when the ball goes out of play over the sideline. Rugby league also has a six-tackle rule: The attacking team has six tackles to advance the ball as far as possible before the opposing team gains possession and does the same. In rugby union, however, possession changes on a more continuous basis. This is an important difference, because in rugby league the defending team commits only a few players to a tackle to maintain a defensive line, whereas more players commit to a tackle in rugby union to contest the ball and play is more continuous through the use of rucks and mauls (where the ball is recycled from a tackled player by teammates, allowing play to continue).

Professionalism in rugby league was introduced in 1898 after the game emerged in 1895; however, in rugby union the International Rugby Board (formed in 1886) only relaxed restrictions making the game openly professional in 1995. The advent of professionalism in the code of rugby union has meant that fitness levels have developed rapidly over the last two decades. Rugby union is played in over 100 countries across six continents; rugby league is played in over 30 countries worldwide.

Energy Requirements and Activity Levels of Rugby Union Players

Forward players (the ball winners; males 180 to 195 cm [5 ft 11 in to 6 ft 5 in.] and 100 to 120 kg [220 to 265 lb]; females 65 to 75 kg [143 to 165 lb]) are generally taller and heavier and possess greater proportions of body fat than back players (the so-called ball carriers; males 170 to 185 cm [5 ft 6 in. to 6 ft 1 in.] and 80 to 95 kg [176 to 209 lb]; females 55 to 65 kg [121 to 143 lb]). However, the physical characteristics of forwards are changing; they are becoming heavier largely as a result of higher levels of muscularity (Duthie, Pyne & Hooper 2003).

ATHLETE'S PERSPECTIVE: Pacing in Rugby Union

Joe Roff
Former Australian rugby union footballer

Joe Roff represented Australia's Wallabies on 86 occasions, of which 62 were consecutive wins from 1996 to 2001. Roff played in the 1999 World Cup–winning team and Tri Nation tournament winning teams in 2000 and 2001. He played as a full back, winger and centre for Australia. In his final match he was captain of Oxford in the 2007 varsity match against Cambridge.

Comments directed at me throughout my own playing career, which for some reason were often framed as criticism, often revolved around the notion that 'you looked like you were cruising out there'. I probably was. That notion that you give 100 per cent in a match over 80 minutes is an ideal; however, in reality it is more accurate to say that you choose when you give 100 per cent to give yourself the best chance of winning. This is relevant to individuals, teams and competitions.

I am trying to recall a time in my 10 years of professional rugby in which a coach told me to pace myself. I cannot. Contact sports such as rugby give little formal attention to pacing, perhaps through a lack of understanding. In a holistic sense, coaches often talk about the need for a fast start. This is generally tied to the value of establishing momentum in the match.

Contact sports at an elite level are focused on building pressure. Without understanding the notion of pacing, individuals and teams 'blow out'. This leaves them exposed, and consequently, there is a great focus on exploiting these moments in a match, often in the last 10 minutes of the first half and the last 20 minutes of the second half, when the highest level of fatigue exists.

There is a reactive element to pacing strategies in contact sports. While in principle pacing strategies are set, this is often refined within the context of the match and in relation to the way the match unfolds. Often, the pacing strategy is determined within the match itself. This includes notions of slowing the match down or speeding it up and using strategies to pace it at the desired level.

The most successful athletes are the players who are described as 'having time' on the field. These are generally the players who have an innate understanding of the notion of pacing and the value of conserving energy in a repeat-effort environment. They also have an appreciation of the impact of acceleration and deceleration in a contact sport and especially in a fatiguing environment.

In absolute terms, forwards have been found to demonstrate superior aerobic and anaerobic capacities. Backs have been found to be superior sprinters over 20 to 50 m, and when body weight is taken into account, they also have relatively better endurance (aerobic) fitness than forwards. Because of the heterogeneous nature of a rugby union team's line-up, the physical characteristics of players are wide ranging. For example, among forward players, the hooker might be 10 kg (22 lb) lighter than the props (who generally weight 95 to 110 kg [209 to 243 lb]) and 10 to 15 cm (4 to 6 in.) shorter than locks (who might be around 190 to 195 cm [6 ft 2 in. to 6 ft 4 in.] tall). These size and shape differences relate to their roles in the team. The shorter and heavier build of the hooker and props helps them scrummage in the front row of the scrum, whereas the tall lock plays a supporting role by pushing them forward from behind. In turn, the lock plays the vital role in the line-out by jumping to catch the ball. This time the props play the supporting role by helping to lift the lock into the air.

There is some evidence that rugby union players possess relatively lower aerobic fitness than soccer and field hockey players; their maximal aerobic capacity (maximal oxygen uptake or $\dot{V}O_2$max) varies from around 51 to 59 ml/kg/min in high-standard players (Duthie, Pyne & Hooper 2003). Anaerobic energy requirements are substantial in rugby because players are required to undertake multiple sprints during a match and forwards must exhibit high levels of strength and power in scrums, rucks and mauls. Front-row forwards produce 1,200-1,700 N of force during scrums, which can last 5 to 20 seconds (Morton 1978; Quarrie & Wilson 2000).

In addition to the diversity of the physical and physiological attributes within a team, many other factors influence the intensity and duration of play, including the following:

- Competition level
- Nature of the playing positions, individual players' capacities and their patterns of play
- Frequent and significant stoppages by the officials, which can amount to 60 per cent of the match duration
- Environmental conditions
- Team tactics

Taken together, these factors make it extremely difficult to determine whether rugby union players pace their activity during a match.

Relevance of Pacing in Rugby Union

The relevance of pacing in rugby union matches may be questionable considering that the ball is generally in play for only 30 minutes or so. The ball is out of play for the remaining 50 minutes of the match because of injury stoppages, conversions and penalties (Duthie, Pyne & Hooper 2003; McLean 1992). Also, rugby union players typically spend the majority of the match in low- to moderate-intensity activity (elite forwards, 86 to 88 per cent of the match; elite backs, 94 to 96 per cent of the match). This suggests that they have ample time to recover between high-intensity efforts (Duthie, Pyne & Hooper 2005; Roberts et al. 2008). For example, forward players might spend only around 15 per cent of their time in very intense activities such as scrums, rucks and mauls (Carter 1996; Treadwell 1988).

If any pacing of effort is required during a rugby union match, it would be by the forward players. Back players appear to rarely become fatigued and so have little need to pace themselves. They undertake 50 to 60 per cent less overall work and demonstrate lower heart rates and movement patterns than forward players do. Moreover, although backs do spend more time performing intense running (30 seconds or so more per match), most of these efforts are sprints of only a few seconds in duration (Deutsch, Kearney & Rehrer 2002). Backs also have more time to recover following sprints, and because they have good endurance, they recover quickly (Duthie, Pyne & Hooper 2003, 2005; Roberts et al. 2008). In contrast, props and locks (forward players) exhibit more continuous involvement in play and undertake more moderate- to high-intensity activity than backs do, perhaps because of their closer proximity to the ball during play (Deutsch, Kearney & Rehrer 2002; Docherty, Wenger & Neary 1988: Duthie, Pyne & Hooper 2005; Roberts et al. 2008; Treadwell 1988).

Studies have reported that forward players perform around 6 to 7 minutes more of high-intensity activity than back players largely as a result of spending more time in static exertion (scrums, mauls, line-outs and tackles) (Duthie, Pyne & Hooper 2005; Roberts et al. 2008). Consequently, forward players spend over 55 per cent of the match with their hearts beating at around 85 to 95 per cent of their maximal rates, whereas this is more like 34 to 40 per cent in back players (Deutsch et al. 1998). Critically, forward players use their anaerobic capacity at more frequent intervals than back players do, but are less able to recover because they (1) have shorter recovery periods between passages of play (e.g., 20 seconds vs. 100 seconds for backs; Duthie, Pyne & Hooper 2005); (2) work, on average, at a greater relative exercise intensity; and (3) have relatively lower levels of endurance fitness. This suggests that forwards would become fatigued during intense periods of a match and subsequently have to pace themselves for a portion of the match.

Rugby union players have been observed to cover 4 to 7 km (2.5 to 4.3 miles) during matches, which is considerably less than the 8 to 13 km (5 to 8 miles) performed by soccer players (Cunniffe et al. 2009; Duthie, Pyne & Hooper 2005; Roberts et al. 2008). A few studies that measured activity periods during rugby union matches found approximately 135 to 185 activity periods; however, 85 per cent of them lasted less than 15 seconds, and 70 per cent of them lasted only 4 to 10 seconds. Recovery between activities is generally around 40 seconds or less, and work-to-rest ratios are often between 1 to 1-1.9 or 1-1.9 to 1 suggesting that players work and then rest for similar quantities of time. However, in a study of International Five Nation players, many rest periods were more than four times longer than the work periods (McLean 1992; Menchinelli, Morandini & De Angelis 1992; Morton 1978; Treadwell 1988).

These findings suggest that although rugby players are frequently active during matches, the regular and relatively long periods of recovery limit the development of fatigue and so lessen the need for them to pace themselves. This argument is supported by the fact that only moderate levels of blood lactate (around 3 to 7 mmol/L with peaks under 10 mmol/L) have been measured in matches, suggesting low to moderate levels of anaerobic energy contribution (Duthie, Pyne & Hooper 2003). In addition, a recent study of elite English rugby union matches over two seasons reported no differences in the volume of high-intensity activity completed by individual players throughout each match following an analysis of 10-minute periods across each match (Roberts et al. 2008). Another study reported that both back and forward players recorded greater running distances during the second half of an elite-standard match, and although it was an out of season, the match was still highly competitive (Cunniffe et al. 2009). Taken together, these studies suggest that fatigue would rarely develop during matches to the extent that second half performance is compromised, as happens in soccer. Therefore, in summary, it would appear that pacing is not a significant aspect of rugby union match play, although forward players might need to pace their activity at times, when a number of consecutive high-intensity phases of play occur with little respite between them.

Rugby Sevens

A variation of rugby union called rugby sevens has been added to the Olympic sport programme for 2016. This variant of rugby union has just seven players from each side on a full-size pitch at one time and is played over two 7-minute halves. There are either 1-minute or 2-minute (in finals) half-time rest periods and an extra 5 minutes of play if the match is tied after normal time. Each team has five substitutes but can use only

COACH'S PERSPECTIVE: Pacing in Rugby Union

Jake White
2007 rugby union World Cup–winning coach

Jake White was head coach of the "Springboks" South Africa national side from 2004 to 2007, which won the 2007 rugby union World Cup and was ranked number one in the world that year. He also coached the 2004 Tri Nations title-winning Springbok team and the 2002 under-21 World Cup–winning Springbok team. While head coach of the University of Canberra Brumbies team from 2011 to 2013, White coached the side to runner-up position in the Super Rugby competition involving top club sides from Australia, New Zealand and South Africa.

In world-class rugby matches, the ball might be in play for only 30 minutes, giving plenty of time for players to recover most of the time. However, there can be sustained passages of play that are very fatiguing. We train for the worst. In training sessions, the players complete, say, 3×3-minute drills, where they might pick up a medicine ball and try to get past a defender 5 m out from the touch line. The defender pushes against them to make them work hard, but having crossed the line, the attacker then sprints 10 m and runs back and repeats the 5 m drive to the touch line, and so on. Drills are carefully constructed to ensure that what we do in training is harder than what the players come up against in a match. This means they do not have to pace their effort in the match; they know they can last and maintain high-intensity play when needed.

Players work at high intensity sometimes by strategy and sometimes by circumstance. Sometimes the coach tells the team to start at a frenetic pace for 3 to 4 minutes, which might not have an immediate impact, but it will later in the match if the opposition are not well conditioned. In the 2003 World Cup semifinal, Australia played New Zealand and did something unexpected. They kicked off, gained possession and played with the ball for 2 minutes. They did the same in the second half. This unexpectedly high pace of play was a deliberate attempt to unsettle New Zealand.

The coach will set a tempo in training for the match; for example, players will practise walking slowly up to the opposition's 22-yard line before rushing the opposition in a wave of play. You need to be able to play very 'direct' at times, meaning that you pass to the ball carrier, who runs into the tackle; the ball is then recycled, and the same play is then repeated. All of a sudden the players switch to 'normal' play, in which they pass, say, three times before the last ball carrier runs into a tackle situation. We practise when to play direct and when to play normal and when to switch again; this keeps the opposition guessing, destroying any chance of an even-paced, predictable tempo. Sometimes you deliberately play 'normal' style for a planned number of times so the opposition get lulled into thinking there is a predictable pattern developing, and they stop thinking. Then you suddenly switch to a direct style of play to catch them out.

I like the teams I coach to outwork the opposition, working them hard, pressuring them so they make defensive decisions under fatigue. We try to keep them guessing by changing the tempo (pace) of the match, to provide no rhythm for them to pace themselves with. Pace for me is not just about managing physical fatigue; it is also about asking the opposing team's players to make frequent decisions. This decision making can lead to mental fatigue and mistakes.

You can predict that some teams will play at a certain tempo. Pacific Island teams love to play at high tempo, running the ball like a sevens match, whereas South Africans tend to kick more ball and look to maul. Sometimes you deliberately slow down activity to disrupt the opposition, even before play begins. For example, the All Blacks (New Zealand team) get fired up before the match doing the Haka (the team's trademark traditional dance), so I asked the South African team to wear their tracksuit bottoms and take their time in taking them off after the Haka finished. This delay was designed to subdue the All Black players' mood somewhat and potentially frustrate them. At times you need to slow the match down to kill it off—for example, when you have a lead or when the team needs to regain its composure—so players can regroup and start to play their set pieces again. In this situation the captain and senior players might shout 'Banker' to each other, meaning play direct, pass, carry, go to ground, recycle the ball, pass, carry and so on. You need to choose the right players to do this, as some players just instinctively play the normal style of play, even when banker has been communicated, which is risky; or they carry the ball too far and become isolated and probably lose the ball.

The environment can play a role in the pace of the team. If you play the Bulls in the Super Rugby tournament at altitude, then you might start slower than normal and walk to line-outs. Or if you are playing in a tournament, then you will have to rotate players as they fatigue or pick up injuries when playing a high frequency of matches in a shorter-than-normal time frame. Personally, I would not want a player to ever coast through a match. Sometimes you hear that players might have saved themselves during a league match when they have an international match to play soon after, but that is rare and not something I have seen in any of my players.

three of them during a match. The physical requirements of rugby sevens differ significantly from those of the 15-a-side game, which has some concerned that it is becoming a separate sport rather than a developmental step for players who could use a couple of years of rugby sevens to develop their running and passing skills for the 15-player game.

Pacing is much more likely to play a significant role in rugby sevens than in the common game. In a study of 19 international-standard male rugby sevens players it was found that they covered 5 per cent less distance during the second half of sevens games. In addition, compared to their performances in the first half, the players also demonstrated a 14 and 16 per cent decline, respectively, in their ability to produce moderate and high accelerations over each minute of the second half (Higham et al. 2012). These findings suggest that, unlike the players in the 15-a-side game, rugby sevens players experience progressively worsening fatigue over the match. Therefore, it is highly likely that rugby sevens players pace their efforts over the course of a match. Pacing is therefore an area in which further studies would inform coaching theory and practice.

Energy Requirements and Activity Levels of Rugby League Players

Rugby league matches are of the same duration as rugby union matches, but because of the differences in rules and regulations, they are played very differently. Rugby league players cover greater distances in matches (8.5 to 10 km, or 5.2 to 6.2 miles), and forward players cover greater distances than backs do (Meir, Colla & Milligan 2001). This difference between codes is no doubt related to the fact that the ball stays in play for longer in rugby league matches: 50 minutes versus 30 minutes or so in rugby union (Brewer & Davis 1995; Duthie, Pyne & Hooper 2003).

Rugby league players also appear to be less varied in height and weight than rugby union players are. A study of players competing for selection in the Australian National Rugby League competition found selected players to measure approximately 170 to 190 cm (5 ft 7 in. to 6 ft 2 in.) in height and 88 to 104 kg (194 to 229 lb) in weight. Rugby league players demonstrate good levels of aerobic fitness (a predicted $\dot{V}O_2$max of around

55 ml/kg/min) and during matches exercise at around 75 to 80 per cent of their $\dot{V}O_2$max on average. They also possess well-developed sprinting abilities (Coutts, Reaburn & Abt 2003; Gabbett, Jenkins & Abernethy 2011; Gabbett, Kelly & Pezet 2007).).

Well-trained rugby league players spend more time playing at a moderate or high intensity than at a low intensity during matches. However, only moderately high blood lactate levels of 5 to 8 mmol/L have been measured during breaks in match play, which would suggest that the anaerobic energy contribution during matches is not high (Coutts, Reaburn & Abt 2003). A likely reason for this is that work-to-rest ratios of between 1:7 and 1:28 in terms of high-intensity work periods versus low-intensity rest periods have been observed in rugby league matches (Meir, Colla & Milligan 2001).

Some of the factors that influence the intensity and duration of play in rugby union apply to rugby league as well. These factors—such as patterns of play and stoppages by officials—undoubtedly contribute to the low work-to-rest ratio.

Therefore, although intense activity does occur frequently during rugby league matches, these efforts are short in duration and are followed by a significant period during which the players can recover. In fact, it is likely that the overall anaerobic energy contribution is small in terms of the total energy expenditure required during rugby league matches, because the total amount of time players are involved in high-intensity activity might be only 9 to 13 per cent of the match (Meir, Arthur & Forrest 1993).

Relevance of Pacing in Rugby League

The scientific evidence to date suggests that pacing may not be a significant factor during rugby league matches. For example, a study of 37 elite rugby league players showed that most sprint efforts (67 per cent) covered only 20 m and were generally (67.5% of the time) followed by a long recovery of over 5 minutes (Gabbett 2012). Finally, although no studies have specifically investigated pacing in rugby league, one study did report that the heart rate values and the estimated energy expenditure of rugby league players, during a competitive match, did not change between the first and second halves. This suggests that fatigue did not progressively develop over the match (Coutts, Reaburn & Abt 2003).

In summary, there appears to be little evidence to suggest that rugby league players pace their activity during matches. The nature of the game allows them sufficient time to recover between efforts so they can maintain their physical playing capability over the course of a match. However, because relatively few studies have been carried out to date related to pacing in rugby league, a definitive conclusion as to whether players pace themselves is not possible. It is highly likely that experienced players intuitively manage their energy by taking advantage of the ample rest periods that occur naturally within the course of the match, which in essence is a form of pacing.

chapter 13

Squash and Tennis

Squash and tennis are high-speed racket sports involving two players competing against each other in singles matches or four players competing in pairs in doubles matches. Both sports are pan-global. Around 150 national squash associations are members of the World Squash Federation (Wallbutton n.d.). Tennis has over 200 member national associations worldwide.

History of Squash and Tennis

Many historians believe that squash and tennis originated from real tennis, a game that evolved from various ball games played in the streets of France in the 12th century. During this period, the French played *la paume* ('the palm of the hand'), which developed later into *jeu de paume*, or real tennis (Wallbutton n.d.). Originally, balls were slapped around roofs, awnings and doorways. Then fishing nets were strung up in courtyards, and players used gloved hands to hit the ball over them. Monasteries are thought to have adopted the game, and monks may have added webbing to the glove and then extended the glove by adding a stick to resemble a racket. In the 15th century, the Dutch invented the first racket. Over the years, a dozen or so European countries adopted tennis as a national sport, which was played in enclosed areas (Zug n.d.). By the end of the 16th century, real tennis had become well established in Europe; 'tennis balles' were even mentioned in Shakespeare's 1599 play *Henry V*. However, the popularity of tennis then eroded for a variety of reasons. It had gained a reputation for involving gambling and violence; the Italian painter Caravaggio infamously killed a man at a court in Rome in 1606. Tennis was also to suffer under English puritanism and the Napoleonic wars, although it remained popular in royal circles.

Lawn tennis as we know it today evolved from a game invented in 1873 in Great Britain as an outdoor version of real tennis (Zug n.d). The popularity of the game grew, and in March 1913 the International Lawn Tennis Federation (ILTF) was founded in Paris with 15 member countries (International Tennis Federation n.d.). In 1977 the ILTF became simply the International Tennis Federation (ITF). Tennis was reintroduced as an Olympic sport at the 1988 Olympic Games, having returned to the competition programme after a 64-year absence.

In today's form of the game, men's and women's tennis matches are generally played over three sets. However, in men's tennis five-set matches are frequently played, including the four Grand Slam tournaments. Matches can vary hugely in length from short-lived three-set matches taking perhaps 30 minutes to 5 hours or more over five-set matches. A few five-set matches have even lasted beyond 6 hours; the longest match recorded was 11 hours and 5 minutes when John Isner defeated Nicolas Mahut over a three-day match at Wimbledon in 2010!

In the early part of the 19th century, a derivative of squash, called rackets, reputedly emerged as a variant of real tennis. The origin of the game of rackets has been attributed to a game arising from the Fleet Prison in London where prisoners hit a hard ball against walls with a makeshift stretched tennis bat. Working-class men played the game in tavern yards and alleys. Roofless racket courts began to be built, and in 1830 the first roofed court was built at the Royal Artillery barracks in Woolwich. Additional indoor courts followed at the Marylebone Cricket Club (1844) and Prince's Club (1853). The game also gained a foothold in the British colonies around this time; indoor courts were established in Canada, India, America and Australia.

Squash, as we know it today, originated at Harrow School in England, around 1830 (Wallbutton n.d.). It began as a modified form of rackets, designed to be easier to play with a soft rubber ball and shorter racket; it was initially known as 'baby racquets' (Zugg n.d.). Doubles in squash began in Philadelphia, USA, in 1907. By the 1920s a number of nations had developed national squash associations, and national championships had also been established. International competition began to be formalized, particularly after World War II.

Squash is now played in over 185 countries. The modern form of the game takes place in an enclosed four-walled court, generally indoors. In major competitions, however, the court can be set up in unique surroundings—sometimes even outdoors to make the sport more appealing to sponsors and fans. Matches consist of games played to 11 points, and players must win three games to win a match. At the international level, short matches may take only 40 minutes, but long matches can take as long as 105 minutes.

This chapter briefly describes some of the physical characteristics and requirements of squash and tennis and looks at why and how players might pace themselves during match play. To date, no research studies have specifically investigated pacing strategies in these sports, although there has been interest in analysing shifts in momentum in squash, which does relate to pacing in many respects. An example of this type of analysis is provided later in the chapter.

Key Factors in Determining a Pacing Strategy for Squash and Tennis

Many factors potentially affect how players approach matches in squash or tennis. This section addresses court surfaces, match duration, nutrition and hydration, injury management and training and competition periodisation.

Court surfaces affect the playing style and tactics players adopt and, hence, potentially, the pacing of matches. Court surfaces are particularly variable in tennis, where players compete on clay, grass and hard courts. Clay courts in tennis are notoriously difficult to hit winning shots on, because the ball bounces higher from topspin shots and travels more slowly off the court than it does on hard or grass surfaces. As a consequence, players tend to stand farther back on clay courts than they do on other court surfaces. This gives them more time to hit the shot, which is often under shoulder height, and to generate maximal power for a groundstroke. In contrast, grass courts play faster and lower, so players are more able to hit winning shots; consequently, rallies are shorter. Tennis and squash players' approaches to matches on different court surfaces differ depending on whether they expect rallies to be longer or shorter and how aggressively they intend to play during the match. When they anticipate longer matches with frequent extended rallies, they may well adopt pacing strategies to lessen the development of fatigue and a related decrease in skill level.

When players are closely matched in skill level, squash and tennis matches can last a long time irrespective of the type of court surface. Elite players prepare for the worst-case scenario (a long, arduous match), but hope for a short, straightforward victory.

A critical aspect for players to consider is their energy requirement during matches and the nutritional strategy needed for maximising their chances of meeting that requirement. For example, energy expenditures of 7.4 ± 1.3 and 10.8 ± 1.8 calories per minute have been reported in women's and men's tennis matches, respectively, regardless of the playing surface (Ranchordas et al. 2013). To maintain their ability to produce energy from carbohydrate oxidation, elite players take carbohydrate drinks and snacks onto the court to ingest periodically during matches. This nutritional strategy counters the potential for muscle and liver glycogen (carbohydrate) and blood glucose levels to fall too low during match play. It is recommended that tennis players consume 30 to 60 grams (1 to 2 oz) of carbohydrate per hour of play, which is the same recommendation prescribed for carbohydrate intake during a 2- to 3-hour triathlon! High daily carbohydrate intakes of 6 to 10 grams per kilogram of body mass per day are also recommended for tennis players, which suggests that they experience considerable energy expenditure during training and competition. The Australian Institute of Sport (n.d.) recommends that squash players have a high carbohydrate intake to support skill maintenance during match play. These recommendations imply that players are at risk of developing fatigue during match play and provide some evidence that they might indeed have to pace their efforts during matches to manage their energy reserves.

The need to manage energy reserves is not surprising given that, during training phases, elite squash and tennis players might exercise 4 to 6 hours per day. Moreover, while competing in tournaments, they spend considerable time in matches and pre-match practices. Based on our current understanding of how low carbohydrate levels in the body affect pacing in humans, we can propose that if the carbohydrate levels of elite squash and tennis players were insufficient to meet the required energy demands during a match, the brain's central motor drive, motor coordination and executive function (decision making) would be affected, as would the force-producing capability of their muscles. The requirement for a high carbohydrate intake in both squash and tennis, to meet the energy demands of training and longer matches, therefore seems to suggest that pacing is a consideration for players in these sports.

Dehydration is another threat to performance during match play in squash and tennis. During tournament matches, sweat losses of 1.3 to 2.4 litres per hour have been observed in male squash players (Brown, Weigland & Winter 1998). This study also revealed that, during matches, most players were not able to replace the fluid they lost. This was probably influenced by the rules of squash, which restrict players' drinking opportunities to the short breaks between games. Consequently, the players in this study lost between 1.3 and 2.2 per cent of their body weight during the match. This is a concern because losing more than 2 per cent of one's body weight during matches affects performance (Australian Institute of Sport n.d.). Tennis players are also at risk of dehydration during matches. It has been reported that tennis players can sweat between 2.5 and 3 litres of fluid per hour during match play in hot and humid conditions (Bergeron 2003; Bergeron, Armstrong & Maresh 1995; Bergeron et al. 1995). It is plausible that the high sweat rates evident in both of these sports could induce sufficient cardiac strain that a player would consider changing the pace of match play—perhaps by adopting a less aggressive match strategy.

A related issue is muscle cramping, which is not uncommon during long squash and tennis matches played in hot conditions. Muscle cramps are thought to arise from increased mineral losses, such as sodium depletion, as a result of high sweat rates (Bergeron, Armstrong & Maresh 1995; Bergeron et al. 1995). A player suffering muscle cramps will want to shorten the length of rallies and match time—a pacing strategy born of necessity. Ranchordas and colleagues (2013) recommend that tennis players drink 200 ml (6.8 oz) of fluid every changeover when playing in temperatures less than 27 °C (80.6 °F), but to increase to 400 ml (13.5 oz) of fluid at temperatures beyond that to reduce the risk of dehydration and muscle cramps.

Because players are most at risk of dehydration, muscle cramping, glycogen depletion and a heat-related decline in performance at latter stages of squash and tennis tournaments, appropriate nutritional practices are most important at this point (Kovacs 2006b). Emerging evidence from scientific studies suggests that tennis match-play evokes pronounced physiological, neuromuscular and psychological perturbation, which might well become exaggerated after consecutive days of match-play (Reid & Duffield 2014). Another factor that affects playing ability towards the end of tournaments is an increased incidence and progression of soft tissue injuries. Unfortunately, as players progress through tournaments, they might suffer from increasing soft tissue (muscle, tendon, ligament and skin) damage and related acute pain, inflammation and soreness. Markers of muscle damage and stress hormones have been shown to increase after 2 to 3 days of match play demonstrating that a significant internal physiological strain had been experienced (Ojala & Hakkinen 2013). Notably, in the men's 2013 and 2014 Australian Open finals both saw injuries to players (Andy Murray with painful blisters and Rafael Nadal with a back injury). Players may well need to apply a pacing strategy to their match tactics at the end of a tournament to mitigate against increasing physical discomfort and the potential for a more severe injury.

A final point to consider is that professional squash and tennis tournament calendars are almost yearlong. As a result, players need to plan to peak for certain competitions and organise their calendars and preparations accordingly. This periodisation of the training and competition schedule over a year is in effect a form of pacing that regulates the demands on the physical and mental capacities of players.

Pacing in Squash

Squash consists of short, high-intensity bouts of exercise that are typically 5 to 20 seconds long interspersed with rest periods of less than 10 seconds. The dominant shot is the drive, particularly down the side wall, with the addition of volleys and drop shots to exploit advantages. The precise placement of the shot, often hard and low and close to the side wall, is a key requirement of match play. Accurate shot making allows the player to dominate the T (the area of the court where the lines that separate the front and back of the court intersect with the half-court line—considered the prime position for getting to and returning the opponent's next shot). A recent study of the World Team Championships, Slovenian National Championships and a local tournament found that match winners invariably spent a greater proportion of their total playing time in the T area, except when the match was closely contested, in which case players spent similar amounts of time at the T. The researchers concluded that time in the T indicated dominance of rallies (Vuckovic et al. 2009). Studies by a number of researchers (Hughes & Franks 1994; Murray & Hughes 2001; Vuckovic et al. 2009) suggested that successful players prevail in matches through a combination of the following:

- Placing shots accurately
- Setting up a winning shot with a previous shot
- Playing forward of the opposing player
- Moving faster sideways and generally with higher accelerations
- Playing with effective movement

All of these tactics deny the opponent time and space.

ATHLETE'S PERSPECTIVE: Applying Pacing in Squash

Nick Matthew
Number-one world ranking, 2011

PSA World Open squash champion 2013, 2011 and 2010

Commonwealth Games gold medallist, singles, 2010; Commonwealth Games gold medalist, doubles, 2010

Australian Open champion, 2010; British Open champion 2009 and 2006; US Open champion, 2007

A fast-start/slow-finish pacing strategy might be possible if you win 3–0; otherwise, you would lose the match! A slow-start/fast-finish pace is not a workable strategy in squash because if you lose the early games, you will be on the back foot (at a disadvantage). To adopt an even pace or level of effort in a squash match, you would need to warm up well to start at a high tempo and then maintain your style, be consistent, but also adapt to the opponent or court conditions. Humidity reduces the intensity you can maintain. A version of a variable pacing strategy is most commonly used in squash. You need to be in control, taking conditions into account and adapting to them, but not simply reacting—you need to dictate the situation.

You play to your strengths. If you like a slower pace, you need accuracy of shot and to be able to float the ball. A fast pace allows you to take the ball early. I favour a fast-paced, high-tempo style, but opponents adapt to what you do, so over the years I have developed speeds within speeds, and I use the different gears to keep opponents guessing and reacting. It's good to vary speeds. You need the right gear for the right opponent, especially in the early rounds where you want a short, 40-minute win. Varying the tempo works well—play fast to take the ball early; then slow things down with a deception shot. My game is about pace. I like to take the ball early, I like to use volleys, but subtleties within pace are important and I am still trying to evolve ways to do this, to this day.

At this level, I am more aware of when pacing is not working—I can recognise it and adjust. When I was younger, I could be a game and a half down before recognising it. Momentum shifts in matches, and I know when to put my foot down. Like, at the start of a game following one you have just won—this is when you need to match your opponents, because if they have anything about them they will up the pace, so you have to as well. You look for that second goal, to put it in football terms. You need to be proactive; otherwise, you are reacting and you are not in control. You can have a few bad rallies, but what matters is how quickly you recognise what's happening and adapt.

In training, I practise with my strengths, work on my pace, how I want to play. You have to know your playing style. Be respectful of your opponent, but play to your own strengths. When preparing the week before a tournament, out on the competition court, you might notice that it has a high roof, so you think about using high lobs. Or you target points on the walls where your shots will come off, as each court plays differently. You take the tournament a day at a time. If you are playing a late match, then you do not think about your next match until the next day, so you can relax and sleep that night. Then at practice the next morning you prepare for your opponent and go over your 3-point plan, thinking about your strengths, what you will implement in the match, and what your opponent is good at. Then you can switch off for a few hours. With 2 hours to

> continued

> continued

go, I switch on—I begin to pack my match bag and go over the 3-point plan. I have mental space in the match both to execute the plan and to adapt it during the match. If I recognise it is not working, I do something that will work. I no longer feel scared to make those decisions. I feel calm in matches even when the pressure is on.

The danger of pacing yourself for a 2-hour match is that you can lose it in half that time. You need to play to what is in front of you. When I was younger, I learned how to play fast. There were many pressure sessions, times when I'd get into oxygen debt, times when it seemed like the longer I could stay on court, the better. If I was under pressure in a match, I played faster! But as I have gotten older, I have realised that you have to maintain the shot making. You can play fast, but if the quality of the shot is not good, then you tire and lose, unless the opponent has poor fitness. Now, I pace. Now, I am calmer and can assess situations better.

Energy Requirements and Activity Levels of Squash Players

A study investigating English players from international to part-time talented players revealed that the higher-standard players demonstrated a shorter total time to complete 10 sprint efforts interspersed with 20 seconds of recovery than lower-standard players. The study found that higher standard players possessed a greater repeated-sprint ability, a faster sprint time and greater change-of-direction speed, which illustrates that the modern game requires a greater level of anaerobic fitness than was previously required (Wilkinson et al. 2012). The players' maximal aerobic capacity ($\dot{V}O_2$max) did not differ among the playing levels; all players possessed high levels of aerobic fitness. This seems to indicate that high aerobic and anaerobic thresholds are a requirement in squash (Brown, Weigland & Winter 1998). Male elite squash players have been measured with $\dot{V}O_2$max values of around 56 to 64 ml/kg/min, whereas female players have been measured at 49 to 53 ml/kg/min (Gillam et al. 1990; Girard et al. 2005; Wilkinson et al. 2012). These values are quite high, although not in comparison to those of athletes in endurance sports.

Research describing the physical and physiological characteristics of squash players is constrained by the fact that they have generally been measured in a laboratory setting rather than during match play. However, in a recent study, players wore portable gas (oxygen) analysers and portable heart rate monitors while playing competitive squash games. In this study, 11 national to elite standard players undertook three simulated matches. Their oxygen uptakes reached around 86 per cent of maximum, and their heart rates reached 92 per cent of maximum (Girard, Chevalier et al. 2007). Many players exhibited high rates of oxygen consumption during 25 per cent or more of the match, demonstrating a high aerobic energy requirement during a significant proportion of matches. This occurred despite the relatively short rallies, because the recovery periods between points were short and so did not allow much time for recovery. Indeed, the actual playing time in this study averaged around 70 per cent of the total match time. The average rally was 18.6 seconds long, although 35 per cent of all rallies lasted less than 10 seconds and 33 per cent lasted over 21 seconds. The researchers concluded that the sport requires high-intensity aerobic activity. However, they also found that the anaerobic energy system is used extensively because moderate blood lactate concentrations (around 8 mmol/L) were observed after each game, demonstrating that players frequently exercised beyond their critical power.

COACH'S PERSPECTIVE: Applying Pacing in Squash

Chris Robertson
Performance director, England Squash

English National coach: January 2011–present

Welsh National coach: 1994–2011

Former champion Australian, South African, Dutch, and European Open

Former World junior champion

A fast-start/slow-finish pacing strategy might work if you could build up a lead, then ease off once you have the lead. Adopting an even pace or effort throughout would suit players with big engines (high levels of aerobic fitness) who can work at a high tempo throughout. That kind of player, even if losing, can keep the opponent working until he tires. A varied pacing strategy is the most relevant pacing strategy for squash.

It is rare to beat someone at the top level in 40 minutes, and sometimes it can take as long as 1 hour and 45 minutes. You need consistency—it's about a telling effect over the match, speed of shot (fast and accurate shots which keep the opponent working hard to get to the shots in time) takes its toll on the opponent. You can tell, set by set, if it is having an effect. Speed has a number of dimensions—you have to move in fast to play the ball early, to hit harder and change direction quickly.

The physical dimension is much harder than it was 10 years ago; the players are better athletes. It is no longer an aerobic game with long, slow rallies and players grinding out wins as the norm. It is all about high pace now, but the best athletes can play like this with accuracy. They can maintain a high pace and deal with the cumulative effect of fatigue over the course of the tournament. A high pace gives your opponent less time to make a decision, and this is more and more effective as the opponent tires. You are taking time off the opponent, his feet get tired and he loses racket head control.

As a player you begin at a certain pace, but it is not until you get into the match for a while that you will know if that pace is right. You can't tell until you get so far. You take the opponent on, but if the opponent answers, then you have to adapt. If you do not recognise that, then you continue and start to fatigue without getting the points you need. You need to ask yourself, did I do something well enough at pace, or was the opponent fitter than anticipated?

Squash is about always working against your opponent, and the quality of shot. If a player can play well at a high pace and play technically well, even at a slow pace, and then inject pace at the right time, he will be formidable. You need the quality of shot as otherwise you will simply tire and lose the point, which is a poor strategy unless your opponent tires more easily and makes more mistakes than you do.

When in control at a high tempo, high pace, you have the best pacing strategy to get your opponent off the court quickly. When you get under pressure, you may need to slow the pace, be defensive, but then inject pace again when the opportunity arises. You need a good engine (high aerobic fitness) to do this. If you have high pace and full control, you can maintain this for 40 minutes, but if it is a longer game—say, 60 minutes—then you cannot maintain the high pace, so there will be ebbs and flows in tempo.

A pacing strategy prior to a game, from a coach's perspective, involves analysing the matchups, looking at the strengths and weaknesses of the player you coach

> continued

> continued

and those of the opponent. If they are even, physically, then you need to take opportunities in the match as they come.

Court temperature and the amount of work each player has done in previous rounds are important factors to consider if the match is going to be close. Five rounds are played in a tournament, so there is cumulative fatigue, and many modern players find it very hard to recover because of the high tempo of matches. Split rounds mean there is often a rest day between rounds. This helps players recover, but this schedule is not beneficial for those who recover and deal with fatigue well from round to round.

Another strategy is not to play at a high pace if it is not needed. It's better to play at a lower pace against a weaker opponent—you may stay on court 15 minutes longer, but it will not hurt you; it's easy.

You need to know you are in shape when you come to the event; nowadays, you need to be in your best shape to win. After a match you regenerate; then begin to look at the opponent for the next round. You look at the opponent's draw and previous results to judge what shape he is in. After morning practice and lunch, you prepare for the afternoon or evening match. Begin the pre-match strategy; decide the tempo. It varies among players as to when the final pre-match strategy is set, but it is at least 2 hours before.

Courts can vary as far as being air-conditioned or not, the amount of heat and humidity, the court surface and the type of walls. If the ball travels faster because of the conditions, then it comes back to the middle more, and games take longer.

You can only hydrate when you finish a game. You might play for 30 minutes and then have 2 minutes to take on fluid. What you do before the match is therefore critical, especially when preparing for a hard and very tiring, dynamic match.

There is a higher tempo in the modern game. Rackets now generate pace without much backswing, so you can take less time to play a shot and play it faster. Physically, squash has moved from an aerobically dominant sport to a higher-paced, change-of-direction sport. The points system has also changed from 15 to 11 points per game to make the sport more dynamic and attractive to watch.

Relevance of Pacing in Squash

The short recovery periods in squash result in depleted creatine phosphate stores. As a result, anaerobic glycolysis is required during very intense rallies to provide energy at sufficient rates for muscle contractions, causing moderate to high levels of lactic acid production. During matches, the frequent requirement for a high rate of energy production can deplete the anaerobic capacity and lead to fatigue. These factors suggest that squash players have to pace their efforts at times during match play as part of their ongoing game strategy. In addition, squash players can suffer significant heat stress when they play in hot and humid conditions, particularly during outdoor events (where no air conditioning is available). For example, fluid losses of 2.4 litres per hour have been observed in British national-level players (Brown, Weigland & Winter 1998). All of these factors suggest that players must pace themselves during games to avoid premature exhaustion. However, because of the complexity of match play, pacing strategies may not be obvious.

Figure 13.1 provides a momentum analysis of an elite senior men's match (i.e., an analysis of where players begin to decisively gain the upper hand over a series

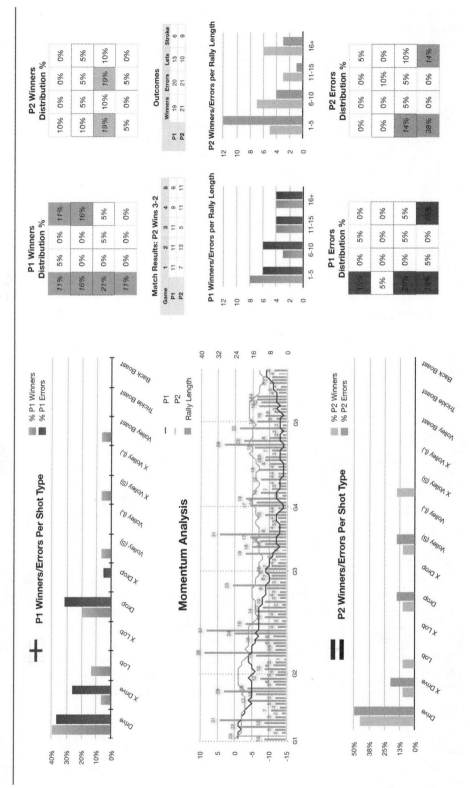

Figure 13.1 English squash match report.

P1 = player 1, P2 = player 2; the boxes in the 4 × 4 quadrants (Winners Distribution % and Errors % Distribution) represent areas of the squash court.

Courtesy of Mandie Tromp, Performance Analyst, English Institute of Sport.

of points). The following interpretation of this match is by Mandie Tromp (performance analyst to England Squash at the English Institute of Sport):

> Momentum is calculated by keeping a 'running score' of each rally-ending shot. In figure 13.1 each player has his own graphed line based on his own shots, and each player starts at 0. Players get +1 point for a winner and –1 point for an error. A let is 0 points, and a stroke, considered an error, is also –1 point. In this match, the most obvious indicator that it was a long and arduous one is that it lasted five games. Looking at the momentum analysis graph, you can see that it's a very flat profile during the bulk of the match, with neither player pulling away from the other in games 1 through 3. Games 2 and 5 are short games, with player 2 clearly dominating as shown by the score in these games. However, from the start of game 4, player 2 pulls away from his opponent, after a long game 3 in which there were a number of long rallies, five of which had between 20 and 40 shots. This takes its toll on player 1, and even though player 1 wins that game, in game 5 the gap widens and player 2 finishes the match swiftly (11–4). This is demonstrated by the rapidly rising momentum score at the end of the match.

Pacing in squash is complex because matches are unpredictable. The outcomes from a number of rallies influence whether a player persists in a particular match strategy. The expert opinions of world champion squash players Nick Matthew (number-one world player) and Chris Robertson (performance director, England Squash) presented in the perspectives in this chapter offer fascinating insights into the relevance of pacing in squash.

Pacing in Tennis

Pacing in tennis, as in squash, has not been specifically researched. Additionally, the physiological aspects of tennis play vary dramatically because the game is unpredictable because of the individual nature of point length, shot selection, strategy, match duration, weather and opponents (Kovacs 2006a). It could be argued that pacing in tennis is only required during long, arduous matches, particularly when environmental conditions—namely, heat and humidity—become a major consideration. In very physically challenging matches, players may even concede a set they are losing to save themselves physically (and mentally) for the next set. Players might also try to extend the length of rallies to tire an opponent. This section looks at some of the physical and physiological characteristics of tennis to demonstrate that pacing is undertaken during matches at certain times.

Male tennis players are typically 1.81 ± 0.09 m (5 ft 11 in. ± 3.5 in.) tall and weigh 77 ± 7 kg (170 ± 15 lb), whereas female players are typically 1.67 ± 0.05 m (5 ft 6 in. ± 2 in.) tall and weigh 59 ± 6 kg (130 ± 13 lb) (Ranchordas et al. 2013). Tennis is an intermittent sport with brief periods of play interspersed with recovery periods between points and games. This can mean that players are actively playing for only 15 per cent of a match (Ranchordas et al. 2013). A tennis player's energy expenditure during matches is difficult to predict because it is affected by court surface, style of play (serve and volley or baseline), phase of play (service or return game), environment (ambient temperature and humidity) and tournament standard. For the men, Grand Slam tournaments require five-set matches rather than three-set matches.

One reason pacing is not obvious in tennis is that the sport is punctuated by frequent and significant recovery periods. For example, 20 seconds of recovery are allowed between points, 90 seconds are allowed during changeovers every two games (or after only one game at the beginning of each set) and 120 seconds are allowed between sets. These regular recovery periods give players time to physically recover during matches in most instances.

If a rally is relatively short, a 20-second recovery period between points is sufficient for another near-maximal effort during the next point. The serving player can attempt to raise the pace of a game by electing not to take the full 20-second rest between points; however, the returning player can choose not to be ready to play and so undermine the effectiveness of this tactic. Players also rise from their chairs at changeovers before they are required to, to put pressure on their opponent to do so as well and thus deprive them of recovery time. Line calls can also be challenged by players a number of times per set, which can also slow play down. In addition, players can take injury and comfort breaks. The ethical issues of injury and comfort breaks have been debated during some high-profile matches in which players have been perceived to be using them to gain additional recovery time.

The regularity and duration of breaks in tennis enables players to use high-intensity, explosive movements during each point because, although they are using up their anaerobic stores, they can recover between points. Indeed, in most elite-level matches players spend two to five times as much time resting as playing; individual points last between 3 and 15 seconds, or approximately 8 seconds on average (Kovacs 2006a). On clay courts, attacking players might spend only 15 to 26 per cent of the match playing tennis, and baseline players might spend 33 to 43 per cent of the match playing. This suggests that there is a greater need to consider pacing in baseline-oriented matches, in which rally lengths and recovery periods are proportionately longer and shorter, respectively (Bernadi et al. 1998).

As mentioned earlier, the playing surface also makes a difference in the way tennis is played and indeed which players are successful, although the very best players in the world seem increasingly capable of adapting their games to play the highest standard of tennis on any surface. Clay court matches tend to produce longer rallies and larger percentages of playing times (25 per cent) compared to hard court matches (21 per cent; Christmass et al. 1998; Fernandez-Fernandez, Sanz-Rivas & Mendez-Villanueva 2009; Fernandez-Fernandez et al. 2007, 2008; Girard et al. 2006; Martin et al. 2011; Mendez-Villanueva et al. 2007; Smekal et al. 2001). In contrast, grass court tennis is known for shorter rallies because of the faster and low-bounce characteristics of the grass surface. Grass court tennis has also been perceived to produce a higher-paced game in which serve and volley tennis is a highly successful tactic. However, changes in tennis ball and grass technology have resulted in baseline rallies becoming increasingly common even on grass courts, because the bounce is higher and more consistent and the courts play slower.

Energy Requirements and Activity Levels of Tennis Players

During the 2012 Australian Open, Novak Djokovic and Rafael Nadal played over 120 hours of tennis across 13 days involving six singles matches and then played each other in the final, which lasted 5 hours and 53 minutes. In the final they competed in 369 points and according to the Hawkeye tournament data, covered in-point distances of 6.6 km (Djokovic) and 6.2 km (Nadal) and reached speeds exceeding 20 km/h. The players also hit over 1,000 groundstrokes at average velocities over 95 km/h with more than 40 per cent of points involving more than eight shots (Reid & Duffield 2014). These data demonstrate the extreme stresses and strains that elite tennis players experience. To date, this level of match intensity has proven difficult to replicate in scientific studies; however, the availability of technologies like the Hawkeye system and Global Positioning Satellite systems, which can provide data during tournament match play, is beginning to greatly enhance our understanding of the physical requirements of tennis. For example, in an unpublished study which used GPS to measure the movement patterns of players undertaking matches on consecutive days, the investigators found a reduction of approximately 15 per cent in the overall movement patterns from the first to fourth day of the study, which they surmised to be representative of either cumulative fatigue or a change in the player's game style or a combination of the two (Reid & Duffield 2014).

Typical heart rate responses for tennis players during singles play have been reported to be 60 to 80 per cent of their maximal heart rate with oxygen consumption approximating 60 to 70 per cent of their $\dot{V}O_2$max (Reid & Duffield 2014). Fourteen professional tennis players in one clay court tournament and two hard court tournaments exhibited average heart rates around 75 to 78 per cent of maximum (Hornery et al. 2007a). Tennis players possess good levels of aerobic fitness, and this is reflected in their maximal aerobic capacity ($\dot{V}O_2$max) values, which have been reported to range from 44 to 69 ml/kg/min, with average values of over 55 ml/kg/min. However, tennis has been described as a predominantly anaerobic sport in general (Green et al. 2003; Kovacs 2006a).

Tennis players must have good levels of aerobic fitness, both to provide some of the energy needed during points and to allow for recovery between points. The aerobic energy system restores creatine phosphate during the rest periods between points and games, which ensures that sufficient creatine phosphate is available for the anaerobic energy production needed for intense and explosive tennis points. Thus, anaerobic glycolysis is not extensively required to produce energy during match play, because creatine phosphate levels are continually replenished between points. Therefore, because the requirement for anaerobic glycolysis is limited during match play, only low to moderate levels of blood lactate (1.5 to 6 mmol/L) are observed in tennis matches (Bergeron et al. 1991; Christmass et al. 1998; Ferrauti et al. 2001; Reilly & Palmer 1994). Also, the blood lactate that is produced does not accumulate in the blood because it is removed almost continually during the numerous resting periods by the aerobic energy system, which uses it as fuel for further energy production.

Relevance of Pacing in Tennis

Evidence suggests that as tennis players tire during long matches, their playing techniques and movement mechanics are affected (Myers et al. 1999), reducing ball velocity and shot accuracy and adversely affecting their 'feel', or proprioceptive ability (Davey, Thorpe & Williams 2002, 2003; Myers et al. 1999). Various studies have also shown reductions in running speed, jumping ability and maximal voluntary strength in the leg muscles (quadriceps), during and following one hour (involving 10 minutes of effective tennis play) to two hours of match-play (Ferrauti, Pluim & Weber 2001; Girard et al. 2006; Girard et al. 2008; Girard et al. 2014; Ojala & Hakkinen 2013). These findings highlight that a loss in neuromuscular function of the lower body can occur during match-play. It has also been shown that a loss of leg strength (from a maximal voluntary muscle contraction test) can worsen over consecutive days of match-play and following matches in hot conditions (Ojala & Hakkinen 2013; Periard, Girard & Racinais 2014). All of this can lead to more conservative playing tactics and an increase in the prevalence of injury (Kovacs 2006a). Interestingly, the serve has been identified as the stroke most affected by fatigue, and the consistency of the ball toss might be partly to blame. One study observed that toss consistency decreased as the match time and players' levels of dehydration increased during competitive match play (Davey, Thorpe & Williams 2002; Hornery et al. 2007a). To mitigate against a deterioration in skill level due to fatigue, a player might well choose to take more recovery between points and changeovers. In support of this point, a recent review of the development of fatigue in tennis concluded that players adjust their game strategy (pacing), and resultant shot-making, to accommodate for any deterioration in physiological function (Reid & Duffield 2014).

Rally duration has been reported to be related to rectal temperature (a measure of core body temperature), thermal perception and skin temperature in tennis players (Morante & Brotherhood 2008). These findings indicate that players perceive a significant thermal load and related discomfort during matches when playing many long rallies in hot conditions. To alleviate these deleterious effects, at least to some degree, professional tennis players try to maximise their recovery time between points and, if playing in the sun, seek shade whenever possible. A study which compared player's responses to playing a match in a cool condition (approximately 19°C wet-bulb-globe temperature or WBGT) versus playing a match in a hot condition (approximately 34°C WBGT) found that player's rectal and thigh skin temperatures, heart rate, and feelings of thermal comfort, thermal sensation and perceived exertion were all elevated when playing in the hot condition. This coincided with the players taking approximately 10 seconds longer recovery between points in the hot match, which meant a 3-4% reduction in effective playing time during the match and a longer overall match time (Periard et al. 2014). The investigators concluded that the players adopted a behavioural change to minimize or offset the difficult environmental conditions. These adjustments in the match-play characteristics suggest that the players changed the pace of their match-play when experiencing severe heat stress. Tennis players may also attempt to change the pace of the match in other ways such as serving and volleying or attempting groundstroke winners more frequently to reduce the length of rallies. Players also drink carbohydrate–electrolyte drinks during changeovers so they can regulate against thermal strain and cramping as effectively as possible by not amassing large sweat and sodium (salt) losses.

Researchers have reported that tennis players expend a significant number of calories (energy) during matches. Energy expenditure during 60-minute women's and men's matches has been estimated to be 440 and 649 calories, respectively, rising to 1,107 and 1,622 calories, respectively, for a 150-minute match and 3,244 calories for a men's five-set, 300-minute match (Ranchordas et al. 2013). Ferrauti and colleagues (2003) investigated the blood glucose responses of elite standard players during tournament play and estimated that their endogenous glycogen stores (glycogen stored within the body) were sufficient for only approximately 100 minutes of match play. To mitigate against the depletion of the muscles' carbohydrate (glycogen) stores during matches, players consume carbohydrate solutions and foodstuffs (gels, bars, bananas) at regular intervals, a strategy that appears to be effective in matches lasting around 2 hours.

Vergauwen, Brouns and Hespel (1998) demonstrated that taking a carbohydrate supplement during 2 hours of simulated match play can maintain the velocity and accuracy of players' strokes and reduce errors and the percentage of balls not reached. However, Ranchordas and colleagues (2013) proposed, from a review of nutritional strategies in tennis, that muscle glycogen (carbohydrate) depletion is likely to be a key contributing factor to fatigue during prolonged tennis matches (longer than 2 hours). This suggests that the carbohydrate intake of tennis players is insufficient to maintain or restore glycogen levels during longer matches.

Taken together, the somewhat limited scientific evidence suggests that fatigue in tennis matches lasting more than 100 minutes is likely to be partly due to a reduction in the muscles' carbohydrate stores, and that this might lead to a reduction in movement (or so-called motor) control and skill execution as a result of lowered blood glucose levels. The consuming of foodstuffs containing carbohydrate during matches will mitigate against this during 2-hour matches, but not necessarily during longer matches.

It has also been observed that professional tennis players, despite regularly drinking carbohydrate drinks, demonstrate moderate dehydration and develop high internal body temperatures during matches, and that these responses coincide with and might negatively affect the service action (Hornery et al. 2007a). A loss of control of technique (or motor function), albeit in a moderate way such as this, is further evidence of fatigue. Therefore, when players detect that their service technique is deteriorating, they might well 'pace' themselves by taking the full period of time allowed between points and games to try to recover their skill level.

In summary, it is likely that functional tennis skills are affected by severe fatigue during long, arduous matches in extremely hot and humid conditions (Hornery et al. 2007b). In these conditions a decrease in running speed might result and lead to suboptimal stroke preparation and a reduction in the 'weight' (i.e., velocity) of shots (Ferrauti et al.

2001). The decrease in running speed could be argued to be due to the brain reducing the level of muscle activation to protect the tired and hot (hyperthermic) player from suffering further heat stress or to avoid injury; however, only a few scientific studies to date provide any evidence of a centrally (brain) controlled pacing response during prolonged tennis playing (Girard, Racinais et al. 2007; Girard et al. 2008). However, it is plausible that a deterioration in running speed and technical skill might result from a gradual depletion of carbohydrate stores in the muscles, arising from the lengthy duration of the match coupled with a high internal body temperature. This would increase the body's overall energy expenditure and the player's perception of effort. Such physiological events would concern tennis players who might consciously or subconsciously pace their efforts during and between points to maintain their playing standards. The scientific evidence currently available is, however, sparse. There is clearly a need for further studies to explore whether pacing is a major factor in tennis.

chapter 14

Basketball

Since its reputed invention in 1891 by Dr James Naismith, the game of basketball has developed into one of the top 10 sports in the world. Basketball is typically played indoors on a wooden court. At almost all levels, the game is contested over four quarters; however, the precise amount of playing time varies with the type and level of competition. For example, the duration of each quarter can be 10 minutes (International Basketball Federation, FIBA), 12 minutes (National Basketball Association [NBA], USA), or even 8 minutes in U.S. high school varsity games; U.S. college basketball is played over two 20-minute halves. Recovery periods at half-time are usually 15 minutes long (FIBA, NBA, NCAA rules), but only 10 minutes long in U.S. high schools. Because the clock is stopped when players are inactive (e.g., during timeouts and free throws), games can take 2 hours to complete. At any time, five players per team are on the court. Unlimited substitutions are allowed, although they must be made during breaks in play. Timeouts can be called by coaches, but only on a limited number of occasions, and they generally last less than 1 minute (or 100 seconds in the NBA). A basketball court in international games is 91.9 feet (28 m) long and 49.2 feet (15 m) wide, although in NBA and NCAA games the dimensions are slightly larger.

To ensure that the game is played in an offensive manner, limits are typically placed on how long a team can take to cross the halfway line. This limit is 8 seconds for FIBA and NBA games and 10 seconds in men's NCAA and boys' and girls' U.S. high school games. Teams are also required to attempt a shot within 24 seconds in FIBA and NBA games, or within 30 or 35 seconds in women's and men's NCAA games, respectively. Finally, possession while being guarded can be limited to 5 seconds, and time in the free-throw lane is restricted to 3 seconds for the attacking players. These rules ensure that the game is played at a fast tempo and that there is frequent end-to-end action.

Key Factors in Determining a Pacing Strategy for Basketball

Elite basketball teams such as the Australian Institute of Sport women's and men's programmes train one to three times a day and up to six days a week (Australian Institute of Sport n.a.). In the United States, a 20-hour rule has been introduced for NCAA teams that allows them to undertake up to 20 hours of team activity for practices each week, which does not include competitive games. These examples demonstrate how physically demanding the training for high-performing basketball teams is. Training practices involve a mix of skill and technical development as well as strength and conditioning.

Simulated playing practices can be 1 to 2 hours long, and like competitive games, involve significant amounts of time exercising at a severe level of exercise intensity. Players frequently undertake sprinting and jumping activity as well as multiple explosive changes of direction, which use and deplete their anaerobic capacity.

During competitive games, these high-intensity anaerobic activities occur with high frequency. Thus, there are plenty of opportunities for the exercising muscles' store of phosphocreatine to become depleted. Recall from chapters 3 and 5 that the phosphocreatine store is used to produce energy rapidly during maximal exercise over a few seconds in duration. Once used, the phosphocreatine store can then only be replenished when the player is exercising below a severe exercise intensity, also known as critical power (see chapter 5). The question is: Do basketball players, following a maximal sprint, spend sufficient time jogging, walking or standing for their phosphocreatine stores to fully recover before the next maximal sprint—on every occasion throughout the game? If the answer is yes, then there would seem to be little need for players to pace their activity during a game. However, given the high-speed nature of basketball, it would seem unlikely that players would not need to pace their activity—at times—during games. Unfortunately, to date, there is little evidence from scientific investigation to provide a conclusive answer, largely because of the dearth of studies specifically examining this question.

A number of other factors might cause basketball players to contemplate or adopt a pacing strategy during a basketball game. First, players need to consider their energy intake, which because of their physical size and training volume is significant. As a starting point, players should consume 5 to 7 grams of carbohydrate per kilogram of body mass per day, to guard against decreased performance in training or competition (Australian Institute of Sport n.d.). Players' recovery nutrition for the first 2 or 3 hours after training or competition has been recommended to be approximately 1 to 2 grams of carbohydrate per kilogram of body mass per hour to replenish muscle and liver glycogen (carbohydrate) stores (Gatorade Sport Science Institute n.d.). Failing to follow these guidelines might result in players starting games with suboptimal glycogen (carbohydrate) stores, which might affect their ability to exercise at a sufficiently high intensity for the duration of the game. During games, it has also been suggested that players need to consume 30 to 60 grams (1 to 2 oz) of carbohydrate per hour to help maintain their performance in the fourth quarter (Gatorade Sport Science Institute n.d.). That being said, provided that players fully replenish their muscle and liver glycogen stores prior to a game, it is unlikely that these stores would become exhausted during just one basketball game and lead to dramatically reduced activity on court.

Many basketball players begin games without having fully replenished their glycogen stores since their previous games because of poor eating practices, especially when games are played in short succession. Recovering between games is particularly difficult when teams play multiple games either on the road or in tournaments. In these situations it is not uncommon for teams to be playing up to four games per week with some games on back-to-back days. Under these circumstances players' recovery practices can easily be compromised by late finishing times, unfamiliar environments (e.g., uncomfortable beds) and a lack of access to good nutrition and medical support. These factors lessen players' ability to recover between games and lead to progressive feelings of general fatigue and muscle soreness, potentially affecting their playing strategies and performances over a series of games. As a result, teams may elect to pace their play perhaps through a greater use of half-court defence rather than full-court defence to manage their dwindling energy reserves, general fatigue, soreness and injuries.

To date, pacing in basketball has not been specifically investigated. Therefore, this chapter examines the physical requirements of the game as well as studies that have looked at whether basketball players change their activity levels during games as a result of fatigue or other factors. Based on evidence from scientific studies and the view of a world-class coach, conclusions are drawn as to whether basketball players pace their efforts during a single game or during a sequence of games played in close succession.

Energy Requirements and Activity Levels of Basketball Players

Male college and junior elite players have been reported to range from 1.82 to 2.00 m (6 ft to 6 ft 7 in.) tall and weigh 74 to 103 kg (163 to 227 lb); however, senior elite players in the NBA average around 2.00 m (6 ft 7 in.) in height and 100 kg (220 lb) in mass (Gillam 1985; Montgomery, Pyne & Minahan 2010). A study of 60 elite Serbian basketball players found that centres were heavier and taller than guards and forwards and had a higher percentage of body fat (Ostojic, Mazic & Dikic 2006). Female college players in the United States have been reported to average around 1.77 m (5 ft 10 in.) in height and 70 kg (154 lb) in mass (Lamonte et al. 1999). Women NBA players average around 1.83 m (6 ft) and 60 kg (132 lb); however, individual players can be much larger. For example, Lauren Jackson, a leading player from Australia, is reputedly 1.98 m (6 ft 6 in.) tall and weighs around 85 kg (187 lb).

Players cover approximately 4500 to 5000 m (2.8 to 3.1 miles) during a 40-minute game and exhibit a variety of multidirectional movements involving running with (dribbling) and without the ball and jumping (Crisafulli et al. 2002). Explosive jumps might be completed up to 50 times per game with high-intensity runs undertaken every 20 seconds or so (McInnes et al. 1995; Montgomery, Pyne & Minahan 2010). However, players also spend significant time walking and shuffling (albeit sometimes at a high intensity). Abdelkrim, Fazaa and Ati (2007) observed that during games, players spent 41 per cent of their time undertaking specific game movements, including shuffling, 5.3 per cent of their time sprinting, and 22 per cent of their time doing low- to moderate-intensity running. It has been estimated that basketball players complete around 1,000 discrete movements during games with movements changing every 2 or 3 seconds or so (Abdelkrim, Fazaa & Ati 2007; McInnes et al. 1995).

Because of the start-and-stop nature of the game and the frequent short, explosive efforts, basketball has been conventionally categorised as an anaerobic sport with anaerobic conditioning emphasised in training practices (Crisafulli et al. 2002; Gillam 1985; Narazaki et al. 2009). This belief is supported by a few studies that have revealed that male and female varsity-level players consume relatively moderate levels of oxygen during play (28 to 37 ml/kg/min). The implication is that between hard efforts players have low to moderate periods of inactivity in which to recover (Ainsworth et al. 2000; Narazaki, Berg & Shinohara 2006). This might suggest that basketball players do not need to pace their activity; rather, the game itself sets the pace (or tempo), and the players can meet that challenge without significant fatigue. However, evidence suggests that the aerobic fitness levels of basketball players, as well as their height and weight, are increasing, which would also suggest that physical stress is increasing in the modern game. These trends were shown in a study that compared elite female basketball players over a 10-year period (Smith & Thomas 1991).

Relevance of Pacing in Basketball

Basketball requires frequent movements and end-to-end forays, so it would seem logical to assume that the aerobic energy system is highly active throughout games and that, as a result, players should indeed possess a high degree of aerobic fitness. However, a number of factors might explain why there is still some debate about the relative degree of aerobic and anaerobic conditioning required by basketball players. First, studies providing compelling evidence either way are few. Second, the maximal oxygen uptake ($\dot{V}O_2$max) values of players have generally been estimated from non-basketball-specific tests, such as treadmill running and running up and down a 20 m track at increasing speeds to exhaustion. These tests can be misleading because the type of exercise bears little resemblance to basketball, and basketball players are relatively large people whose size likely limits their endurance running capacity anyway.

Sport scientists know that the specificity of exercise is important when attempting to measure an athlete's physiological responses to their sport. Put simply, a basketball player will appear to be relatively inefficient compared to a long-distance runner and have a mediocre maximal oxygen uptake when running on a treadmill, because basketball players do not complete a great deal of straight line running in their training and are much larger athletes than runners. However, if you could measure a basketball player's oxygen uptake during a basketball game and compare it to that of a long-distance runner playing basketball, the basketball player would appear much more efficient in this situation.

In general, studies evaluating the aerobic energy requirements of basketball players have not measured their oxygen uptake directly during games. Instead, they have measured their heart rate responses and then estimated the oxygen consumption from that. This estimation of oxygen uptake has been necessary because players cannot wear portable oxygen analysers during official games, although they can sometimes wear heart rate monitors or smart sensors to measure their heart rates. Unfortunately, this method tends to overestimate oxygen consumption.

A complication for sport scientists is that when basketball players undertake movements in which their muscles are contracting—for example, when holding a static position on court (e.g., guarding or dribbling the ball in place)—their heart rates will likely be higher than during dynamic leg exercise (such as running), which means oxygen values estimated from heart rate responses are likely to be inflated in these situations. In addition, a player's heart rate can be affected by psychological arousal and anxiety, which might also result in an overestimation of their oxygen uptake at times during a game. For example, a player may have a high heart rate while simply standing and watching an opponent score critically important points during free throws. Nonetheless, the predictive software that measures real-time heart rate and uses it to calculate oxygen consumption has revealed that it can detect moderate to large changes (greater than 6 per cent) in oxygen consumption (Montgomery, Pyne & Minahan 2010). Sport scientists are now using this technology to estimate players' oxygen consumption and energy expenditure during games.

The assessment of the anaerobic energy contribution during basketball is also limited in scope and application to date. A number of studies have measured blood lactate responses during games to indicate players' anaerobic energy contributions. However, blood lactate responses should be interpreted with caution because they represent no more than a gross, indirect estimate of what is happening in the exercising muscles during exercise. Also, because blood samples in many basketball studies have been taken only at the end of each quarter, the values obtained are not representative of a whole quarter of play.

Another factor that might explain why some studies suggest that fatigue is not an issue during games while other studies suggest that it might be is that large differences exist in the physical stresses exhibited by players during basketball games. Montgomery, Pyne and Minahan (2010) studied the demands of 11 elite junior basketball players ages 18 to 20, who were 1.90 to 1.92 m (around 6 ft 3 in.) tall, weighed 73 to 103 kg (161 to 227 lb) and possessed high levels of aerobic fitness ($\dot{V}O_2$max approximately 67 to 70 ml/kg/min). Over three competitive games they found that heart rate averaged 155 to 169 beats per minute, depending on the player, which approximated to about 54 to 86 per cent of the players' maximal aerobic capacity ($\dot{V}O_2$max), which indicated that some players were exercising at much higher levels than others were. Interestingly, the same study also revealed large differences in average exercise intensities among 5-on-5 play, half-court scrimmage practice drills and actual game play. Game play was the most intense, resulting in significantly greater average heart rates and predicted oxygen uptake values. This brings into question the game specificity of some basketball practices.

A number of studies have reported that competitive basketball yields both relatively high blood lactate concentrations, indicative of a significant anaerobic energy demand, as well as relatively high heart rate responses, which might indicate a high aerobic energy

COACH'S PERSPECTIVE: Pacing in Basketball

Carrie Graf, OAM

Head coach, Canberra Capitals women's professional basketball team, 2008/2009 Six-time coach of the Women's National Basketball League champions in Australia

Head coach, Opals Australian Women's National Basketball team, 2009–2012 (the team won the bronze medal at the 2012 Olympic Games)

Assistant coach, Opals Australian Women's National Basketball team, 1996 and 2000 Olympic Games (the team won a silver medal at the 2000 Olympic Games and a bronze medal at the 1996 Olympic Games)

Managing fatigue is part of a basketball game, and the coach uses substitutions and timeouts strategically at times to rest fatigued players. The coach sometimes encourages players to give a maximum effort; however, it is critical to identify when a player is becoming fatigued. Say a player has been up-tempo for 6 minutes, and in the 6th minute, she is fatigued and the coach has not anticipated this. This last minute can be critical as fatigued players are more likely to make poor decisions. Errors can occur leading to points being rapidly scored against you. It is not always easy to see fatigue in women players, as some do not sweat greatly or look red-faced—you have to look at their playing decisions and skill execution. Some players simply go all-out all the time, 'hell for leather', and need to be substituted to recover.

The depth of the team is critical in basketball; the more depth there is on the team, the more the coach can rotate players freely. Sometimes your best player is not only your best offensive player but also your best defensive player, and so you will try to rest her when it will not damage the team performance. The coach, where possible, also tries to make sure the best offensive player is matched against an opponent who is not as good during defensive spells. This limits the need for high-intensity play as much as possible in defence and allows for up-tempo offence. The better players and more experienced players pace themselves by reading the game and knowing when to up their tempo; this may even be a subconscious trait. They rest intelligently during play. The game has structured breaks, there are frequent, short stoppages in-play and timeouts—and the professional game is now played over quarters (with breaks between them). Players can elect a slower build-up after a score to slow the tempo down. All these factors can aid recovery and are used strategically.

The playing style of the team affects the need for players to adopt a particular tempo, or pace. A half-court organised structure creates a slow build-up at a controlled tempo, so the pacing is set naturally by the playing strategy. Some coaches adopt a full-court defence to force the opposition into errors and so the team quickly regains possession. An up-tempo team strategy would be to adopt full-court defence and a 'run and gun' attack (quickly attacking and taking a shot). The coach has to read the momentum of the game. If the team loses momentum, then players might start to rush and make poor decisions and errors. At that point the coach can call a timeout to slow the game down again. This allows players to take back control of the tempo and what they should be doing.

Momentum affects physical fatigue and decision making. Playing up-tempo (at a fast pace) throughout a game of basketball is only possible if the players have superior conditioning and the team has sufficient depth of talent. Therefore, as a player tires, another player of sufficient talent can be substituted so the team

> continued

> *continued*

performance is not compromised. Coaches in the United States have a tendency to recruit to the tempo they want their team to play—an up-tempo style of play requires the drafting of up-tempo players. The other approach is to look at the talent you have in the team and work out what style of play is possible given the team's strength and weaknesses, including their physical capacities.

Tournament play, in which seven games might be played over a 2-week period, requires players to pace their efforts. The coach will try to rest star players, in terms of minutes on court, where possible. Even in seasonal play, some teams compete in a number of games on the road in a short time frame; for example, 34 games in 12 weeks might be played in the United States. This resembles a tournament situation.

demand (Abdelkrim, Fazaa & Ati 2007; McInnes et al. 1995; Rodriguez-Alonso et al. 2003). Taken together, these findings suggest that basketball players undertake exercise at a severe intensity during games. Some have suggested that there has been an increase in the aerobic energy demand of games in recent years, which has been attributed to the changes in the rules of basketball (Abdelkrim, Fazaa & Ati 2007). For example, as a result of the 8- to 24-second rule (which states that teams must cross the half-court line within 8 seconds of acquiring possession and must take a shot within 24 seconds of acquiring possession), teams can no longer adopt long offensive tactical systems but rather must rely on creative play involving a large number of varying movement patterns at rapidly changing exercise intensities. These frequently changing movement patterns limit the time available for players to recover during play. But does all this mean that modern players now have to pace themselves during games?

Narazaki and colleagues (2009) measured the oxygen uptake of six female and six male NCAA Division II players during 20-minute practice games with coaches and referees present to simulate competitive game play. The players wore portable expired gas analysers to measure oxygen consumption as they played. The researchers found that the players spent 34 per cent of their game time running and jumping, 9 per cent standing and the remainder walking. They also found that players exercised at 65 to 68 per cent of their maximal oxygen uptake ($\dot{V}O_2max$), and their heart rates averaged around 168 to 170 beats per minute, or just under 90 per cent of their maximal heart rates. The players reported their perceived exertion to be hard to very hard, which demonstrates that they possessed good fitness levels given the cardiorespiratory strain they experienced.

The heart rate values in Narazaki and colleagues' study (2009) are similar to those observed during practices and official games in a number of other studies (Abdelkrim, Fazaa & Ati 2007; McInnes et al. 1995; Ramsey et al. 1970; Rodriguez-Alonso et al. 2003). Heart rate values for elite male players have been measured at well over 190 beats per minute at times during games (McCardle 1995; Ramsey et al. 1970). Also, blood lactate values between 3 and 11 mmol/L and 3.5 and 8 mmol/L in males and female international players, respectively, have been recorded, which supports the argument that players do experience severe-intensity exercise at times during games (Abdelkrim, Fazaa & Ati 2007; McInnes et al. 1995; Rodriguez-Alonso et al. 2003).

Finally, players in the guard position appear to be most at risk of fatigue during games and therefore the most likely to pace themselves during games. Studies have shown that guards and forward players tend to spend more time in high-intensity activity than centres do. Guards have also demonstrated greater physical strain during games, exhibiting higher heart rate and blood lactate values than centres (Abdelkrim, Fazaa & Ati 2007). A study of 60 elite Serbian basketball players revealed that guards tended to be older and more experienced in terms of game play than forwards and centres (Ostojic, Mazic & Dikic 2006). This is interesting, because the greater game experience might allow guards to pace their activity more effectively during games to cope with the higher-intensity playing periods they face.

McInnes and colleagues (1995) analysed a number of players during games and reported no differences in movement characteristics during any of the four quarters of play. They argued that because they did not observe a reduction in playing intensity, significant fatigue was not evident. However, a number of other studies have reported findings that suggest that fatigue is evident during basketball games, which implies that players do pace themselves during games.

A study of a national basketball competition found that distances covered in a game at either a moderate or high speed decreased markedly during the second half, as did the players' blood lactate and heart rate responses (Janeira & Maia 1998). Blood lactate responses were also found to be lower at the end of the game compared to at half-time in a study of 38 elite under-19-year-old Tunisian players. Moreover, the amount of time spent in high-intensity activity was less during the last quarter of each half (Abdelkrim, Fazaa & Ati 2007). The investigators compared their study participants to the senior elite Australian players in McInnes and colleagues' (1995) study and debated whether the greater amount of high-intensity activity demonstrated by the Australian players was the result of their superior aerobic fitness, which allowed them to recover from intense effort more quickly during games. By implication, this suggest that fatigue is very much a part of a basketball game and that pacing would thus be highly likely.

Narazaki and colleagues (2009) also observed that players' blood lactate values fell by 12 per cent following 10 minutes of play, but then remained at a similar level when remeasured after 15 and 20 minutes of play. They also observed reductions in the duration of active movements, including running and jumping, in the final 5 minutes of each 20-minute playing period. They suggested that this might be due to the players pacing their efforts during play, either subconsciously or consciously, to maximise performance and minimise fatigue. A reduction in players' activity during the final stages of games might therefore be an attempt to 'manage' the final minutes of possession by reducing the proportion of straight play and fast breaks (Abdelkrim, Fazaa & Ati 2007). In this situation, the tempo of play is being deliberately slowed down. Whether this is due to fatigue or tactics intended to reduce opportunities for the opposing team to score is, of course, debatable. However, it seems likely that fatigue would be a cause of reduced activity level in some players during games in general. International women's basketball coach Carrie Graf, who provides the coach's view for this chapter, certainly supports this assertion.

There is some evidence that competitive basketball games in close succession can lead to cumulative fatigue and hinder subsequent competition performance (Montgomery et al. 2008). The researchers found that during a three-day tournament-style basketball competition the sprint, agility and vertical jumping performances of the players deteriorated to a small or moderate degree, despite their undertaking various recovery techniques. The players also reported increases in feelings of general fatigue and muscle soreness. The researchers concluded that repeated high-intensity basketball games over several days could lead to significant fatigue. Therefore, it would appear that during a tournament, or an intensive series of games on the road, players might well choose to pace their activity on court, to preserve their physical capacities by limiting muscle damage and general fatigue.

In summary, there appears to be evidence that basketball is a sport that requires players to pace their activity. The physical demands of the game are such that players do tire at certain times. They recover on court by pacing themselves or by being substituted by the coach. Players are also at risk of cumulative fatigue when they play multiple games in quick succession. This is because recovery practices, such as having good-quality sleep and nutrition, can be affected when frequently playing games on the road. Thus, players might well need to pace their efforts on court when starting a game in an already fatigued or sore state.

During games, basketball coaches intuitively perceive players' fatigue from decreases in their skill levels or in the quality of their decision making. Sport scientists, employed to support professional and national basketball teams, also attempt to detect player fatigue by discerning changes in their activity patterns and physiological responses during games using video-based techniques and smart technologies. Therefore, it is an anomaly that there are few published scientific studies specifically addressing the importance of pacing in this sport. Evidently, further research is warranted in this area to enhance coach, support staff and player education.

Preface

Foster, C., Snyder, AC, Thompson, NN., Green, MA., Foley, M, et al (1993). Effect of pacing strategy on cycle time trial performance. *Medicine and Science in Sports and Exercise.* 25: 383-388.

Foster, C., Schrager, M., Snyder, A.C., Thompson, N.N. (1994) Pacing strategy and athletic performance. *Sports Medicine.* 17(2), 77-85).

St Clair Gibson, A., de Koning JJ., Thompson KG., Roberts WO., Micklewright D., Raglin J., Foster C. (2013) Crawling to the finish line: why do endurance runners collapse? : implications for understanding of mechanisms underlying pacing and fatigue. *Sports Medicine,* 43(6):413-24

Stone, M.R., Thomas, K., Wilkinson, M., Jones, A.M., St Clair Gibson., A., Thompson, K.G. Effects of deception on exercise performance: implications for determinants of fatigue in humans. *Medicine & Science in Sports & Exercise,* 2012. 44(3): p. 534-541.

Ulmer, HV. (1996) Concept of an extracellular regulation of muscular metabolic rate during heavy exercise in humans by psychophysiological feedback. *Experientia,* 52: 416-420.

Chapter 1

Abbis, C.R. & Laursen, P. (2008). Describing and understanding pacing strategies during athletic competition. *Sports Medicine* 38, 239-253.

Abbis, C.R., Burnett, A., Nosaka, K., Green, J.P., Foster, J.K. & Laursen, P. (2009). Effect of hot versus cold climates on power output, muscle activation and perceived exertion during a dynamic 100-km cycling trial. *Journal of Sports Sciences* 27, 1-9.

Adams, W.C. & Bernauer, E.M. (1968). The effects of selected pace variations on the oxygen requirement of running a 4:37 mile. *Research Quarterly* 16, 977-981.

Amann, M., Eldridge, M.W., Lovering, A.T., Stickland, M.K., Pagelow, D.F. & Dempsey, J.A. (2006). Arterial oxygenation influences central motor output and exercise performance via effects on peripheral locomotor muscle fatigue in humans. *Journal of Physiology* 575, 937-952.

Amann, M., Proctor, L.T., Sebranek, J.J, Eldridge, M.W., Pegelow, D.F. & Dempsey, J.J. (2008). Somatosensory feedback from the limbs exerts inhibitor influences on central neural drive during whole body exercise. *Journal of Applied Physiology* 105, 1714-1724.

Ansley, L., Robson, P.J. & St Clair Gibson, A. (2004). Anticipatory pacing strategies during supramaximal exercise lasting longer than 30s. *Medicine & Science in Sports & Exercise* 36, 309-314.

Bath, D., Turner, L.A., Bosch, A.N. et al. (2012). The effect of a second runner on pacing strategy and RPE during a running time trial. *International Journals of Sports Physiology and Performance* 7, 26-32.

Corbett, J., Barwood, M.J. & Parkhouse, K. (2009). Effect of task familiarization on distribution of energy during a 2000m cycling time trial. *British Journal of Sports Medicine* 43, 770-774.

Cordain, L., Gotshall, R.W., Eaton, S.B. & Eaton, S.B. III. (1998). Physical activity, energy expenditure and fitness: An evolutionary perspective. *International Journal of Sports Medicine* 19, 328-335.

Crewe, H., Tucker, R. & Noakes, T.D. (2008). The rate of increase in rating of perceived exertion predicts the duration of exercise to fatigue at a fixed power output in different environmental conditions. *European Journal of Applied Physiology* 103, 569-577.

Daniels, J. & Oldridge, N. (1970). The effects of alternate exposure to altitude and sea level on world-class middle distance runners. *Medicine and Science in Sports* 2, 107-112.

de Koning, J.J., Bobbert, M.F. & Foster, C. (1999). Determination of optimal pacing strategy in track cycling with an energy flow model. *Journal of Science, Medicine and Sport* 2, 266-277.

de Koning, J.J., Foster, C., Lampen, J., Hettinga, F. & Bobbert, M.F. (2005). Experimental evaluation of the power balance model of speed skating. *Journal of Applied Physiology* 98, 227-233.

de Koning, J.J., Foster, C., Bakkum, A. et al. (2011a). Regulation of pacing strategy during athletic competition. *PLOS ONE* 6, e15863.

de Koning, J.J. Foster, C., Lucia, A., Bobbert, M.F., Hettinga, F.J. & Porcari, J.P. (2011b). Using modeling to understand how athletes in different disciplines solve the same problem: Swimming vs. running vs. speed skating. *International Journal of Sports Physiology and Performance* 6, 276-280.

de Koning, J.J., Foster, C. & Hettinga, F. (2011). Exploring the pacing landscape. *Medicine & Science in Sports & Exercise* 43, 1027.

Eaton, S.B., Konner, M. & Shostak, M. (1988). Stone agers in the fast lane: Chronic degenerative diseases in evolutionary perspective. *American Journal of Medicine* 84, 739-749.

Eston, R.G., Faulkner, J.A., St Clair Gibson, A., Noakes, T. & Parfitt, G. (2007). The effect of antecedent fatiguing activity on the relationship between perceived exertion and the physiological activity during a constant load task. *Psychophysiology* 44, 779-786.

Faulkner, J., Parfitt, G. & Eston, R. (2008). The rating of perceived exertion during competitive running scales with time. *Psychophysiology* 45, 977-985.

Foster, C., Snyder, A.C., Thompson, N.N., Green, M.A., Foley, M. & Schrager, M. (1993). Effect of pacing strategy on cycle time trial performance. *Medicine & Science in Sports & Exercise* 25, 383-388.

Foster, C., Schrager, M., Snyder, A.C. & Thompson, N.N. (1994). Pacing strategy and athletic performance. *Sports Medicine* 17, 77-85.

Foster, C., de Koning, J.J., Hettinga, F. et al. (2004). Effect of competitive distance on energy expenditure during simulated competition. *International Journal of Sports Medicine* 25, 198-204.

Foster, C., Hoyos, J., Earnest, C. & Lucia, A. (2005). Regulation of energy expenditure during prolonged athletic competition. *Medicine & Science in Sports & Exercise* 37, 670-675.

Foster, C., Hendrickson, K.J., Peyer, K. et al. (2009). Pattern of developing the performance template. *British Journal of Sports Medicine* 43, 765-769.

Foster, C., de Koning, J.J., Bischel, S., Casolino, E., Malterer, K., O'Brien, K., Rodríguez-Marroyo, J., Splinter, A., Thiel, C. & Van Tunen, J. (2012). Pacing strategies for endurance performance. In I. Mujika (Ed.), *Endurance Training – Science and Practice* (pp. 85-98). Vitoria-Gasteiz, Basque Country: Iñigo Mujika S.L.U.

Foster, C., Porcari, J.P., de Koning, J.J. et al. (2012). Exercise training for performance and health. *Deutsche Zeitschrift fur Sportmedizin* 63, 69-74.

Hettinga, F.J., de Koning, J.J., Broersen, F.T., van Geffen, P. & Foster, C. (2006). Pacing strategy and the occurrence of fatigue in 4000m cycling time trials. *Medicine & Science in Sports & Exercise* 38, 1484-1491.

Hulleman, M., de Koning, J.J., Hettinga, F.J. & Foster, C. (2007). The effect of extrinsic motivation on cycle time trial performance. *Medicine & Science in Sports & Exercise* 39, 709-715.

Johnson, B.D., Joseph, T., Wright G. et al. (2009). Rapidity of responding to a hypoxic challenge during exercise. *European Journal of Applied Physiology* 106, 493-499.

Jones, A.M., Wilkerson, D.P., DiMenna, F., Fulford, J. & Poole, D.C. (2008). Muscle metabolic responses above and below the 'critical power' assessed using ^{31}P-MRS. *American Journal of Physiology* 294, R585-593.

Joseph, T., Johnson, B., Battista, R.A. et al. (2008). Perception of fatigue during simulated competition. *Medicine & Science in Sports & Exercise* 40, 381-386.

Karlsson, J. & Saltin, B. (1970). Lactate, ATP and CP in working muscles during exhaustive exercise in man. *Journal of Applied Physiology* 29, 598-602.

Karlsson, J. & Saltin, B. (1971). Diet, muscle glycogen and endurance performance. *Journal of Applied Physiology* 31, 203-206.

Lambert, E.V., St Clair Gibson, A. & Noakes, T.D. (2005). Complex systems model of fatigue: Integrative control of peripheral physiological systems during exercise in humans. *British Journal of Sports Medicine* 39, 52-62.

Leger, L.A. & Ferguson, R.J. (1974). Effect of pacing on oxygen uptake and peak lactate for a mile run. *European Journal of Applied Physiology* 32, 251-257.

Martin, L., Lambeth-Mansell, A., Beretta-Azevedo, L., Holmes, L.A., Wright, R. & St Clair Gibson, A. (2012). Even between lap pacing despite higher within lap variation during mountain biking. *International Journal of Sports Physiology and Performance* (In press).

Mauger, A.R., Jones, A.M. & Williams, C.A. (2011). The effect of non-contingent and accurate performance feedback on pacing and time trial performance in a 4-km track cycling. *British Journal of Sports Medicine* 45, 225-229.

Micklewright, D., Papadopoulous, E., Swart, J. & Noakes, T.D. (2010). Previous experience influences pacing during 20-km time trial cycling. *British Journal of Sports Medicine* 44, 952-960.

Noakes, T.D., St Clair Gibson, A. & Lambert, E.V. (2004). From catastrophe to complexity: A novel model of integrative central neural regulation of effort and fatigue during exercise in humans. *British Journal of Sports Medicine* 38, 511-514.

Noakes, T.D., Lambert, M.I. & Hauman, R. (2009). Which lap is slowest? An analysis of 32 world mile record performances. *British Journal of Sports Medicine* 43, 760-764.

Padilla, S., Mujika, I., Angulo, F. & Goiriena, J.J. (2000). Scientific approach to the 1-h cycling world record: A case study. *Journal of Applied Physiology* 89, 1522-1527.

Rauch, H., St Clair Gibson, A., Lambert, E.V. & Noakes, T.D. (2005). A signaling role for muscle glycogen in the regulation of pace during prolonged exercise. *British Journal of Sports Medicine* 39, 34-38.

Roelands, B., de Koning, J., Foster, C., Hettinga, F. & Meeusen, R. (2013). Neurophysiological determinants of theoretical concepts and mechanisms involved in pacing. *Sports Medicine* 43 (5), 301-311.

Robertson, E., Pyne, D., Hopkins, W. & Anson, J. (2009). Analysis of lap times in international swimming competitions. *Journal of Sports Sciences* 27, 387-395.

Robinson, S., Robinson, D.L., Mountjoy, R.J. & Bullard, R.W. (1958). Influence of fatigue on the efficiency of men during exhausting runs. *Journal of Applied Physiology* 12, 197-201.

St Clair Gibson, A. & Noakes, T.D. (2004). Evidence for complex system regulation and dynamic neural regulation of skeletal muscle recruitment during exercise in humans. *British Journal of Sports Medicine* 38, 797-806.

St Clair Gibson, A., Lambert, E.V., Rauch, L.H.G., Tucker, R., Baden D.A., Foster, C. & Noakes, T.D. (2006). The role of information processing between the brain and peripheral physiological systems in pacing and perception of effort. *Sports Medicine* 36, 705-722.

St Clair Gibson, A. & Foster, C. (2007). The role of self-talk in the awareness of physiological state and physical performance. *Sports Medicine* 37, 1029-1044.

St Clair Gibson, A., de Koning, J., Thompson, K.G., Roberts, W.O., Micklewright, D., Raglin, J. & Foster, C. (2013). Crawling to the finish line—Why do endurance runners collapse? Implications for understanding the mechanisms underlying fatigue and pacing. *Sports Medicine* 43, 413-424.

Skibba, P.F., Chidnok, W., Vanhatalo, A. & Jones, A.M. (2012). Modeling the expenditure and reconstitution of work capacity above critical power. *Medicine & Science in Sports & Exercise* 44, 1526-1532.

Studdel-Numbers, K.L. & Wall-Scheffler, C.M. (2009). Optimal running speed and the evolution of hominine hunting strategies. *Journal of Human Evolution* 56, 355-360.

Swart, J., Lamberts, R.P., Lambert, M.I., Woolrich, R.W., Johnston, S. & Noakes, T.D. (2009a). Exercising with reserve: Exercise regulation by perceived exertion in relation to duration of exercise and knowledge of endpoint. *British Journal of Sports Medicine* 43, 775-778.

Swart, J., Lamberts, R.P., Lambert, M.I., St Clair Gibson, A., Lambert, E.V., Skowno, J. & Noakes, T.D. (2009b). Exercising with reserve: Evidence

that the central nervous system regulates prolonged exercise performance. *British Journal of Sports Medicine* 43, 782-788.

Thiel, C., Foster, C., Banzer, W. & de Koning, J.J. (2012). Pacing in Olympic track races: Competitive tactics versus best performance strategy. *Journal of Sports Sciences.* dx.doi.org/10.1080/02 640414.2012.701759.

Tucker, R., Lambert, M.I. & Noakes, T.D. (2006). An analysis of pacing strategies during men's world-record performances in track athletes. *International Journal of Sports Physiology and Performance* 1, 233-245.

Tucker, R., Kayser, B., Rae, E., Rauch, L., Bosch, A. & Noakes, T.D. (2007). Hyperoxia improves 20km cycling time trial performance by increasing muscle activation levels while perceived exertion stays the same. *European Journal of Applied Physiology* 101, 771-781.

Tucker, R. & Noakes, T.D. (2009). The physiological regulation of pacing strategy during exercise: A critical role. *British Journal of Sports Medicine* 43, e1-9.

Ulmer, H.V. (1996). Concept of an extracellular regulation of muscular metabolic rate during heavy exercise by psychophysiological feedback. *Experientia* 52, 416-420.

van Ingen Schenau, G.J., de Koning, J.J. & de Groot, G. (1992). The distribution of anaerobic energy in 1000 and 4000 meter cycling bouts. *International Journal of Sports Medicine* 13, 447-451.

Wilber, R.L. & Pitsiladis, Y.P. (2012). Kenyan and Ethiopian distance runners: What makes them so good? *International Journal of Sports Physiology and Performance* 7, 92-102.

Chapter 2

Abbiss, C.R. & Laursen, P.B. (2008). Describing and understanding pacing strategies during athletic competition. *Sports Medicine* 38, 239-252.

Atkinson, G., Peacock, O. & Law, M. (2007). Acceptability of power variation during a simulated time trial. *International Journal of Sports Medicine* 28, 157-163.

Atkinson, G., Peacock, O. & Passfield, L. (2007). Variable versus constant power strategies during cycling time-trials: Prediction of time savings using an up-to-date mathematical model. *Journal of Sports Science* 25 (9), 1001-1009.

Bar-Or, O. (1987) The Wingate anaerobic test: an update on methodology, reliability and validity. *Sports Medicine*, 4: 391-394.

Billat, V., Wesfried, E., Kapfer, C., Koralsztein, J. & Meyer, Y. (2006). Nonlinear dynamics of heart rate and oxygen uptake in exhaustive 10,000 m runs: Influence of constant vs freely paced. *Journal of Physiological Science* 56, 103-111.

Brickley, G., Green, S., Jenkins, D.G., McEinery, M., Wishart, C., Doust J.D. & Williams, C.A. (2007). Muscle metabolism during constant- and alternating-intensity exercise around critical power. *International Journal of Sports Medicine* 28 (4), 300-305.

Burnley, M. & Jones, A.M. (2007). Oxygen uptake kinetics as a determinant of sports performance. *European Journal of Sport Science* 7 (2), 63-79.

Cheetham, M.E., Boobis, L.H., Brooks, S., Williams, C. (1986) Human muscle metabolism during sprint running. *Journal of Applied Physiology*, 61: 54-60, 1986.

Corbett, J., Barwood, M.J. & Parkhouse, K. (2009). Effect of task familiarisation on distribution of energy during a 2000 m cycling time trial. *British Journal of Sports Medicine* 43 (10), 770-774.

Esteve-Lanao, J., Lucia, A., de Koning, J.J. & Foster, C. (2008). How do humans control physiological strain during strenuous endurance exercise? *PLOS ONE* 3 (8), e2943. doi: 10.1371/journal.pone.0002943.

Foster, C., de Koning, J.J., Bischel, S., Casolino, E., Malterer, K., O'Brien, K., Rodríguez-Marroyo, J., Splinter, A., Thiel, C. & Van Tunen, J. (2012). Pacing strategies for endurance performance. In I. Mujika (Ed.), *Endurance Training – Science and Practice* (pp. 85-98). Vitoria-Gasteiz, Basque Country: Iñigo Mujika S.L.U.

Foster, C., de Koning, J.J., Hettinga, F., Lampen, J., Dodge, C., Bobbert, M. & Porcari, J.P. (2004). Effect of competitive distance on energy expenditure during simulated competition. *International Journal of Sports Medicine* 25 (3), 198-204.

Foster, C., Schrager, M., Snyder, A.C. & Thompson, N.N. (1994). Pacing strategy and athletic performance. *Sports Medicine* 17 (2), 77-85.

Foster, C., Snyder, A.C., Thompson, N.N., Green, M.A., Foley, M. & Schrager, M. (1993). Effect of pacing strategy on cycle time trial performance. *Medicine & Science in Sports & Exercise* 25, 383-388.

Fukuba, Y. & Whipp, B.J. (1999). A metabolic limit on the ability to make up for lost time in endurance events. *Journal of Applied Physiology* 87 (2), 853-861.

Garland, S.W. (2005). An analysis of the pacing strategy adopted by elite competitors in 2000 m rowing. *British Journal of Sports Medicine* 39 (1), 39-42.

Hettinga, F.J., de Koning, J.J., Broersen, F.T., Van Geffen, P. & Foster, C. (2006). Pacing strategy and the occurrence of fatigue in 4000 m cycling time trials. *Medicine & Science in Sports & Exercise* 38 (8), 1484-1491.

Liedl, M.A., Swain D.P. & Branch J.D. (1999). Physiological effects of constant versus variable power during endurance cycling. *Medicine & Science in Sports & Exercise* 31 (10), 1472-1477.

Mattern, C.O., Kenefick, R.W., Kertzer, R. & Quinn, T.J. (2001). Impact of starting strategy on cycling performance. *International Journal of Sports Medicine* 22 (5), 350-355.

McCartney, N., Heigenhauser, GJF., Sargent, A.J., Jones, N.L. (1983). A constant velocity cycle ergometer for the study of dynamic muscle function. Journal of Applied Physiology, 55: 212-217.

Padilla, S., Mukia, I., Orban Anos, J., Santisteban, J., Angula, F. & Goiriena, J.J. (2001). Exercise intensity and load during mass-start stage races in professional road cycling. *Medicine & Science in Sports & Exercise* 33 (5), 796-802.

Palmer, G.S., Borghouts, L.B., Noakes, T.D. & Hawley, J.A. (1999). Metabolic and performance responses to constant-load vs. variable-intensity exercise in trained cyclists. *Journal of Applied Physiology* 87 (3), 1186-1196.

Palmer, G.S., Noakes, T.D. & Hawley, J.A. (1997). Effects of steady-state versus stochastic exercise on subsequent cycling performance. *Medicine & Science in Sports & Exercise* 29 (5), 684-687.

Rauch, H.G.L., St Clair Gibson, A., Lambert, E.V. & Noakes T.D. (2005). A signalling role for muscle glycogen in the regulation of pace during prolonged exercise. *British Journal of Sports Medicine* 39 (1), 34-38.

Schabort, E J., Hawley, J.A., Hopkins, W.G. & Blum, H. (1999). High reliability of performance of well-trained rowers on a rowing ergometer. *Journal of Sports Sciences* 17 (8), 627-632.

Schumacher, Y.O., Ahlgrim, C., Prettin, S. & Pottgiesser, T. (2011). Physiology, power output, and racing strategy of a race across America finisher. *Medicine & Science in Sports & Exercise* 43 (45), 885-889.

Stevinson, C.D. & Biddle, S.J. (1998). Cognitive orientations in marathon running and 'hitting the wall'. *British Journal of Sports Medicine* 32, 229-235.

Stone, M.R., Thomas, K., Wilkinson, M., Jones, A.M., St Clair Gibson, A. & Thompson, K. G. (2012). Effects of deception on exercise performance: Implications for determinants of fatigue in humans. *Medicine & Science in Sports & Exercise* 44 (3), 534-541.

Stone, M.R., Thomas, K., Wilkinson, M., St Clair Gibson, A. & Thompson K.G. (2011). Consistency of perceptual and metabolic responses to a laboratory-based simulated 4,000-m cycling time trial. *European Journal of Applied Physiology* 111, 1807-1813.

Theurel, J. & Lepers, R. (2008). Neuromuscular fatigue is greater following highly variable versus constant intensity endurance cycling. *European Journal of Applied Physiology* 103, 461-468.

Thomas, K., Stone, M.R., Thompson, K.G., St Clair Gibson, A. & Ansley, L. (2012a). Reproducibility of pacing strategy during simulated 20-km cycling time trials in well-trained cyclists. *European Journal of Applied Physiology* 112 (1), 223-229.

Thomas, K., Stone, M., Thompson, K.G., St Clair Gibson, A. & Ansley, L. (2012b). The effect of self- even- and variable-pacing strategies on perceived exertion and the physiological response to exercise. *European Journal of Applied Physiology* 112 (8), 3069-3078.

Thompson, K.G., MacLaren, D.P., Lees, A. & Atkinson, G. (2003). The effect of even, positive and negative pacing on metabolic, kinematic and temporal variables during breaststroke swimming. *European Journal of Applied Physiology* 88 (4), 438-443.

Vogt, S., Schumacher, Y.O., Roecker, K., Dickhuth, H.-H., Schoberer, U., Schmid, A. & Heinrich, A. (2007). Performance profile during the Tour de France. *International Journal of Sports Medicine* 28, 756-761.

Wilberg, R.B. and Pratt, J. (1988) A survey of race profiles of cyclists in the pursuit and kilo track events. Canadian Journal of Sport Sciences. 13(4): 208-13.

Withers, R.T., Sherman, W.M., Clark, D.G., Esselbach, P.C., Nolan, S.R., et al. (1991) Muscle metabolism during 30, 60 and 90s of maximal cycling on an air-braked erometer. European Journal of Applied Physiology and Occupational Physiology, 63: 354-362.

Chapter 3

Amann, M. (2011). Central and peripheral fatigue: Interaction during cycling exercise in humans. *Medicine & Science in Sports & Exercise* 43 (11), 2039-2045.

Amann, M. & Dempsey, J.A. (2008). Locomotor muscle fatigue modifies central motor drive in healthy humans and imposes a limitation to exercise performance. *Journal of Physiology* 586 (1), 13-24.

Amann, M., Eldridge, M.W., Lovering, A.T., Stickland, M.K., Pegelow, D.F. & Dempsey, J.A. (2006). Arterial oxygenation influences central motor output and exercise performance via effects on peripheral locomotor muscle fatigue in humans. *Journal of Physiology* 575 (Part 3): 937-952.

Amann, M., Proctor, L.T., Sebranek, J.J., Pegelow, D.F. & Dempsey, J.A. (2009). Opioid-mediated muscle afferents inhibit central motor drive and limit peripheral muscle fatigue in humans. *Journal of Physiology* 587, 271-283.

Amann, M., Romer, L.M., Subudhi, A.W., Pegelow, D.F. & Dempsey, J.A. (2007). Severity of arterial hypoxaemia affects the relative contributions of peripheral muscle fatigue to exercise performance in healthy humans. *Journal of Physiology* 581 (Part 1), 389-403.

Ansley, L., Robson P.J. et al. (2004). Anticipatory pacing strategies during supramaximal exercise lasting longer than 30 s. *Medicine & Science in Sports & Exercise* 36 (2), 309-314.

Basset, D.R. & Howley, E.T. (2000). Limiting factors for maximum oxygen uptake and determinants of endurance performance. *Medicine & Science in Sports & Exercise* 32 (1), 70-84.

de Koning, J.J., Foster, C., Bakkum, A., Kloppenburg, S., Thiel, C., Joseph, T., Cohen, J. & Porcari, J.P. (2011). Regulation of pacing strategy during athletic competition. *PLOS ONE* 6 (1), 1-6.

Foster, C., de Koning, J.J., Hettinga, F. et al. (2003). Pattern of energy expenditure during simulated competition. *Medicine & Science in Sports & Exercise* 35, 826-831.

Foster, C., Schrager, M., Snyder, A.C. & Thompson, N.N. (1994). Pacing strategy and athletic performance. *Sports Medicine* 17 (2), 77-85.

Foster, C., Snyder, A.C, Thompson, N.N., Green, M.A., Foley, M. et al. (1993). Effect of pacing strategy on cycle time trial performance. *Medicine & Science in Sports & Exercise* 25, 383-388.

Galloway, S.D.R. & Maughan, R.J. (1997). Effects of ambient temperature on the capacity to perform prolonged cycle exercise in man. *Medicine & Science in Sports & Exercise* 29, 1240-1249.

Henslin-Harris, K.B., Foster, C., de Koning, J.J., Dodge, C., Wright, G.A. & Porcari, J.P. (2013). Rapidity of response to hypoxic conditions during exercise. *International Journal of Sports Physiology and Performance* 8, 330-335.

Hill, A.V., Long, C.V.H. & Lupton, H. (1924). Muscular exercise, lactic acid and the supply and utilisastion of oxygen: Parts VII-VIII. *Proceedings of the Royal. Society of. London. B* 97 (682), 155-176.

Hopkins, W.G. (2009). The improbable central governor of maximal endurance performance. *Sportscience* 13, 9-12.

Hunter, A.M., St Clair Gibson, A., Lambert, M.I., Nobbs, L. & Noakes, T.D. (2003). Effects of supramaximal exercise on the electromyographic signal. *British Journal of Sports Medicine* 7, 296–299.

Jones, A.M. & Burnley, M. 2009. Oxygen uptake kinetics: An underappreciated determinant of exercise performance. *International Journal of Sports Physiology and Performance* 4, 524-532.

Joyner, M.J. & Coyle, F. (2008). Endurance exercise performance: The physiology of champions. *Journal of Physiology* 586, 35-44.

Kayser, B., Narici, M., Binzoni, T., Grassi, B. & Cerretelli, P. (1994). Fatigue and exhaustion in chronic hypobaric hypoxia: Influence of exercising muscle mass. *Journal of Applied Physiology* 76, 634–640.

Keller, J.B. (1974). Optimal velocity in a race. *American Mathematical Monthly* 81 (5), 475-480.

Levine, B.D. (2008). $\dot{V}O_2$ max: What we do know, and what we still need to know? *Journal of Physiology* 586 (1), 25-34.

Marino, F.E., Lambert, M.I. & Noakes, T.D. (2004). Superior performance of African runners in warm humid but not in cool environmental conditions. *Journal of Applied Physiology* 96, 124-130.

Nielsen, B. (1996). Olympics in Atlanta: A fight against physics. *Medicine & Science in Sports & Exercise* 28, 665-668.

Nielsen, B., Savard, G., Richter, E.A., Hargreaves, M. & Saltin, B. (1990). Muscle blood flow and muscle metabolism during exercise and heat stress. *Journal of Applied Physiology* 69, 1040-1046.

Noakes, T.D. (2011). Time to move beyond a brainless exercise physiology: The evidence for complex regulation of human exercise performance. *Applied Physiology Nutrition and Metabolism* 36 (1), 23-35.

Noakes, T.D. & St Clair Gibson, A. (2004). Logical limitations to the 'catastrophe' models of fatigue during exercise in humans. *British Journal of Sports Medicine* 38, 648-649.

Nummela, A., Vurorimaa, T. & Rusko, H. (1992). Changes in force production, blood lactate and EMG activity in the 400-m sprint. *Journal of Sport Science* 107, 217-228.

Peltonen, J.E., Rantamaki, J., Niittymaki, S.P.T. et al. (1997). Effects of oxygen fraction in inspired air on force production and electromyogram activity during ergometer rowing. *European Journal of Applied Physiology* 76, 495-503.

Rauch, H.G., St Clair Gibson, A., Lambert, E.V. et al. (2005). A signalling role for muscle glycogen in the regulation of pace during exercise. *British Journal of Sports Medicine* 39, 34-38.

Shephard, R.J. (2009). Is it time to retire the central governor? *Sports Medicine* 39 (9), 709-721.

Skorski, S., Faude, O., Rausch, K. & Meyer, T. (2013). Reproducibility of pacing profiles in competitive swimmers. *International Journal of Sports Medicine* 34, 152-157.

St Clair Gibson, A., de Koning, J.J., Thompson, K.G., Roberts, W.O., Micklewright, D., Raglin, J. & Foster, C. (2013). Crawling to the finish line: Why do endurance runners collapse? Implications for understanding of mechanisms underlying pacing and fatigue. *Sports Medicine* 43 (6), 413-424.

St Clair Gibson, A. & Noakes, T.D. (2004). Evidence for complex system integration and dynamic neural regulation of skeletal muscle recruitment during exercise in humans. *British Journal of Sports Medicine* 38, 797-806.

Stiles, P. (1920). Types of fatigue. *American Journal of Public Health* 10 (8), 653-656.

Tatterson, A.J. et al. (2000). Effects of heat stress on physiological responses and exercise performance in elite cyclists. *Journal of Science and Medicine in Sport* 3, 186-193.

Taylor, A.D., Bronks, R., Smith, P. & Humphries, B. (1997). Myoelectric evidence of peripheral muscle fatigue during exercise in severe hypoxia: Some references to m. vastus lateralis myosin heavy chain composition. *European Journal of Applied Physiology and Occupational Physiology* 75 (2), 151-159.

Triplett, N. (1898). The dynamogenic factors in pacemaking and competition. *American Journal of Psychology* 9 (4), 507-533.

Tucker, R., Kayser, B., Rae, E., Rauch, L., Bosch, A. & Noakes, T. (2007). Hyperoxia improves 20-km cycling time trial performance by increasing muscle activation levels while perceived exertion stays the same. *European Journal of Applied Physiology* 101, 771-781.

Tucker, R. & Noakes, T.D. (2009). The physiological regulation of pacing strategy during exercise: A critical review. *British Journal of Sports Medicine* 43, 1-9.

Tucker, R. et al. (2006). The rate of heat storage mediates an anticipatory reduction in exercise intensity during cycling at a fixed rating of perceived exertion. *Journal of Physiology* 574, 905-915.

Ulmer, H.V. (1996). Concept of an extracellular regulation of muscular metabolic rate during heavy exercise in humans by psychophysiological feedback. *Experientia* 52, 416-420.

Wagner, P.D. (2010). Limiting factors of exercise performance. *Deutsche Zeitschrift Fur Sportmedizin* 61 (5), 108-111.

Chapter 4

Ader, R. & Cohen, N. (1975). Behaviorally conditioned immunosuppression. *Psychosomatic Medicine* 37, 333-340.

Ahsen, A. (1984). ISM: The triple code model for imagery and psychophysiology. *Journal of Mental Imagery* 8 (4), 15-42.

Aitchison, C., Turner, L.A., Ansley, L., Thompson, K.G., Micklewright, D.P. & St Clair Gibson, A. (2013). The inner dialogue and its relationship to RPE during different running intensities. *Perceptual and Motor Skills* 117 (1), 1-20.

Al-Rahamneh, H.Q. & Eston, R.G. (2011). Prediction of maximal oxygen uptake from the ratings of perceived exertion during a graded and ramp exercise test in able-bodied and persons with paraplegia. *Archives of Physical Medicine and Rehabilitation* 92, 277-283.

Albertus, Y. (2008). Critical analysis of techniques for normalising electromyographic data. PhD thesis, University of Cape Town, Cape Town, South Africa.

Amann, M., Eldridge, M.W., Lovering, A.T., Stickland, M.K., Pegelow, D.F. & Dempsey, J.A. (2006). Arterial oxygenation influences central motor output and exercise performance via effects on peripheral locomotor muscle fatigue in humans. *Journal of Physiology* 575, 937-952.

Amanzio M. & Benedetti, F. (1999). Neuropharmacological dissection of placebo analgesia: Expectation-activated opioid systems versus conditioning-activated specific subsystems. *Journal of Neuroscience* 19, 484-494.

Baden, D.A., McLean, T.L., Tucker, R., Noakes, T.D. & St Clair Gibson, A. (2005). Effect of anticipation during unknown or unexpected exercise duration on rating of perceived exertion, affect, and physiological function. *British Journal of Sports Medicine* 39, 742-746.

Bargh, J., Chen, M. & Burrows, L. (1996). Automaticity of social behavior: Direct effects of trait construct and stereotype activation on action. *Journal of Personality and Social Psychology* 71, 230-244.

Bath, D., Turner, L.A., Bosch, A.N., Tucker, R., Lambert, E.V., Thompson, K.G. & St Clair Gibson A. (2011). The effect of a second runner on pacing strategy and RPE during a running time trial. *International Journal of Sports Physiology and Performance* 7 (1), 26-32.

Beedie, C.J. (2007). Placebo effects in competitive sport: Qualitative data. *Journal of Sports Science and Medicine* 6, 21-28.

Beedie C.J. & Lane A.M. (2012). The role of glucose in self-control: Another look at the evidence and an alternative conceptualization. *Personality and Social Psychology Review* 16, 143-153.

Benedetti, F., Mayberg, H.S., Wager, T.D., Stohler, C.S. & Zubieta, J.K. (2005). Neurobiological mechanisms of the placebo effect. *Journal of Neuroscience* 25(45), 10390-10402.

Bennett, C.M., Baird, A.A., Miller, M.B. & Wolford, G.L. (2010). Neural correlates of interspecies perspective taking in the post-mortem Atlantic salmon: An argument for proper multiple comparisons correction. *Journal of Serendipitous and Unexpected Results* 1, 1-5.

Bettendorff, L., Sallanin-Moulin, M., Toret, M., Wins, P., Margineanu, I. & Schoffeniels, E. (1996). Paradoxical sleep deprivation increases the content of glutamate and glutamine in rat cerebral cortex. Laboratory of Neurochemistry, University of Liège, Belgium.

Boecker, H., Sprenger, T., Spilker, M.E., Henriksen, G., Koppenhoefer, M., Wagner, K.J., Valet, M., Berthele, A. & Tolle, T.R. (2008). The runner's high: Opioidergic mechanisms in the human brain. *Cerebral Cortex* 18 (11), 2523-2531.

Borg, G.A. (1998). *Borg's perceived exertion and pain scales.* Champaign, IL: Human Kinetics.

Borg, G.A. (1982). Psychophysical bases of perceived exertion. *Medicine & Science in Sports & Exercise* 14 (5), 377-381

Boulevard Entertainment. (2006). *The history of Ferrari: The definitive story.* Boulevard Entertainment Ltd.

Burton, D. & Naylor, S. (2002). The Jekyll/Hyde nature of goals: Revisiting and updating goal setting. In: Horn, T.S. (Ed.), *Advances in sports psychology.* Champaign, IL: Human Kinetics, 459-499.

Button, K.S., Ioannidis, J.P.A., Mokrysz, C., Nosek, B.A., Flint, J., Robinson, E.S.J. & Munafò, M.R. (2013). Power failure: Why small sample size undermines the reliability of neuroscience. *Nature Reviews Neuroscience* 14, 365-376.

Carter, C.S., Braver, T.S., Barch, D.M., Botvinick, M.M., Noll, D. & Cohen, J.D. (1998). Anterior cingulate cortex, error detection, and the online monitoring of performance. *Science* 280, 747-749.

Chakalis, E. & Lowe, G. (1992). Positive effects of subliminal stimulation of memory. *Perceptual & Motor Skills* 74 (3), 956-958.

Chang, C.Y., Ke, D.S. & Chen, J.Y. (2009). Essential fatty acids and human brain. *Acta Neurologica Taiwanica* 18 (4), 231-241.

Clough, P.J., Earle, K. & Sewell, D. (2002). Mental toughness: The concept and its measurement. In: Cockerill, I. (Ed.), *Solutions in sport psychology.* London: Thomson, 32-43.

Colloca, L. & Benedetti, F. (2005). Placebos and painkillers: Is mind as real as matter? *Nature Reviews Neuroscience* 6, 545-552.

Colloca, L., Lopiano, L., Lanotte, M. & Benedetti, F. (2004). Overt versus covert treatment for pain, anxiety and Parkinson's disease. *Lancet Neurology* 3, 679-684.

Cook, H. (1985). Effects of subliminal symbiotic gratification and the magic of believing on achievement. *Psychoanalytic Psychology* 2, 365-371.

Coquart, J.B.J., Eston, R., Nycza, M., Grosboise, J-M. & Garcin, M. (2012). Estimation of maximal oxygen uptake from ratings of perceived exertion elicited during sub-maximal tests in competitive cyclists. *Archives of Medical Science* (Torino) 171, 165-172.

Crewe, H., Tucker, R. & Noakes, T.D. (2008). The rate of increase in rating of perceived exertion predicts the duration of exercise to fatigue at a fixed power output in different environmental conditions. *European Journal of Applied Physiology* 103, 569-577.

Cumming, J. & Ramsey, R. (2009). Imagery interventions in sport. In: Mellalieu, S.D. & Hanton, S. (Eds.), *Advances in applied sport psychology: A review.* Oxford: Routledge.

Davidson, R. & Schwartz, G. (1976). The psychobiology of relaxation and related states: A multiprocess theory. In: Mostofsky, D.I. (Ed.), *Behavior control and the modification of physiological activity.* New York: The Free Press, 200-233.

Davies, R.C., Rowlands, A.V. & Eston, R.G. (2008). The prediction of maximal oxygen uptake from sub-maximal ratings of perceived exertion elicited during the multistage fitness test. *British Journal of Sports Medicine* 42:, 1006-1010.

Davis, N.J. (2013). Neurodoping: Brain stimulation as a performance-enhancing measure. *Sports Medicine.* 43 (8), 649-653

DeWall, C.N., Baumeister, R.F., Stillman, T. & Gailliot, M.T. (2007). Violence restrained: Effects of self-regulatory capacity and its depletion on aggressive behavior. *Journal of Experimental Social Psychology*, 43, 62-76.

Dijksterhuis, A., Chartrand, T.L. & Aarts, H. (2005). The relation between perception and motivation. In: Bargh J.A. (Ed.), *Handbook of automaticity.* Philadelphia: Psychology Press.

Doyen, S., Klein, O., Pichon, C-L. & Cleeremans, A. (2012). Behavioral priming: It's all in the mind, but whose mind? *PLOS ONE* 7 (1), e29081. doi:10.1371/journal.pone.0029081

Edwards, A. & Polman, R. (2012). *Pacing in sport and exercise: A psychophysiological perspective. Sports and athletics preparation, performance and psychology.* New York: Nova Science.

Eston, R. (2012). Use of ratings of perceived exertion in sports. *International Journal of Sports Physiology and Performance* 7, 175-182.

Eston, R. (2012). Use of ratings of perceived exertion (RPE) in sports (invited commentary). *International Journal of Sports Physiology and Performance* 7, 175-182.

Eston, R., Evans, H., Faulkner, J., Lambrick, D., Al-Rahamneh, H. & Parfitt G. A. (2012). Perceptually regulated, graded exercise test predicts peak oxygen uptake during treadmill exercise in active and sedentary participants. *European Journal of Applied Physiology.* doi:10.1007/s00421-012-2326-8

Eston, R., Stansfield, R., Westoby, P. & Parfitt, G. (2012). Effect of deception and expected exercise duration on psychological and physiological variables during treadmill running and cycling. *Psychophysiology* 49, 462-469.

Faulkner, J., Parfitt, G. & Eston, R. (2008). The rating of perceived exertion during competitive running scales with time. *Psychophysiology* 45, 977-985.

Fitzgerald, C.T. & Carter, L.P. (2012). Possible role for glutamic acid decarboxylase in fibromyalgia symptoms: A conceptual model for chronic pain. *Medical Hypotheses* 77, 409-415.

Gailliot, M.T., Peruche, B.M., Plant., E.A. & Baumeister, R.F. (2009). Stereotypes and prejudice in the blood: Sucrose drinks reduce prejudice and stereotyping. *Journal of Experimental Social Psychology* 45, 288-290.

Gardner, F.L. & Moore, Z.E. (2006). *Clinical sport psychology.* Champaign, IL: Human Kinetics.

Goode, K.T. & Roth, D.L. (1993). Factor analysis of cognitions during running: Association with mood change. *Journal of Sport and Exercise Psychology* 15, 375-389.

Hagger, M.S., Wood, C., Stiff, C. & Chatzisarantis, N.L. (2010). Ego depletion and the strength model of self-control: A meta-analysis. *Psychological Bulletin* 136 (4), 495-525.

Hampson, D.B., St Clair Gibson, A., Lambert, M.I. & Noakes, T.D. (2001). The influence of sensory cues on the perception of exertion during exercise and central regulation of exercise performance. *Sports Medicine* 31, 935-952.

Hanin, Y.L. (1980). A study of anxiety in sports. In: Straub, W.F. (Ed.), *Sport psychology: An analysis of athlete behavior.* Ithaca, NY: Mouvement, 236-249.

Hardy, J. (2006). Speaking clearly: A critical review of the self-talk literature. *Psychology of Sport and Exercise* 7, 81-97.

Hardy, J., Oliver, E. & Tod, D. (2009). A framework for the study of self-talk in sport. In Mellalieu, S.D. & Hanton, S. (Eds.), *Advances in applied sport psychology: A review.* Oxford: Routledge.

Herbert, R. & Gandevia, S. (1996). Muscle activation in unilateral and bilateral efforts assessed by motor nerve and cortical stimulation. 80, 1351–1356.

Hill, A.V., Long, C.N.H. & Lupton, H. (1924). Muscular exercise, lactic acid, and the supply and utilisation of oxygen. *Proceedings of the Royal Society B: Biological Sciences* 96 (679), 438.

Hilty, L., Jancke, L., Luechinger, R., Boutellier, U. & Lutz, K. (2011a). Limitation of physical performance in a muscle fatiguing hand grip exercise is mediated by thalamo-insular activity. *Human Brain Mapping* 32, 2151-2160.

Hilty, L., Langer, N., Pascual-Marqui, R., Boutellier, U. & Lutz, K. (2011b). Fatigue-induced increase in intra-cortical communication between mid/anterior insular and motor cortex during cycling exercise. *European Journal of Neuroscience* 34, 2035-2042.

Holmes P.S. & Collins, D.J. (2001). The PETTLEP approach to motor imagery: A functional equivalence model for sport psychologists. *Journal of Applied Sport Psychology* 13, 60-83.

Horstman, D.H., Morgan, W.P., Cymerman, A. & Stokes, J. (1979). Perception of effort during constant work to self-imposed exhaustion. *Perceptual Motor Skills* 48 (3 Part 2): 1111-1126.

Jacobson, E. (1930). Action currents from muscular contractions during conscious. *American Journal of Physiology* 91, 567-608.

Johnson, B.D., Joseph, T., Wright, G., Battista, R.A., Dodge, C., Balweg, A., de Koning, J.J., & Foster, C. (2009). Rapidity of responding to a hypoxic challenge during exercise. European *Journal of Applied Physiology*, 106, 493-499.

Karlsson, A.K.(1999). Autonomic dysreflexia. *Spinal Cord*, 37 (6), 383-391.

Kingston, K. & Wilson, K. (2009). The application of goal setting in sport. In: Mellalieu, S. & Hanton, S. (Eds.), *Advances in applied sport psychology: A review.* Oxford: Routledge.

Kingston, K. & Wilson, K. (2009). The application of goal setting in sport. In: Mellalieu, S. & Hanton S. (Eds.), *Literature reviews in applied sport psychology.* NY: Routledge.

Kirsch, I. & Sapirstein, G. (1998). Listening to Prozac but hearing placebo: A meta-analysis of antidepressant medication. *Prevention and treatment*, vol. I, article 0002a, available at http://journals.apa.org/prevention/volume1/pre0010002a.html

Levine, J.D., Gordon, N.C. & Fields, H.L. (1978). The mechanisms of placebo analgesia. *Lancet* 2, 654-657.

Liebert, R.M. & Morris, L.W. (1967). Cognitive and emotional components of test anxiety: A distinction and some initial data. *Psychological Reports* 20 (3), 975-978.

Locke, E.A., Shaw, K.N., Saari, L.M. & Latham, G.P. (1981). Goal setting and task performance: 1969, 1980. *Psychological Bulletin* 90, 125-152.

Lopresti, A.L., Hood, S.D. & Drummond, P.D. (2013). A review of lifestyle factors that contribute to important pathways associated with major depression: Diet, sleep and exercise. *Journal of Affective Disorders* 148 (1), 12-27.

Magnay, J. (2012, June 24). Paralympics 2012: Athletes warned about the dangers of self-harming to boost performance. *The Telegraph*.

Marcora, S.M. & Staiano, W. (2010). The limit to exercise tolerance in humans: Mind over muscle? *European Journal of Applied Physiology* 109 (4), 763-770.

Marcora, S.M., Staiano, W. & Manning, V. (2009). Mental fatigue impairs physical performance in humans. *Journal of Applied Physiology* 106 (3), 857-864.

Marsh, D.R. & Weaver, L.C. (2004). Autonomic dysreflexia, induced by noxious or innocuous stimulation, does not depend on changes in dorsal horn substance. *Journal of Neurotrauma* 21 (6), 817-828.

Martin, J.J., Craib, M. & Mitchell, V. (1995). The relationships of anxiety and self-attention to running economy in competitive male distance runners. *Journal of Sports Science* 13 (5), 371-376.

Martin, V. (2012). The motivational versus metabolic effects of carbohydrates on self-control. *Psychological Science* 23, 1130-1137.

Masters, K.S. & Ogles, B.M. (1998). Cognitive strategies relate to injury, motivation, and performance among marathon runners: Results from two studies. *Journal of Applied Sport Psychology* 10, 281-296.

Mehta, J.P., Verber, M.D., Wieser, J.A., Schmit, B.D. & Schindler-Ivens, S.M. (2009). A novel technique for examining human brain activity associated with pedaling using fMRI. *Journal of Neuroscience Methods* 179 (2), 230-239.

Merton, P. (1954). Voluntary strength and fatigue. *Journal of Physiology* 123, 553-564.

Molden, D.C., Hui, C.M., Noreen, E.E., Meier, B.P., Scholer, A.A., D'Agostino, P.R. &Morgan, W.P. (1978, April). The mind of the marathoner. *Psychology Today*, pp. 38-40, 43, 45-46, 49.

Molden, D.C., Hui, C.M., Noreen, E.E., Meler, B.P., Scholer, A.A., D'Agostino, P.R., & Martin, V. (2012). The motivational versus metabolic effects of carbohydrates on self-control. *Psychological Science*, 23(10), 1130-1137.

Morgan, W.P. & Pollock, M.L. (1977). Psychologic characterization of the elite distance runner. *Annals of the New York Academy of Sciences* 301, 382-403.

Murphy, S.M., Nordin, S.M. & Cumming, J. (2008). Imagery in sport, exercise and dance. In: Horn, T. (Ed.), *Advances in sport psychology*, 3rd ed. Champaign, IL: Human Kinetics, 297-324.

Noakes, T.D. (1997). 1996 J.B. Wolffe Memorial Lecture. Challenging beliefs: Ex Africa semper aliquid novi. *Medicine & Science in Sports & Exercise* 29 (5), 571-590.

Noakes, T.D. (2012). Time to move beyond a brainless exercise physiology: The evidence for complex regulation of human exercise performance. *Applied Physiology, Nutrition, and Metabolism* 36, 23-35.

Okano, A.H., Fontes, E.B., Montenegro, R.A., Farinatti, P., Cyrino, E.S., Li, L.M. Bikson, M. & Noakes, T. (2013). Brain stimulation modulates the autonomic nervous system, rating of perceived exertion and performance during maximal exercise. British Journal of Sports Medicine. Doi: 10.1136/bjsports-2012-091658

Painelli, V.S., Nicastro, H. & Lancha, A.H. Jr. (2010). Carbohydrate mouth rinse: Does it improve endurance exercise performance? *Nutrition Journal* 9, 33.

Parfitt, G., Evans, H. & Eston, R.G. (2012). Perceptually-regulated training at RPE13 is pleasant and improves physical health. *Medicine & Science in Sports & Exercise* 44, 1613-1618.

Parker, K.A. (1982). Effects of subliminal symbiotic stimulation on academic performance: Further evidence on the adaptation-enhancing effects of oneness fantasies. *Journal of Counseling Psychology* 29 (1), 19-28.

Paul, M., Gargh K. & Sandhu, J.D. (2012). Role of biofeedback in optimizing psychomotor performance in sports. *Asian Journal of Sports Medicine* 3 (1), 29-40.

Paulus, M.P., Flagan, T., Simmons, A.N., Gillis, K., Kotturi, S., Thom, N., Johnson, D.C., VanOrden, K.F., Davenport, P.W. & Swain, J.L. (2011). Subjecting elite athletes to inspiratory breathing load reveals behavioural and neural signatures of optimal performers in extreme environments. *PLOS ONE* 7, e29394. doi:10.1371/journal.pone.0029394

Pires, F.O., Lima-Silva, A.E., Bertuzzi, R., Casarini, D.H., Kiss, M.A., Lambert, M.I. & Noakes, T.D. (2011). The influence of peripheral afferent signals on the rating of perceived exertion and time to exhaustion during exercise at different intensities. *Psychophysiology* 48, 1284-1290.

Rasmussen, P., Stie, H., Nybo, L. & Nielsen, B. (2004). Heat induced fatigue and changes of the EEG is not related to reduced perfusion of the brain during prolonged exercise in humans. *Journal of Thermal Biology* 29, 731-737.

Reeve, J. (2009). *Understanding motivation and emotion* (5th ed.). Hoboken, NJ: Wiley.

Schomer, H.H. (1987). Mental strategy training programme for marathon runners. *International Journal of Sport Psychology* 18, 133-151.

Shabbir, F., Patel, A., Mattison, C., Bose, S., Krishnamohan, R., Sweeney, E., Sandhu, S., Nel, W., Rais, A., Sandhu, R., Ngu, N. & Sharma S. (2013). Effects of diet on serotonergic neurotransmission in depression. *Neurochemistry International* 62, 324-329.

Sloniger, M.A., Cureton, K.J., Prior, B.M. & Evans, E.M. (1997a). Anaerobic capacity and muscle activation during horizontal and uphill running. *Journal of Applied Physiology* 83, 262-269.

Sloniger, M.A., Cureton, K.J., Prior, B.M. & Evans, E.M. (1997b). Lower extremity muscle activation during horizontal and uphill running. *Journal of Applied Physiology* 83, 2073-2079.

Suinn, R.M. (1980). Psychology and sports performance: Principles and applications. In: Suinn, R. (Ed.), *Psychology in sports: Methods and applications*. Minneapolis, MN: Burgess International, 26-36.

Swart, J., Lamberts, R.P., Lambert, M.I., Lambert, E.V., Woolrich, R.W., Johnston, S. & Noakes, T.D. (2009). Exercising with reserve: Exercise regulation by perceived exertion in relation to duration of exercise and knowledge of endpoint. *British Journal of Sports Medicine* 43, 775-781.

Tammen, V.V. (1996). Elite middle and long distance runners associative/dissociative coping. *Journal of Applied Sport Psychology* 8, 1-8.

Tanaka, M. & Watanabe, Y. (2012). Supra spinal regulation of physical fatigue. *Neuroscience & Biobehavioral Reviews* 36, 727-734.

Tucker, R. (2009). The anticipatory regulation of performance: The physiological basis for pacing strategies and the development of a perception-based model for exercise performance. *British Journal of Sports Medicine* 43, 392-400.

Tucker, R., Rauch, L.H., Harley, Y.X.R. & Noakes, T.D. (2004). Impaired exercise performance in the heat is associated with an anticipatory reduction in skeletal muscle recruitment. *Pflügers Archiv: European Journal of Physiology* 448, 422-430.

Valles, M., Benito, J., Portell, E. & Vidal, J. (2005). Cerebral hemorrhage due to autonomic dysreflexia in a spinal cord injury patient. *Spinal Cord* 43, 738-740.

Vogt, W. (1999). *Breaking the chain: Drugs and cycling, The true story* (trans. William Fotheringham). London: Random House/Yellow Jersey Press.

Williamson, J.W., Fadel, P.J. & Mitchell, J.H. (2006). New insights into central cardiovascular control during exercise in humans: A central command update. *Experimental Physiology* 91, 51-58.

Yerkes, R.M. & Dodson, J.D. (1908). The relation of strength of stimulus to rapidity of habit formation. *Journal of Comparative Neurology and Psychology* 18, 459-482.

Chapter 5

Abbiss, C.R. & Laursen, P.B. (2008). Describing and understanding pacing strategies during athletic competition. *Sports Medicine* 38, 239-252.

Aisbett, B., Le Rossignol, P., McConell, G., Abbiss, C. & Snow, R. (2009). Influence of all-out and fast start on 5-min cycling time trial performance. *Medicine & Science in Sports & Exercise* 41 (10), 1965-1971.

Atkinson, G. & Brunskill, A. (2000). Pacing strategies during a cycling time trial with simulated headwinds and tailwinds. *Ergonomics* 43 (10), 1449-1460.

Balsom, P.D., Gaitanos, G.C., Soderlund, K. & Ekblom, B. (1999). High-intensity exercise and muscle glycogen availability in humans. *Acta Physiologica Scandanavia* 165, 337-345.

Bemben, M.G. & Lamont, H.S. (2005). Creatine supplementation and exercise performance: recent findings. *Sports Medicine* 35 (2), 107-125.

Burnley, M., Doust, J.H. & Jones, A.M. (2005). Effects of prior warm-up regime on severe-intensity cycling performance. *Medicine & Science in Sports & Exercise* 37, 838-845.

Burnley, M. & Jones, A.M. (2007). Oxygen uptake kinetics as a determinant of sports performance. *European Journal of Sport Science* 7 (2), 63-79.

Cangley, P., Passfield, L., Carter, H. & Bailey, M. (2010). The effect of variable gradients on pacing in cycling time-trials. *International Journal of Sports Medicine* 32, 132-136.

Carr, A.J., Gore, C.J. & Dawson, B. (2011). Induced alkalosis and caffeine supplementation: Effects on 2,000-m rowing performance. *International Journal of Sport Nutrition and Exercise Metabolism* 21 (5), 357-364.

Carr, A.J., Hopkins, W.G. & Gore, C.J. (2011). Effects of acute alkalosis and acidosis on performance: A meta-analysis. *Sports Medicine* 41 (10), 801-814.

Christensen, E.H. (1939). Untersuchungen uber die Verbrennungsvorgange bei langdauernder, scwherer Muskelarbeit. *Skandinavisches Archiv für Physiologie* 81, 152-161.

Coyle, E.F. (1995). Integration of the physiological factors determining endurance performance ability. *Exercise and Sport Sciences Reviews* 23, 25-63.

Coyle, E.F., Coggan, A.R., Hemmert, M.K. & Ivy, J.L. (1986). Muscle glycogen utilization during prolonged strenuous exercise when fed carbohydrate. *Journal of Applied Physiology* 61, 165-172.

Coyle, E.F., Coggan, A.R., Hopper, M. & Walters, T.J. (1988). Determinants of endurance in well-trained cyclists. *Journal of Applied Physiology* 64, 2622-2630.

Coyle, E.F., Hagberg, J.M., Hurley, B.F., Martin, W.H., Ehsani, A.A. & Holloszy, J.O. (1983). Carbohydrate feeding during prolonged strenuous exercise can delay fatigue. *Journal of Applied Physiology* 55, 230-235.

de Koning, J.J., Bobbert, M.F. & Foster C. (1999). Determination of optimal pacing strategy in track cycling with an energy flow model. *Journal of Science and Medicine in Sport* 2 (3), 266-277.

de Koning, J.J., Foster, C., Bakkum, A., Kloppenburg, S., Thiel, C., Joseph, T., Cohen, J. & Porcari, J.P. (2011). Regulation of pacing strategy during athletic competition. *PLOS ONE* 6 (1), e15863.

Ely, M.R., Cheuvront, S.N., Roberts, W.O. & Montain, S.J. (2007). Impact of weather on marathon-running performance. *Medicine & Science in Sports & Exercise* 39, 487-493.

Foster, C. & Daniels, J. (1975). Running by the numbers. *Runner's World* 10, 14-17.

Foster, C., de Koning, J.J., Bischel, S., Casolino, E., Malterer, K., O'Brien, K., Rodríguez-Marroyo, J., Splinter, A., Thiel, C. & Van Tunen, J. (2012). Pacing strategies for endurance performance. In I. Mujika (Ed.), *Endurance Training – Science and Practice* (pp. 85-98). Vitoria-Gasteiz, Basque Country: Iñigo Mujika S.L.U.

Foster, C., Schrager, M., Snyder, A.C. & Thompson, N.N. (1994). Pacing strategy and athletic performance. *Sports Medicine* 17 (2), 77-85.

Foster, C., Snyder, A.C., Thompson, N.N., Green, M.A., Foley, M. & Schrager, M. (1993). Effect of pacing strategy on cycle time trial performance. *Medicine & Science in Sports and Exercise* 25, 383-388.

Foster, C., de Koning, J.J., Hettinga, F., Lampen, J., La Clair, K.L., Dodge, C., Bobbert, M., Porcari, J.P. (2003) Pattern of energy expenditure during simulated competition. *Medicine and Science in Sports and Exercise* 35, 826-831.

Galloway, S.D.R. & Maughan, R.J. (1997). Effects of ambient temperature on the capacity to perform prolonged cycle exercise in man. *Medicine & Science in Sports & Exercise* 29, 1240-1249.

Hargreaves, M. (2008). Physiological limits to exercise performance in the heat. *Journal of Science and Medicine in Sport* 11 (1), 66-71.

Hulleman, M., de Koning, J.J., Hettinga, F. & Foster, C. (2007). The effect of intrinsic motivation on cycle time trial performance. *Medicine & Science in Sports & Exercise* 39 (4), 709-715.

Jones, A.M. & Burnley, M. (2009). Oxygen uptake kinetics: An underappreciated determinant of exercise performance. *International Journal of Sports Physiology and Performance* 4, 524-532.

Jones, A.M., Wilkerson, D.P., Vanhatalo, A. & Burnley, M. (2008). Influence of pacing strategy on O$_2$ uptake and exercise tolerance. *Scandinavian Journal of Medicine & Science in Sports* 18, 615-626.

Joyner, M.J. & Coyle, E.F. (2008). Endurance exercise performance, the physiology of champions. *Journal of Physiology* 586, 35-44.

Karatzaferi, C., de Haan, A., van Mechelen, W. & Sargeant, A.J. (2001). Metabolism changes in single human fibres during brief maximal exercise. *Experimental Physiology* 86, 411-415.

Karlsson, J. & Saltin, B. (1971). Diet, muscle glycogen, and endurance performance. *Journal of Applied Physiology* 31 (2), 203-206.

Keller, J.B. (1974). Optimal velocity in a race. *American Mathematical Monthly* 81 (5), 475-480.

Lambert, M.I., Dugas, J.P., Kirkman, M.C., Mokone., G.G. & Waldeck, M.R. (2004). Changes in running speeds in a 100 km ultramarathon race. *Journal of Sports Science and Medicine* 3, 167-173.

Lemon, P.W. (2002). Dietary creatine supplementation and exercise performance: Why inconsistent results? *Canadian Journal of Applied Physiology* 27 (6), 663-681.

Levels, K., Teunissen, L.P.J., de Haan, A., de Koning, J.J., van Os, B. & Daanen, H.A.N. (2013). Effect of warm-up and pre-cooling on pacing during a 15-km cycling time trial in the heat. *International Journal of Sports Physiology and Performance* 8, 307-311.

Nicol, C., Komi, P.V. & Marconnet, P. (1991). Fatigue effects of marathon running on neuromuscular performances. I. Changes in muscle force and stiffness characteristics. *Scandinavian Journal of Medicine & Science in Sports* 1, 10-17.

Padilla, S., Mujika, I., Angulo, F. & Goiriena, J.J. (2000). Scientific approach to the 1-h cycling world record: A case study. *Journal of Applied Physiology* 89, 1522-1527.

Sargeant, A.J. (2009). Structural and functional determinants of human muscle power. *Experimental Physiology* 92 (2), 323-331.

Sherman, W.M. & Costill, D.L. (1984). The marathon: Dietary manipulation to optimize performance. *American Journal of Sports Medicine* 12, 44-51.

Skiba, P.F., Weerapong, C., Vanhatalo, A. & Jones, A.M. (2012). Modeling the expenditure and reconstitution of work capacity above critical power. *Medicine & Science in Sports & Exercise* 44 (8), 1526-1532.

Sporer, B. & McKenzie, D.C. (2007). Reproducibility of a laboratory based 20-km time trial evaluation in competitive cyclists using the velotron pro ergometer. *International Journal of Sports Medicine* 28 (11), 940-944.

St Clair Gibson, A., de Koning, J.J., Thompson, K.G., Roberts, W.O., Micklewright, D., Raglin, J. & Foster, C. (2013). Crawling to the finish line: Why do endurance runners collapse? Implications for understanding of mechanisms underlying pacing and fatigue. *Sports Medicine*, 43 (6), 413-424.

Stevenson, R. & Thompson, K.G. (2002). Hypohydration, heat and 4000m cycling performance. *Journal of Human Movement Studies* 43 (5), 363-375.

Stone, M.R. (2012). Effects of deception on exercise performance: Implications for determinants of fatigue, PhD thesis, Northumbria University, UK.

Stone, M.R., Thomas, K., Wilkinson, M., Jones, A.M., St Clair Gibson., A. & Thompson, K.G. (2012). Effects of deception on exercise performance: Implications for determinants of fatigue in humans. *Medicine & Science in Sports & Exercise* 44 (3), 534-541.

Swain, D.P. (1997). A model for optimizing cycling performance by varying power on hills and in wind. *Medicine & Science in Sports & Exercise* 29 (8), 1104-1108.

Tatterson, A.J., Hahn, A.G., Martin, D.T. & Febbraio, M.A. (2000). Effects of heat stress on physiological responses and exercise performance in elite cyclists. *Journal of Science and Medicine in Sport* 3, 186-193.

Thompson, K.G. & Haljand, R. (2000). An analysis of selected kinematic variables in national-elite male and female 100 m and 200 m breaststroke swimmers. *Journal of Sports Sciences* 18, 421-431.

Thompson, K.G., MacLaren, D.M., Atkinson, G. & Lees, A. (2003). The effect of even, positive and negative pacing on metabolic, kinematic and temporal variables during breaststroke swimming. *European Journal of Applied Physiology* 88 (4), 438-443.

Townshend, A.D., Worringham, C. J. & Stewart, I.B. (2010). Spontaneous pacing during overground hill running. *Medicine & Science in Sports & Exercise* 42 (1), 160-169.

Trapasso, L.M. & Cooper, J.D. (1989). Record performances at the Boston Marathon: Biometeorological factors. *International Journal of Biometeorology* 33, 233-237.

Tucker, R., Lambert, M.I. & Noakes T.D. (2006). An analysis of pacing strategies during men's world-record performances in track athletics. *International Journal of Sports Physiology and Performance* 1, 233-245.

Tucker, R., Marle, T., Lambert, E.L. & Noakes, T.D. (2006). The rate of heat storage mediates an anticipatory reduction in exercise intensity during cycling at a fixed rating of perceived exertion. *Journal of Physiology* 574, 905-915.

van Ingen Schenau, G.J., de Koning, J.J. & de Groot, G. (1992). The distribution of anaerobic energy in 1000 and 4000 metre cycling bouts. *International Journal of Sports Medicine* 13 (6), 447-451.

van Ingen Schenau, G.J., de Koning, J.J. & de Groot, G. (1990). A simulation of speed skating performances based on a power equation. *Medicine & Science in Sports & Exercise* 22 (5), 718-728.

Chapter 6

Arrelano, R., Brown, P., Cappaert, J. & Nelson, R.C. (1994). Analysis of 50 m, 100 m and 200 m freestyle swimmers at the 1992 Olympic Games. *Journal of Applied Biomechanics* 10 (2), 189-199.

Chengalur, S.N. & Brown, P.L. (1992). An analysis of male and female Olympic finalists in 200 m events. *Canadian Journal of Sport Sciences* 17 (2), 104-109.

Chollet, D., Pelayo, P., Tourny, C., Sidney, M. (1996) Comparative analysis of 100 m and 200 m events in the four strokes in top level swimmers. Journal of Human Movement Studies, 31, 25-37.

Coyle, E.F., Sidossis, L.S., Horowitz, J.F. & Beltz, J.D. (1992). Cycling efficiency is related to the percentage of type 1 fibres. *Medicine & Science in Sports & Exercise* 24, 782-788.

Craig, A. and Pendergast, D.R. (1979) Relationships of stroke rate, distance per stroke and velocity in competitive swimming. *Medicine and Science in Sports and Exercise*, 11, 278-283.

D'Aquisto, L.J., Costill, D.L., Gehlson, G.M., Wong-Tai Young, M.A. & Lee, G. (1988). Breaststroke economy, skill and performance: A study of the breaststroke mechanics using a computer based 'velocity-video' system. *Journal of Swimming Research* 4 (2), 9-13.

Holmer, I. (1974a). Energy cost of arm stroke, leg kick and whole stroke in competitive swimming style. *European Journal of Applied Physiology* 33, 105-118.

Holmer, I. (1974b). Propulsive efficiency of breaststroke and freestyle swimming. *European Journal of Applied Physiology* 33, 95-103.

Kennedy, P., Brown, P., Changalur, S.N., Nelson, R.C. (1990) Analysis of male and female Olym-

pic swimmers in the 100 m events. *International Journal of Biomechanics*, 6(2), 187-197.

Keskinen, K.L. (1997a). Reliability of pool testing: Ability of swimmers to swim at predetermined speeds. In *Proceedings of the XVI Congress of the International Society of Biomechanics*, p. 155. Tokyo: University of Tokyo.

Keskinen, K.L. (1997b). Test-retest reliability of pool testing method in swimmers. In *Proceedings of the 2nd Annual Congress of the European College of Sport Sciences, Book of Abstracts 1*, pp. 324-325. Copenhagen: University of Copenhagen.

Lijestrand, G. and Lindhard, J. (1919) Uber das Minutenvolumen des Herzens beim Schwimmen. *Skandinavisches Archiv fur Physiologie*, 39, 64-77.

Lijestrand, G. and Strenstrom, M. (1919) Studien uber die Physiologie des Schwimmens. *Skandinavisches Archiv fur Physiologie*, 39, 1-63.

Madsen, O. and Lohberg, M. (1987) Lowdown on lactates. Swimming Technique, 24(1), 21-24.

Maglischo, E.W. (1993) Swimming even faster. Moutain View, California: Mayfield Publishing Company. 601-614.

Martin, L., Nevill, A.M. & Thompson, K.G. (2007). Diurnal variation in swim performance remains, irrespective of once or twice daily training. *International Journal of Sports Physiology and Performance*. 2, 192-200.

Martin, L. & Thompson, K.G. (1999). Diurnal variation in physiological and kinematic responses to sub maximal swimming. In *Proceedings of the 4th Annual Congress of the European College of Sport Science* (edited by P. Parisi, F. Pigozzi and G. Prinzi), p. 540. Rome: Rome University institute of Motor Sciences.

Martin, L. & Thompson, K.G. (2000). Reproducibility of diurnal variation in swimming. *International Journal of Sports Medicine* 21, 387-392.

Mauger, A.R., Neuloh, J. & Castle, P.C. (2012). Analysis of pacing strategy selection in elite 400 m freestyle swimming. *Medicine & Science in Sports & Exercise*, 44(11), 2205-12.

Pendergast, D.R., Di Prampero, P.E., Craig, A.B. Jr. & Rennie, D.W. (1978). The influence of selected biomechanical factors on the energy cost of swimming. In: Eriksson, B.O. & Furberg, B. (Eds.), *Swimming medicine IV*. Baltimore, MD: University Park Press, 367-378.

Pyne, D.B., Trewin, C.B. & Hopkins, W.G. (2004). Progression and variability of competitive performance of Olympic swimmers. *Journal of Sports Sciences* 22, 613-620.

Robertson, E., Pyne, D., Hopkins, W. & Anson, J. (2009). Analysis of lap times in international swimming competitions. *Journal of Sports Sciences*, 1-9.

Sano, S., Bongbele, J., Chatard, J.C. & Lavoie, J.M. (1990). Evaluation of the maximal aerobic velocity and prediction of performance in backstroke. In: MacLaren, D.P., Reilly, T. & Lees, A. (Eds.), *Biomechanics and medicine in swimming: Swimming science VI* . London: E&F Spon, 285-288.

Skorski, A., Faude, O., Caviezel, S. & Meyer, T. (2013a). Reproducibility of competition pacing profiles in elite swimmers. *International Journal of Sports Physiology and Performance*. 9(2), 217-225.

Skorski, A., Faude, O., Rausch, K. & Meyer, T. (2013b). Reproducibility of pacing profiles in competitive swimmers. *International Journal of Sports Medicine* 34, 152-157.

Stewart, A.M. & Hopkins, W. (2000). Consistency of swimming performance within and between competitions. *Medicine & Science in Sports & Exercise* 32, 997-1001.

Swaine, I. and Reilly, T. (1983) The freely chosen stroke rate in a maximal swim on a biokientic swimbench. *Medicine and Science in Sports and Exercise*, 15(5), 37—375.

Thompson, K.G. & Cooper, S. (2002). Breaststroke performance, selected physiological variables and stroke rate. *Journal of Human Movement Studies* 44 (1), 001-017.

Thompson, K.G. & Garland, S. (2009). Assessment of an international breaststroke swimmer using a race readiness test. *International Journal of Sport Physiology and Performance* 4 (1), 139-143.

Thompson, K.G., Garland, S. & Lothian, F. (2006a). Assessment of an international breaststroke swimmer using the 7 \x\ 200 m step test. *International Journal of Sports Physiology and Performance* 1, 172-175.

Thompson, K.G. Garland, S. & Lothian, F. (2006b). Interpretations from the physiological monitoring of an international swimmer. *International Journal of Sports Science and Coaching* 2 (1), 117-124.

Thompson, K.G. & Haljand, R. (1997a, November). The secrets of competition breaststroke swimming. *Swimming Times*. 26-28.

Thompson, K.G. & Haljand, R. (1997b, December). The secrets of competition butterfly swimming. *Swimming Times*.

Thompson, K.G. & Haljand, R. (2000). An analysis of selected kinematic variables in national-elite male and female 100 m and 200 m breaststroke swimmers. *Journal of Sports Sciences* 18, 421-431.

Thompson, K.G., Haljand, R., Cooper S.M. & Palfrey, L. (2000). The relative importance of selected kinematic variables in swimming performance in elite male and elite female 100 m and 200 m breaststroke swimmers. *Journal of Human Movement Studies* 39, 15-32.

Thompson, K.G., Haljand, R. & Lindley, M. (2004). A comparison of selected kinematic variables between races in national to elite male 200 m breaststroke swimmers. *Journal of Swimming Research* 16, 6-10.

Thompson, K.G., Harrison, A., Dietzig, B. & Cosgrove, M. (2006). Physiological responses to bouts of high intensity exercise two hours apart. *Journal of Human Movement Studies* 51, 77-88.

Thompson, K.G., MacLaren, D.M., Atkinson, G. & Lees, A. (2002). Accuracy of pacing during breaststroke swimming: Using a novel pacing device the Aquapacer. *Journal of Sports Sciences* 20, 537-546.

Thompson, K.G., MacLaren, D.M., Atkinson, G. & Lees, A. (2003). The effect of even, positive and negative pacing metabolic, kinematic and temporal parameters during breaststroke swimming. *European Journal of Applied Physiology* 88 (4-5), 438-443.

Thompson, K.G., MacLaren, D.M., Atkinson, G. & Lees, A. (2004a). The effect of pace manipulation on metabolic, kinematic and temporal variables during breaststroke swimming. *Journal of Sports Sciences* 22 (2), 149-157.

Thompson, K.G., MacLaren, D.M., Atkinson, G. & Lees, A. (2004b). Reliability of metabolic and kinematic responses during breaststroke swimming. *Journal of Human Movement Studies* 46 (1), 35-54.

Thompson, K.G., St Clair Gibson, A. & Howatson, G. (2009). The effect of changing stroke rate during breaststroke swimming. Presentation at American College of Sports Medicine annual congress, 2nd - 5th June, Baltimore, USA.

Vescovi, J. D., Falenchuk, O. Wells, G. D. (2010). Blood lactate concentration and clearance in elite swimmers during competition. In Kjendlie, P-L., Stallman, R-K., & Cabri, J. (Eds.). Biomechanics and Medicine in Swimming XI. (p. 233-235), Norwegian School of Sports Science, Oslo, Norway: Nordbergtrykkas.

Wakayoshi, K., Nomura, T., Takahashi, G., Mutoh, Y. & Miyashito, M. (1992). Analysis of swimming races in the 1989 Pan Pacific Swimming Championships and Japanese 1988 Olympic Trials. In: MacLaren, D., Reilly, T. & Lees, A. (Eds.), *Biomechanics and medicine in swimming VI*. London: E&F Spon, 135-144.

Chapter 7

Abbiss, C.R., Burnett, A., Nosaka, K., Green, J.P., Foster, J.K. & Laursen, P.B. (2010). Effect of hot versus cold climates on power output, muscle activation, and perceived fatigue during a dynamic 100-km cycling trial. *Journal of Sports Sciences* 28 (2), 117-125.

Atkinson, G., Peacock, O. & Passfield, L. (2007). Variable versus constant power strategies during cycling time trials: Prediction of time savings using an up-to-date mathematical model. *Journal of Sports Sciences* 25, 1001-1009

Atkinson, G., Peacock, O., St Clair Gibson, A. & Tucker, R. (2007). Distribution of power output during cycling. *Sports Medicine* 37 (8), 647-667.

Bassett, D.R., Kyle, C.R., Passfield, L., Broker J., Burke, E.R. (1999). Comparing cycling world hour records, 1967, 1996: modeling with empirical data. *Medicine and Science in Sports and Exercise* 31: 1665-1676.

Broker, J.P., Kyle, C.R. & Burke, E.L. (1999). Racing cyclist power requirements in the individual and team Pursuits. *Medicine & Science in Sports & Exercise* 31, 1677-1685.

Cherry, P.W., Lakomy, H.K.A., Nevill, M.E. & Fletcher, R.J. (1997). Constant work cycle exercise: The performance and metabolic effects of all-out and even-paced strategies. *European Journal of Applied Physiology* 75, 22-27.

Corbett, J. (2009). An analysis of the pacing strategies adopted by elite athletes during track cycling. *International Journal of Sports Physiology and Performance* 4, 195-205.

Craig, N.P. and Norton, K.I. (2001). Characteristics of track cycling. *Sports Medicine* 31: 457-468.

de Koning, J.J., Bobbert, M.F. & Foster, C. (1999). Determination of optimal pacing strategy in track cycling with an energy flow model. *Journal of Science and Medicine in Sport* 2 (3), 266-277.

de Koning J.J., Foster C., Lampen J., Hettinga F., Bobbert M.F. (2005). Experimental evaluation of the power balance model of speed skating. *Journal of Applied Physiology* 98: 227-233.

Earnest, C.P., Foster, C., Hoyos, J., Muniesa, C.A., Santalla, A. & Lucia, A. (2009). Time trial exertion traits of cycling's grand tours. *International Journal of Sports Medicine* 30, 240-244.

Ebert, T.R., Martin, D.T., Stephens, B. & Withers, R.T. (2006). Power output during a professional men's road-cycling tour. *International Journal of Sport Physiology and Performance* 1, 324-335.

Fernandez-Garcia, B., Perez-Landaluce, J., Rodriguez-Alonso, M. & Terrados, N. (2000). Intensity of exercise during road cycling pro-cycling competition. *Medicine & Science in Sports & Exercise* 32 (5), 1002-1006.

Foster, C., De Koning, J.J., Bischel, S., Casolino, E., Malterer, K., O'Brien, K., Rodríguez-Marroyo, J., Splinter, A., Thiel, C. & Van Tunen, J. (2012). Pacing strategies for endurance perfor-mance. In I. Mujika (Ed.), *Endurance Training – Science and Practice* (pp. 85-98). Vitoria-Gasteiz, Basque Country: Iñigo Mujika S.L.U.

Foster C., de Koning J.J., Hettinga F., Lampen F., Dodge C., Bobbert M., Porcari J.P. (2004). Effect of competitive distance on energy expenditure during simulated competition. *International Journal of Sports Medicine* 25: 198-204.

Gardner, S.A., Martin, J.C., Martin, D.T., Barras, M. & Jenkins, D.G. (2007). Maximal torque- and power-pedalling rate relationships for elite sprint cyclists in laboratory and field tests. *European Journal of Applied Physiology* 101, 287-292.

Gotshall, R.W., Bauer, T.A. & Fahrner, S.L. (1996). Cycling cadence alters exercise hemodynamics. *International Journal of Sports Medicine* 17 (1), 17-21.

Jeukendrup, A.E. & Martin, J. (2001). Improving cycling performance: How should we spend our time and money. *Sports Medicine* 31 (7), 559-569.

Jeukendrup A.E., Craig N.P., Hawley J.A. (2000). The bioenergetics of world class cycling. *Journal of Science and Medicine in Sport* 3: 414-433.

Joseph T., Johnson B., Battista R.A., Wright G., Dodge C., Porcari J.P., de Koning J.J., Foster C. (2008). Perception of fatigue during simulated competition. *Medicine and Science in Sports and Exercise* 40: 381-386.

Kyle, C.R. (1996). Selecting cycling equipment. In: Burke, E. (Ed.), *High-tech cycling*. Champaign, IL: Human Kinetics, 1-43.

Lucia, A., Earnest, C. & Arribas, C. (2003). The Tour de France: A physiological review. *Scandinavian Journal of Medicine and Science in Sports* 13 (5), 275-283.

Lucia, A., Hoyos, J., Carvajal, A. & Chicharro, J.L. (1999). Heart rate response to professional road cycling: The Tour de France. *International Journal of Sports Medicine* 20 (3), 167-172.

Lucia, A., Hoyos, J. & Chicharro, J.L. (2000). Physiological response to professional road cycling: Climbers vs. time-trialists. *International Journal of Sports Medicine* 21 (7), 505-512.

Lucia, A., Hoyos, J. & Chicharro, J.L. (2001). Preferred pedalling cadence in professional cycling. *Medicine & Science in Sports & Exercise* 33 (8), 1361-1366.

Lucia, A., Hoyos, J., Santalla, A., Perez, M. & Chicharro, J.L. (2002). Kinetics of $\dot{V}O_2$ in professional cyclists. *Medicine & Science in Sports & Exercise* 34, 320-325

Mauger, A.R., Jones, A.M. & Williams, C.A. (2011). The effect of non-contingent and accurate performance feedback on pacing and time trial performance in 4-km track cycling. *British Journal of Sports Medicine* 45, 225-229.

Moritani, T. (2002) Changes in blood volume and oxygenation level in a working muscle during a crank cycle. *Medicine & Science in Sports & Exercise* 34 (3), 520-528.

Mujika, I. & Padilla, S. (2001). Physiological and performance characteristics of male professional road cyclists. *Sports Medicine* 31 (7), 479-487.

Noakes T.D., Lambert M.I., Hauman R. (2009). Which lap is slowest? An analysis of 32 world mile record performances. *British Journal of Sports Medicine* 43: 760-764.

Padilla, S., Mujika, I., Angulo, F. & Goirena, J.J. (2000). Scientific approach to the 1-h cycling world record: A case study. *Journal of Applied Physiology* 89 (4), 1522-1527.

Padilla, S., Mujika, I., Cuesta, G. & Goiriena, J.J. (1999). Level ground and uphill cycling ability in professional road cycling. *Medicine & Science in Sports & Exercise* 31 (6), 878-885.

Padilla, S., Mujika, I., Orbananos, J. & Angulo, F. (2000). Exercise intensity during competition time trials in professional road cycling. *Medicine & Science in Sports & Exercise* 32 (4), 850-856.

Padilla, S., Mujika, I., Santisteban, J., Impellizzeria, F.M. & Goirena, J.J. (2008) Exercise intensity and load during uphill cycling in professional 3-week races. *European Journal of Applied Physiology* 102 (4), 431-438.

Palmer, G.S, Hawley, J.A., Dennis, S.C et al. (1994). Heart rate responses during a 4 d cycle race. *Medicine & Science in Sports & Exercise* 26, 1278-1283.

Renfree, A., West, J., Corbett, M., Rhoden, C. & St Clair Gibson, A. (2012).Complex interplay between determinants of pacing and performance during 20-km time trials. *International Journal of Sports Physiology and Performance* 7 (2), 121-129.International Journal of Sports Physiology and Performance

Santella, A., Earnest, C.P., Marroyo, J.A., Lucia, A. (2012) The Tour de France: An updated physiological review. International Journal of Sport Physiology and Performance, 7, 200-209.

Schumacher, Y.O. & Mueller, P. (2002). The 4,000-m pursuit cycling world record: Theoretical and practical aspects. *Medicine & Science in Sports & Exercise* 34 (6), 1029-1036.

Swaine, D.P. (1997). A model for optimising cycling performance by varying power on hills and in wind. *Medicine & Science in Sports & Exercise* 29, 1104-1108

Swart, J., Lamberts, R.P., Lamberts, M.I., Lambert, E.V., Woolrich, R.W., Johnston, S. & Noakes, T.D. (2009). Exercising with reserve: Exercise regulation by perceived exertion in relation to duration of exercise and knowledge of end-point. *British Journal of Sports Medicine* 43 (10), 775-781.

Takaisha, T., Sugiura, T., Katayama, K., Sato, Y., Shima, N., Yamamoto T., Moritani, T. (2002) Changes in blood volume and oxygenation level in a working muscle during a crank cycle. *Medicine & Science in Sports & Exercise* 34 (3), 520-528.

Tucker R., Marle T., Lambert E.V., Noakes T.D. (2006). The rate of heat storage mediates an anticipatory reduction in exercise intensity during cycling at a fixed rate of perceived exertion. *Journal of Physiology* 574: 905-915.

Vogt, S., Heinrich, L., Schumacher, Y.O., Blum, A., Roecker, K., Dickwuth, H-H. & Schmid, A. (2006). Power output during stage racing in professional road cycling. *Medicine & Science in Sports & Exercise* 38 (1), 147-151.

Chapter 8

Akahane, K., Kimura, T., Ah Cheng, G., Fujiwara, T., Yamamoto, I. & Hachimori, A. (2006). Relationship between balance performance and leg muscle strength in elite and non-elite junior speed skaters. *Journal of Physical Therapy Science* 18, 149-154.

Bullock, N., Martin, D.T. & Zhang, A. (2008). Performance analysis of world class short track speed skating: What does it take to win? *International Journal of Performance Analysis in Sport* 8, 9-10.

de Boer, R.W., Schermerhorn, P., Gademan, J., de Groot, G. & van Ingen Schenau, G.J. (1986). Characteristic stroke mechanics of elite and trained male speed skaters. *International Journal of Biomechanics* 2, 175-186.

de Groot, G., de Boer, R.W. & van Ingen Schenau, G.J. (1985). Power output during cycling and speed skating. In: Winter, D.A., Norman, R.W., Wells, R.P., Hayes, K.C. & Patla, A.E. (Eds.), *Biomechanics IX-B*. Champaign, IL: Human Kinetics, 555-559.

de Groot, G., Hollander, A.P., Sergeant, A.J., van Ingen Schenau, G.J. & de Boer, R.W. (2007). Applied physiology of skating. *Journal of Sports Sciences* 5 (3), 249-259.

de Koning, J.J., Bobbert, M.F. & Foster, C. (1999). Determination of optimal pacing strategy in track cycling with an energy flow model. *Journal of Science and Medicine in Sport* 2, 266-277.

de Koning, J.J., Foster, C., Lampen, J. et al. (2005). Experimental evaluation of the power balance model of speed skating. *Journal of Applied Physiology* 98, 227-233.

de Koning, J.J. & van Ingen Schenau, G.J. (2000). Performance-determining factors in speed skating. In: Zatsiorsky, V.M. (Ed.), Biomechanics in sport: Performance enhancement and injury prevention. *Olympic encyclopedia of sports medicine,* Vol. IX. Oxford, UK: Wiley-Blackwell Science, 232-246.

Ekblom, B., Hermansen, L. & Saltin, B. (1967). Hastighetsakning pa skridskor. *Idrottsfysiologi Rapport* 5.

Farfel, W.S. (1977). *Bewegungssteuerung in sport.* Berlin: Sportverlag.

Foster, C. & de Koning, J.J. (1999). Physiological perspectives in speed skating. In: Gemser, H., de Koning, J.J. & van Ingen Schanau, G.J. (Eds.), *Handbook of competitive speed skating.* Leuwaarden, The Netherlands: Eisma, 117-137.

Foster, C., de Koning, J.J., Rundell, K.W. & Snyder, A.C. (2000). Physiology of speed skating. In: Garrett, W.E. & Kirkendall, D.T. (Eds.), *Exercise and sport science.* Philadelphia: Lippincott Williams and Wilkins, 885-893.

Foster, C., Schrager, M., Snyder, A.C. & Thompson, N.N. (1994). Pacing strategy and athletic performance. *Sports Medicine* 17 (2), 77-85.

Foster, C. & Thompson, N.N. (1990). The physiology of speed skating. In: Casey, M.J., Foster, C. & Hixson, E.G. (Eds.), *Winter sports medicine.* Philadelphia: FA. Davis, 221-240.

Hettinga, F.J., de Koning, J.J. & Foster, C. (2009). V̇O$_2$ response in supramaximal cycling time trial exercise of 750-m to 4,000-m. *Medicine & Science in Sports & Exercise* 41, 230-236.

Holum, D. (1984). *The complete handbook of skating.* Hillside, NJ: Enslow.

Kandou, T.W.A., Houtman, I.L.D., van der Bol, E., de Boer, R.W., de Groot, G. & van Ingen Schenau, G.J. (1987). Comparison of physiology and biomechanics of speed skating with cycling and skate board exercise. *Canadian Journal of Sports Sciences* 12, 31-36.

Kindermann, W. & Keul, J. (1980). Anaerobic supply of energy in high-speed skating. *Deutscher Zeitschriftfur Sportmedizin* 31, 142-147.

Kuhlow, A. (1974). Analysis of competitors in the world speed-skating championship. In: Nelson, R.C. & Morehouse, C.A. (Eds.), *Biomechanics IV.* Baltimore: University Park Press, 258-263.

Maw, S., Proctor, L., Vredenburg, J. & Overend, T. (2003). Influence of starting position on finishing position in World Cup 500-m short track speed skating. *Journal of Sports Sciences* 24, 1239-1246.

Muehlbauer, T., Schindler, C. & Panzer, S. (2010a). Pacing and performance in competitive middle-distance speed skating. *Research Quarterly for Exercise and Sport* 81 (1), 1-6.

Muehlbauer, T., Schindler, C. & Panzer, S. (2010b). Pacing and speed skating performance in competitive long-distance events. *Journal of Strength and Conditioning* 24 (1), 114-119.

Muehlbauer, T., Schindler, C. & Panzer, S. (2010c). Pacing and sprint performance in speed skating during a competitive season. *International Journal of Sport Physiology and Performance* 5, 165-176.

Muehlbauer, T. & Schindler, C. (2011). Relationship between starting and finishing position in short track speed skating races. *European Journal of Sport Science* 11 (4), 225-230.

Rundell, K.W. (1996a). Compromised oxygen uptake in speed skaters during treadmill in-line skating. *Medicine & Science in Sports & Exercise* 28, 120-127.

Rundell, K.W. (1996b). Effects of drafting during short-track speed skating. *Medicine & Science in Sports & Exercise* 28, 765-771.

Seiler, S. (1997). The new Dutch 'slapskates': Will they revolutionize speed skating technique? Sportscience. www.sportsci.org/news/news9703/slapskat.htm

Sovak, D. & Hawes, M.R. (1987). Anthropological status of international calibre speed skaters. *Journal of Sports Sciences* 5 (3), 287-304.

van Ingen Schenau, G.J. (1982). The influence of air friction in speed skating. *Journal of Biomechanics* 15, 449-458.

van Ingen Schenau, G.J., de Boer, R.W., de Groot, G. et al. (1989). Biomechanics of speed skating. In: Vaughan, C.L. (Ed.), *Biomechanics of sport.* Boca Raton, FL: CRC Press, 121-167.

van Ingen Schenau, G.J. & de Groot, G. (1983). On the origin of differences in performance level between elite male and female speed skaters. *Human Movement Science* 2, 115-119.

van Ingen Schenau, G.J., de Groot, G. & de Boer, R.W. (1985). The control of speed in elite female speed skaters. *Journal of Biomechanics* 18, 91-96.

van Ingen Schenau, G.J., de Groot, G. & Hollander, A.P. (1983). Some technical, physiological and anthropometrical aspect of speed skating. *European Journal of Applied Physiology* 50, 343-354.

van Ingen Schenau, G.J., de Koning, J.J., de Boer, R.W., de Groot, G. et al. (1990). A simulation of speed skating based on a power equation. *Medicine & Science in Sports & Exercise* 22, 718-728.

van Ingen Schenau, G.J., de Koning, J.J. & de Groot, G. (1994). Optimisation of sprinting performance in running, cycling and speed skating. *Sports Medicine* 17, 259-275.

Chapter 9

Abbiss, C.R. & Laursen, P.B. (2008). Describing and understanding pacing strategies during athletic competition. *Sports Medicine* 38 (3), 239-252.

Angus, S. (2013). Did recent world record marathon runners employ optimal pacing strategies? *Journal of Sport Sciences*. doi: 10.1080/02640414.2013.803592

Basset, D.R. & Howley, E.T. (2000). Limiting factors for maximum oxygen uptake and determinants of endurance performance. *Medicine & Science in Sports & Exercise* 32 (1), 70-84.

Billat, V., Hamard, L., Koralsztein, J.P. & Morton, R.H. (2009). Differential modeling of anaerobic and aerobic metabolism in the 800-m and 1,500-m run. *Journal of Applied Physiology* 107 (2), 478-487.

Carr, A.J., Gore, C.J & Dawson, B. (2011). Induced alkalosis and caffeine supplementation: Effects on 2,000-m rowing performance. *International Journal of Sport Nutrition and Exercise Metabolism* 21 (5), 357-364.

Carr, A.J., Hopkins, W.G. & Gore, C.J. (2011). Effects of acute alkalosis and acidosis on performance: A meta-analysis. *Sports Medicine* 41 (10), 801-814.

Dawson, B.B., Fitzsimons, M., Green, S., Goodman, C., Carey, M. & Cole, K. (1998). Changes in performance, muscle metabolites, enzymes and fibre types after short sprint training. *European Journal of Applied Physiology* 78, 163-169.

Duffield, R., Dawson, B. & Goodman, C. (2005a). Energy system contribution to 400-metre and 800-metre track running. *Journal of Sports Sciences* 23 (3), 299-307.

Duffield, R., Dawson, B. & Goodman, C. (2005b). Energy system contribution to 1500- and 3000-metre track running. *Journal of Sports Sciences* 23 (10), 993-1002.

Ely, M.R. (2008). Effect of ambient temperature on marathon pacing is dependent on runner ability. *Medicine & Science in Sports & Exercise* 40 (9), 1675-1680.

Gosztyla, A.E., Edwards, D.G., Quinn, T.J. & Kenefick, R.W. (2006). The impact of different pacing strategies on five-kilometer running time trial performance. *Journal of Strength and Conditioning Research* 20 (4), 882-886.

Hill, D.W. (1999). Energy system contributions in middle-distance running events. *Journal of Sports Sciences* 17 (6), 477-483.

James, D.V., Sandals, L.E., Wood, D.M., Draper, S. & Maldonado-Martin, S. (2007). $\dot{V}O_2$ attained during treadmill running: The influence of a specialist (400-m or 800-m) event. *International Journal of Sports Physiology and Performance* 2 (2), 128-136.

Jones, A.M. & Whipp, B.J. 2002. Bioenergetic constraints on tactical decision making in middle distance running. *British Journal of Sports Medicine* 36 (2), 102-104.

Leger, L.A. & R.J. Ferguson, R.J. (1974). Effect of pacing on oxygen uptake and peak lactate for a mile run. *European Journal of Applied Physiology and Occupational Physiology* 32 (3), 251-257.

Lima-Silva, A.E., Bertuzzi, R.C.M., Pires, F.O., Barros, R.V., Gagliardi, J.F., Hammond, J., Kiss, M.A. & Bishop, D.J. (2009). Effect of performance level on pacing strategy during a 10-km running race. *European Journal of Applied Physiology* 108 (5), 1045-1053.

Linderman, J.K. & Gosselink, K.L. (1994). The effects of sodium bicarbonate ingestion on exercise performance. *Sports Medicine* 18 (2), 75-80.

McNaughton, L.R., Siegler, J. & Midgley, A. (2008). Ergogenic effects of sodium bicarbonate. *Current Sports Medicine Reports* 7 (4), 230-236.

Renfree, A. & St Clair Gibson, A. (2013). Influence of different performance levels on pacing strategy during the women's World Championship marathon race. *International Journal of Sports Physiology and Performance* 8, 279-285.

Ross, A., Leveritt, M. & Riek, S. (2001). Neural influences on sprint running: Training adaptations and acute responses. *Sports Medicine* 31 (6), 409-425.

Sandals, L.E., Wood, D.M., Draper, S.B. & James, D.V. (2006). Influence of pacing strategy on oxygen uptake during treadmill middle-distance running. *International Journal of Sports Medicine* 27 (1), 37-42.

Spencer, M.R. & Gastin, P.B. (2001). Energy system contribution during 200- to 1500-m running in highly trained athletes. *Medicine & Science in Sports & Exercise* 33 (1), 157-162.

Svedenhag, J. & Sjödin, B. (1984). Maximal and submaximal oxygen uptakes and blood lactate levels in elite male middle- and long-distance runners. *International Journal of Sports Medicine* 5 (5), 255-261.

Thomas, C., Hanon, C., Perrey, S., Le Chevalier, J-M., Courturier, A. & Vanderwalle, H. (2005). Oxygen uptake response to an 800-m running race. *International Journal of Sports Medicine* 26 (4), 268-273.

Tucker, R., Lambert, M.I. & Noakes, T.D. (2006). An analysis of pacing strategies during men's world-record performances in track athletics. *International Journal of Sports Physiology and Performance* 1 (3), 233-245.

Chapter 10

Abbiss, C.R. & Laursen, P.B. (2008). Describing and understanding pacing strategies during athletic competition. *Sports Medicine* 38 (3), 239-252.

Abbiss, C.R., Quod, M.J., Martin, D.T., Netto, K.J., Nosaka, K., Lee, H., Surriano, R., Bishop,

D. & Laursen, P.B. (2006). Dynamic pacing strategies during the cycle phase of an Ironman triathlon. *Medicine & Science in Sports & Exercise* 38 (4), 726-734.

Atkinson, G., Peacock, O. & Passfield, L. (2007). Variable versus constant power strategies during cycling time trials: Prediction of time savings using an up-to-date mathematical model. *Journal of Sport Sciences* 25, 1001-1009

Australian Institute of Sport. (2014). Triathlon: Characteristics of the sport. Retrieved from www.ausport.gov.au/ais/nutrition/factsheets/sports/triathlon

Bentley, D.J. et al. (2007). The effects of exercise intensity or drafting during swimming on subsequent cycling performance in triathletes. *Journal of Science and Medicine in Sport* 10, 234-243.

Bentley, D.J., Cox, G.R., Green, D. & Laursen, P.B. (2008). Maximising performance in triathlon: Applied physiological and nutritional aspects of elite and non-elite competitions. *Journal of Science and Medicine in Sport* 11, 407-416.

Bernard, T., Hausswirth, C., Le Meur, Y., Bignet, F., Dorel, S. & Brisswalter, J. (2009). Distribution of power output during the cycling stage of a Triathlon World Cup. *Medicine & Science in Sports & Exercise* 41 (6), 1296-1302.

Bernard, T., Vercruyssen, F., Grego, F., Hausswirth, C., Lepers, R., Vallier, J.M. & Brisswalter J. (2003). Effect of cycling cadence on subsequent 3 km running performance in well trained triathletes. *British Journal of Sports Medicine* 37 (2), 154-158; discussion 159.

Burnley, M. & Jones, A.M. (2007). Oxygen uptake kinetics as a determinant of sport performance, *European Journal of Sport Science* 7 (2), 63-79.

Chatard, J.C., Chollet, D. & Millet, G.P. (1998). Performance and drag during drafting swimming in highly trained triathletes. *Medicine & Science in Sports & Exercise* 30, 1276-1280.

Chatard, J.C. & Wilson, B. (2003). Drafting distance in swimming. *Medicine & Science in Sports & Exercise* 35, 1176-1181.

Chollet, D., Hue, O., Auclair, F., Millet, G. & Chatard, J.C. (2000). The effects of drafting on stroking variations during swimming in elite male triathletes. *European Journal of Applied Physiology* 82, 413-417.

Delextrat, A., Tricot, V., Bernard, T., Vercruyssen, F., Hausswirth, C. & Brisswalter, J. (2003). Drafting during swimming improves efficiency during subsequent cycling. *Medicine & Science in Sports & Exercise* 25, 1612-1619.

Gatorade.co.uk. (2014). Triathlon. Retrieved from www.gatorade.co.uk/nutrition-and-training/triathlon

Hausswirth, C., Bernard, T. & Vallier, J.M. (2002). Effect of different running strategies on running performance in Olympic distance triathlon. In: Proceedings of the 7th annual congress of the European College of Sport Sciences, Athens, 24–28 July 2002, p 183 Athens.

Hausswirth, C. & Brisswalter, J. (2008). Strategies for improving performance in long duration events: Olympic distance triathlon. *Sports Medicine* 38 (11), 881-891.

Hausswirth, C., Lehenaff, D., Dreano, P. & Savonen, K. (1999). Effects of cycling alone or in a sheltered position on subsequent running performance during a triathlon. *Medicine & Science in Sports & Exercise* 31, 599-604.

Hausswirth, C., Vallier, J.M., Lehenaff, D., Brisswalter, J., Smith, D., Millet, G. & Dreano, P. (2001). Effect of two drafting modalities in cycling on running performance. *Medicine & Science in Sports & Exercise* 33, 385-390.

Heiden, T. & Burnett, A. (2003). The effect of cycling on muscle activation in the running leg of an Olympic distance triathlon. *Sports Biomechanics* 2, 35-49.

Jeukendrup, A.E., Craig, N.P. & Hawley, J.A. (2000). The bioenergetics of world class cycling. *Journal of Science and Medicine in Sport* 10, 414-433.

Jeukendrup, A.E., Jentjens, R.L. & Moseley, L. (2005). Nutritional considerations in triathlon. *Sports Medicine* 35, 163-181.

Kimber, N.E., Ross, J.J., Mason, S.L. & Speedy, D.B. (2002). Energy balance during an Ironman triathlon in male and female triathletes. *International Journal of Sport Nutrition and Exercise Metabolism* 12 (1), 47-62.

Laursen, P.B., Knez, W.L., Shing, C.M., Langill, R.H., Rhodes, E.C. & Jenkins, D.G. (2005). Relationship between laboratory-measured variables and heart rate during an ultra-endurance triathlon. *Journal of Sports Sciences* 23 (10), 1111-1120.

Laursen, P.B., Rhodes, E.C., Langill, R.H., McKenzie, D.C. & Taunton, J.E. (2002). Relationship of exercise test variables to cycling performance in an Ironman triathlon. *European Journal of Applied Physiology* 87, 433-440.

Le Meur, Y., Bernard, T., Dorel, S., Abbiss, C.R., Honnorat, G., Brisswalter, J. & Hausswirth, C. (2011). Relationships between triathlon performance and pacing strategy during the run in an international competition. *International Journal of Sports Physiology* 6, 183-194.

Le Meur, Y., Hausswirth, C., Dorel, S., Bignet, F., Brisswalter, J. & Bernard, T. (2009). Influence of gender on pacing adopted by elite triathletes during a competition. *European Journal of Applied Physiology* 106 (4), 535-545.

Lepers, R., Theurel, J., Hausswirth, C. & Bernard, T. (2007). Neuromuscular fatigue following constant versus variable-intensity endurance cycling in triathletes. *Journal of Science and Medicine in Sport* 9, 125-136.

McCole, S.D., Claney, K., Conte, J.C., Anderson, R. & Hagberg, J.M. (1990). Energy expenditure during bicycling. *Journal of Applied Physiology* 68 (2), 748-753.

Millet, G.P., Chollet, D. & Chatard, J.C. (2000). Effects of drafting behind a two- or a six-beat kick swimmer in elite female triathletes. *European Journal of Applied Physiology* 82, 465-471.

Mollendorf, J.C., Termin, A.C. 2nd, Oppenheim, E. & Pendergast, D.R. (2004). Effect of swim suit design on passive drag. *Medicine & Science in Sports & Exercise* 36, 1029-1035.

O'Toole, M.L., Douglas, P.S. & Hiller, W.D. (1998). Use of heart rate monitors by endurance athletes: Lessons from triathletes. *Journal of Sports Medicine and Physical Fitness* 38 (3), 181-187.

O'Toole, M.L., Hiller, W.D.B., Douglas, P.S., Pisarello, J.B. & Mullen, J.L. (1987). Cardiovascular responses to prolonged cycling and running. *Annals of Sports Medicine* 3, 124-130.

Pugh, L.G. (1971). The influence of wind resistance in running and walking and the mechanical efficiency of work against horizontal or vertical forces. *Journal of Physiology* 213, 255-256.

St Clair Gibson, A., de Koning, J.J., Thompson, K., Roberts, W.O., Micklewright, D., Raglin, J. & Foster, C. (2013). Crawling to the finish line: Why do endurance runners collapse? Implications for understanding of mechanisms underlying pacing and fatigue. *Sports Medicine* 43 (6), 413-424.

Vercruyssen, F., Brisswalter, J., Hausswirth, C., Bernard, T., Bernard, O. & Vallier, J.M. (2002). Influence of cycling cadence on subsequent running performance in triathletes. *Medicine & Science in Sports & Exercise* 34 (3), 530-536.

Vleck, V.E., Bentley, D.J. & Bürgi, A. (2006). The consequences of swim, cycle, and run performance on overall result in elite Olympic distance triathlon. *International Journal of Sports Medicine* 27 (1), 43-48.

Vleck, V.E., Bentley, D.J., Millet, G.P. & Burgi, A. (2008). Pacing during an elite Olympic distance triathlon: Comparison between male and female competitors. *Journal of Science and Medicine in Sport* 11 (4), 424-432.

Chapter 11

Baudouin, A. & Hawkins, D. (2002). A biomechanical review of factors affecting rowing performance. British Journal of Sports Medicine 36, 396-402.

Brown, M.R., Delau, S. & Desgorces, F.D. (2010). Effort regulation in rowing races depends on performance level and exercise mode. *Journal of Science and Medicine in Sport* 13, 613-617.

Bourdin, M., Messonnier, L., Hager, J-P. & Lacour, J-R. (2004). Peak power output predicts rowing ergometer performance in elite male rowers. *International Journal of Sports Medicine* 25, 368-373.

Carter, J.E.L. (1982a). Body composition of athletes. In: Carter, J.E. (Ed.), *Physical structure of Olympic athletes*. Part I. Basel: Karger, 107-116.

Carter, J.E.L. (1982b). Age and body size. In: Carter, J.E. (Ed.), *Physical structure of Olympic athletes*. Part I. Basel: Karger, 53-79.

Cosgrove, M.J., Wilson, J., Watt, D. & Grant, S.F. (1999). The relationship between selected physiological variables of rowers and rowing performance as determined by a 2000 m ergometer test. *Journal of Sports Sciences* 17, 845-852.

De Campos Melle, F., De Moraes Beryuzzi, R.C., Grangeiro, P.M. & Franchini, E. (2004). Energy systems contributions in 2000 m race simulation: A comparison among rowing ergometers and water. *European Journal of Applied Physiology* 107, 615-619.

Fukunaga, T., Matsuo, A., Yamamoto, K. & Asami, T. (1986). Mechanical efficiency in rowing. *European Journal of Applied Physiology and Occupational Physiology* 55 (5), 471-475.

Garland, S. (2005) An analysis of the pacing strategy adopted by elite competitor in 2000 m rowing. *British Journal of Sports Medicine* 39(1), 39-42.

Gee, T., Berger, N., French, D., Howatson, G. & Thompson, K.G. (2011). Does a bout of strength training affect 2000 m rowing and anaerobic power in rowers? *European Journal of Applied Physiology* 111 (11), 2653-2662.

Gee, T.I., French, D.N., Gibbon, K.C. & Thompson, K.G. (2013). Consistency of pacing and metabolic responses during 2000 m rowing ergometry. *International. Journal of Sport Physiology and Performance* 8, 70-76.

Hagerman, F.C. (1984). Applied physiology of rowing. *Sports Medicine* 1, 303-326.

Hagerman, F.C., Connors, M.C., Gault, J.A., Hagerman, G.R. & Polinski, W.J. (1978). Energy expenditure during simulated rowing. *Journal of Applied Physiology* 45, 87-93.

Ingham, S.A. Whyte, G.P. Jones, K. & Nevill, A.M. (2002). Determinants of 2,000 m rowing ergometer performance in elite rowers. *European Journal of Applied Physiology* 88, 243-246.

Kleshnev, V. (2001). Racing strategy in rowing during Sydney Olympic Games. *Australian Rowing* 24, 20-23.

Muehlbauer, T. & Melges, T. (2011). Pacing patterns in competitive rowing adopted in different race categories. *Journal of Strength and Conditioning* 25 (5), 1293-1298.

Muehlbauer, T., Schindler, C. & Widmer, A. (2010). Pacing patterns and performance during the 2008 Olympic rowing regatta. *European Journal of Sport Science* 10 (5), 291-296.

Renfree, A., Martin, L., Richards, A. & St Clair Gibson, A. (2013). All for one and one for all! Disparity between overall crew's and individual rower's pacing strategies during rowing. *International Journal of Sports Physiology and Performance* 7, 298-300.

Schabort, E.J., Hawley, J.A., Hopkins, W.G. et al. (1999). High reliability of performance of well-trained rowers on a rowing ergometer. *Journal of Sports Sciences* 17, 627-632.

Secher, N. (1990). Rowing, In: Reilly, T. et al. (Eds.), *Physiology of sports.* London: E&F Spon, 259-285.

Shephard, R.J. (1998). Science and medicine of rowing: A review. *Journal of Sports Sciences* 16, 603-620.

Simoes, M., Velosa, A. & Armada-da-Silva, P. (2006). A kinematic analysis of rowing performance during a 2000 m ergometer test. XXIV ISBS Symposium, Salzburg, Austria.

Slater, G.J., Rice, A.J., Mujika, I., Hahn, A.G., Sharpe, K. & Jenkins, D.G. (2005). Physique traits of lightweight rowers and their relationship to competitive success. *British Journal of Sports Medicine* 39, 736-741.

Soper, C. & Hume, P.A. (2004). Reliability of power output during rowing changes with ergometer type and race distance. *Sports Biomechanics* 3, 237-248.

Steinacker, J.M. (1993). Physiological aspects of training in rowing. *International Journal of Sports Medicine* 14, S3-S10.

Chapter 12

Akenhead, R., French, D., Hayes, P. & Thompson, K.G. (2013). Diminutions of acceleration and deceleration output during professional football match play. *Journal of Science and Medicine in Sport.* doi: 10.1016/j.jsams.2012.12.005

Anderson, A. (2005). AFL annual report: Football operations. Melbourne (VIC): Australian Football League.

Aughey, R.J. (2010). Australian football player work rate: Evidence of fatigue and pacing? *International Journal of Sports Physiology and Performance* 5, 394-405.

Bangsbo, J. (1994). The physiology of soccer—with special reference to intense intermittent exercise. *Acta Physiologica Scandinavica* 151 (Suppl. 619).

Brewer, J. & Davis, J. (1995). Applied physiology of rugby league. *Sports Medicine* 20, 129-138.

Carling, C. & Dupont, G. (2011). Are declines in physical performance associated with a reduction in skill-related performance during professional soccer match-play? *Journal of Sports Sciences* 29 (1), 63-71.

Carter, A. (1996). Time and motion analysis and heart rate monitoring of back-row forward in first class rugby union football. In: Hughes, M. (Ed.), *Notational analysis of sport,* 1 and 2. Cardiff, UK: Centre of Notational Analysis, University of Wales, 145-160.

Coutts, A.J., Quinn, J., Hocking, J., Castagna, C. & Rampinini, E. (2009). Match running performance in elite Australian Rules Football. *Journal of Science and Medicine in Sport* 13 (5), 543-548.

Coutts, A., Reaburn, P. & Abt, G. (2003). Heart rate, blood lactate concentration and estimated energy expenditure in a semi-professional rugby league team during a match: A case study. *Journal of Sports Sciences* 21, 97-103.

Cunniffe, B., Proctor, W., Baker, J.S. & Davies, B. (2009). An evaluation of the physiological demands of elite rugby union using GPS tracking software. *Journal of Strength and Conditioning Research* 23 (4), 1195-1203.

Dawson, B., Hopkinson, R., Appleby, B., Stewart, G., Roberts, C. (2004). Player movement patterns and game activities in the Australian Football League. *Journal of Science and Medicine in Sport* 7 (3), 278-291.

Deutsch, M.U., Kearney, G.A. & Rehrer, N.J. (2002). A comparison of competition work rates in elite club and Super 12 rugby. In: Spinks, W., Reilly, T. & Murphy, A. (Eds.), *Science and football IV.* Sydney: The University Press, 126-131.

Deutsch, M.U., Maw, G.J., Jenkins, D. et al. (1998). Heart rate, blood lactate and kinematic data of elite colts (under 19) rugby union players during competition. *Journal of Sports Sciences* 16, 561-570.

Di Salvo, V., Baron, R., Tschan, H., Calderon Montero, F.J., Bachl, N. & Pigozzi, F. (2007). Performance characteristics according to playing position in elite soccer. *International Journal of Sports Medicine* 28 (3), 222-227.

Di Salvo, V., Gregson, W., Atkinson, G., Tordoff, P. & Drust, B. (2009). Analysis of high intensity activity in Premier League soccer. *International Journal of Sports Medicine* 30, 205-212.

Docherty, D., Wenger, H.A. & Neary, P. (1988). Time motion analysis related to the physiological demands of rugby. *Journal of Human Movement Studies* 14, 269-277.

Duffield, R., Coutts, A.J. & Quinn, J. (2009). Core temperature responses and match running performance during intermittent-sprint exercise competition in warm conditions. *Journal of Strength and Conditioning Research* 23 (4), 1238-1244.

Dupont, G., Nedelec, M., McCall, A., McCormack, D., Berthoin, S. & Wisloff, U. (2010). Effect of 2 soccer matches in a week on physical performance and injury rate. *American Journal of Sports Medicine* 38 (9), 1752-1758.

Duthie, G., Pyne, D. & Hooper, S. (2003). Applied physiology and game analysis of rugby union (Review). *Sports Medicine* 33 (13), 973-991.

Duthie, G., Pyne, D. & Hooper, S. (2005). Time motion analysis of 2001 and 2002 Super 12 rugby. *Journal of Sports Sciences* 23 (5), 523-530.

Eckblom, B. (1986). Applied physiology of soccer. *Sports Medicine* 3, 50-60.

Edwards, A.M. & Noakes, T.D. (2009). Dehydration: Cause of fatigue or sign of pacing in elite soccer? *Sports Medicine* 39 (1), 1-13.

ESPN Soccer. (2011, July 11). FIFA: At least 1 billion saw Cup final. Retrieved from http://espn.go.com/sports/soccer/news/_/id/6758280/least-1-billion-saw-part-2010-world-cup-final

Gabbett, T.J. (2012). Sprinting patterns of National Rugby League competition. *Journal of Strength and Conditioning Research* 26 (1), 121-130.

Gabbett, T.J., Jenkins, D.G. & Abernethy, B. (2011). Relative importance of physiological, anthropometric and skill qualities to team selection in professional rugby league. *Journal of Sports Sciences* 29 (13), 1453-1461.

Gabbett, T., Kelly, J. & Pezet, T. (2007). Relationship between physical fitness and playing ability in rugby league players. *Journal of Strength and Conditioning Research* 21 (4), 1126-1133.

Gray, A.J. & Jenkins, D.G. (2010). Match analysis and the physiological demands of Australian football. *Journal of Sports Medicine* 40 (4), 347-360.

Gore, C.J., McSharry, P.E., Hewitt, A.J. & Saunders, P.U. (2008). Preparation for football competition at moderate to high altitude. *Scandinavian Journal of Medicine and Science in Sports* 18 (Suppl. 1), 85-95.

Higham, D.G., Pyne, D.B., Anson, J.M. & Eddy, A. (2012). Movement patterns in rugby sevens: Effects of tournament level, fatigue and substitute players. *Journal of Science and Medicine in Sport* 15, 277-282.

Jacobs, I., Westlin, N., Karlson, J., Rasmusson, M. & Houghton, B. (1982). Muscle glycogen and diet in male soccer players. *European Journal of Applied Physiology* 48, 297-302.

Krustrup, P., Mohr, M., Steensberg, A., Bencke, J., Kjaer, M. & Bangsbo, J. (2003). Muscle metabolites during a football match in relation to a decreased sprinting ability. Communication to the Fifth World Congress of Soccer and Science, Lisbon, Portugal.

Little, T. & Williams, A.G. (2005). Specificity of acceleration, maximum speed, and agility in professional soccer players. *Journal of Strength and Conditioning Research* 19 (1), 76-78.

McLean, D.A. (1992). Analysis of the demands of international rugby union. *Journal of Sports Sciences* 10, 285-296.

Meir, R., Arthur, D. & Forrest, M. (1993). Time and motion analysis of professional rugby league: A case study. *Strength and Conditioning Coach* 3, 24-29.

Meir, R., Colla, P. & Milligan, C. (2001). Impact of the 10-m rule change on professional rugby league: Implications for training. *Strength and Conditioning Journal* 23, 42-46.

Menchinelli, C., Morandini, C. & De Angelis, M. (1992). A functional model of rugby: Determination of the other characteristics of sports performance [Abstract]. *Journal of Sports Sciences* 10, 196-197.

Mero, A. & Komi, P.V. (1987). Electromyographic activity in sprinting at speeds ranging from submaximal to supra-maximal. *Medicine & Science in Sports & Exercise* 19 (3), 266-274.

Mero, A. & Komi, P.V. (1986). Force-, EMG-, and elasticity-velocity relationships at submaximal, maximal and supramaximal running speeds in sprinters. *European Journal of Applied Physiology and Occupational Physiology* 55 (5), 553-561.

Mohr, M., Krustrup, P., Andersson, H., Kirkendal, D. & Bangsbo, J. (2008). Match activities of elite women soccer players at different performance levels. *Journal of Strength and Conditioning Research* 22 (2), 341-349.

Mohr, M., Krustrup, P. & Bangsbo, J. (2005). Fatigue in soccer: A brief review. *Journal of Sports Sciences* 23 (6), 593-599.

Mohr, M., Krustrup, P. & Bangsbo, J. (2003). Match performance of high-standard soccer players with special reference to development of fatigue. *Journal of Sports Science* 21 (7), 519-528.

Mohr, M., Krustrup, P., Nybo, L., Nielsen, J.J. & Bangsbo, J. (2004). Muscle temperature and sprint performance during soccer matches—beneficial effect of re-warm-up at half-time. *Scandinavian Journal of Medicine & Science in Sports* 14 (3), 156-162.Morton A.R. (1978). Applying physiological principles to rugby training. *Sports Coach* 2, 4-9.

Mustafa, K.Y. & Mahmoud, E.A. (1979). Evaporative water loss in African soccer players. *Journal of Sports Medicine and Physical Fitness* 19, 181-183.

Norton, K.I. (2007). Laws of Australian Football discussion paper. Melbourne (VIC): Australian Football League.

Norton, K.I., Craig, N.P. & Olds, T.S. (1999). The evolution of Australian Football. *Journal of Science and Medicine in Sport* 2 (4), 389-404.

Orendurff, M.S., Walker, J.D., Jovanovic, M., Tulchin, K.L., Levy, M. & Hoffmann, D K. (2010). Intensity and duration of intermittent exercise and recovery during a soccer match. *Journal of Strength and Conditioning Research* 24 (10), 2683-2692.

Osgnach, C., Poser, S., Bernardini, R., Rinaldo, R. & di Prampero, P.E. (2010). Energy cost and metabolic power in elite soccer: A new match analysis approach. *Medicine & Science in Sports & Exercise* 42(1), 170-178.

Pyne, D.N., Gardner, A.S., Sheehan, K. et al. (2005). Fitness testing progression in AFL football. *Journal of Science and Medicine in Sport* 8 (3), 321-332.

Quarrie, K.L. & Wilson, B.D. (2000). Force production in the rugby union scrum. *Journal of Sports Sciences* 18, 237-246.

Rampinini, E., Coutts, A.J., Castagna, C., Sassi, R. & Impellizzeri, F.M. (2007). Variation in top level soccer match performance. *International Journal of Sports Medicine* 28, 1018-1024.

Reilly, T., Bangsbo, J. & Franks, A. (2000). Anthropometric and physiological predispositions for elite soccer. *Journal of Sports Sciences* 18, 669-683.

Reilly, T. & Thomas, V. (1976). A motion analysis of work-rate in different positional roles in professional football match-play. *Journal of Human Movement Studies* 2, 87-97.

Roberts, S.P., Trewartha, G., Higgitt, R.J., El-Abd, J. & Stokes, K.A. (2008). The physical demands of elite English rugby union. *Journal of Sports Sciences* 26 (8), 825-833.

Smaros, G. (1980). Energy usage during a football match. In: Vecchiet L. (Ed), *Proceedings of the First International Congress of Sports Medicine Applied to Football*. Rome: D. Guanello, 795-801.

Sporis, G., Jukic, I., Ostojic, M. & Milanovic, D. (2009). Fitness profiling in soccer: Physical and physiologic characteristics of elite players. *Journal of Strength and Conditioning Research* 23 (7), 1947-1953.

Stolen, T., Chamari, K., Castagna, C. & Wisloff, U. (2005). Physiology of soccer: An update. *Sports Medicine* 35 (6), 501-536.

Treadwell, P.J. (1988). Computer aided match analysis of selected ball games (soccer and rugby union). In: Reilly, T., Lees, A., Davids, K. et al. (Eds.), *Science and football*. London: E&F Spon, 282-287.

Wisbey, B., Montgomery, P.G. & Pyne, D.B. (2008). *Quantifying changes in AFL player game demands using GPS tracking: 2007 AFL season*. Florey, ACT: FitSense Australia.

Wisbey, B., Montgomery, P.G., Pyne, D.B. & Rattray, B. (2010). Quantifying movement demands of AFL football using GPS tracking. *Journal of Science and Medicine in Sport* 13, 531-536.

Wisbey, B., Pyne, D.B. & Rattray, B. (2010). *Quantifying change in AFL player game demands using GPS tracking: 2010 AFL season*. Florey, ACT: FitSense Australia.

Wisbey, B., Rattray, B. & Pyne, D.B. (2008). *Quantifying changes in AFL player game demands using GPS tracking: 2008 AFL season*. Florey, ACT: FitSense Australia.

Young, W.B., Newton, R.U., Doyle, T.L.A. et al. (2005). Physiological and anthropometric characteristics of starters and non-starters and playing positions in elite Australian Rules Football: A case study. *Journal of Science and Medicine in Sport* 8 (3), 333-345.

Chapter 13

Australian Institute of Sport. (n.d.). Squash. Retrieved from www.ausport.gov.au/ais/nutrition/factsheets/sports/squash

Bergeron, M.F. (2003). Heat cramps: Fluid and electrolyte challenges during tennis in the heat. *Journal of Science and Medicine in Sport* 66, 19-27.

Bergeron, M.F., Armstrong, L.E. &. Maresh, C.M (1995). Fluid and electrolyte losses during tennis in the heat. *Clinics in Sports Medicine* 114, 23-32.

Bergeron, M.F., Maresh, C.M., Armstrong, K.E., Signorile, J.F., Castellani, J.W., Kenefick, R.W., LaGasse, K.E. & Riebe, D.A. (1995). Fluid electrolyte balance associated with tennis match play in hot environment. *International Journal of Sport Nutrition* 55, 180-193.

Bergeron, M.F., Maresh, C.M., Kraemer, W.J. et al. (1991). Tennis: A physiological profile during match play. *International Journal of Sports Medicine* 12 (5), 474-479.

Bernadi, M., De Vito, G., Falvo, M.E. et al. (1998). Cardiorespiratory adjustment in middle-level tennis players: Are long term cardiovascular adjustments possible? In: Lees, A., Maynard, I., Hughes, M. & Reilly T. (Eds.), *Science and racket sports II*. London: E&F Spon, 20-26.

Brown, D., Weigland, D.A. & Winter, E.M. (1998). Maximum oxygen uptake in junior and senior elite squash players. In: Lees, A., Maynard, I., Hughes, M. & Reilly, T. (Eds.), *Science and racket sports II.* London: E&F Spon, 14-19.

Christmass, M.A., Richmond, S.E., Cable, N.T., Arthur, P.G. & Hartmann, P.E. (1998). Exercise intensity and metabolic response in singles tennis. *Journal of Sport Sciences* 16, 739-747.

Davey, P.R., Thorpe, R.D. & Williams, C. (2002). Fatigue decreases skilled performance. *Journal of Sport Sciences* 20, 311-318.

Davey, P.R., Thorpe, R.D. & Williams, C. (2003). Simulated tennis match play in a controlled environment. *Journal of Sport Sciences* 21, 459-467.

Fernandez-Fernandez, J., Mendez-Villanueva, A., Fernandez-Garcia, B. & Terrados, N. (2007). Match activity and physiological responses during a junior female singles tennis tournament. *British Journal of Sports Medicine* 41, 711-716.

Fernandez-Fernandez, J., Sanz-Rivas, D., Fernandez-Garcia, B. & Mendez-Villanueva, A. (2008). Match activity and physiological load during a clay-court tennis tournament in elite female players. *Journal of Sports Sciences* 226 (14), 1589-1595.

Fernandez-Fernandez, J., Sanz-Rivas, D. & Mendez-Villanueva, A. (2009). A review of the activity profile and physiological demands of tennis match play. *Strength and Conditioning Journal* 223 (2), 604-610.

Ferrauti, A., Bergeron, M.F., Pluim, B.M. et al. (2001). Physiological responses in tennis and running with similar oxygen uptake. *European Journal of Applied Physiology* 85, 27-33.

Ferrauti, A., Pluim, B.M., Busch, T. & Weber, K. (2003). Blood glucose responses and incidence of hypoglycaemia in elite tennis under practice and tournament conditions. *Journal of Science and Medicine in Sport* 66, 28-39.

Ferrauti, A., Pluim, B.M. & Weber, K. (2001). The effect of recovery duration on running speed and stroke quality during intermittent training drills in elite tennis players. *Journal of Sports Sciences* 19, 235-242.

Gillam, I., Siviour, C., Ellis, L. & Brown, P. (1990). The on-court energy demands of squash on elite level players. In: Draper, J. (Ed.), *Third report on National Sport Research program.* Canberra: Australian Sports Commission, 1-22.

Girard, O., Chevalier, R., Harbrard, M., Sciberras, P., Hot, P. & Millet, G.P. (2007). Game analysis and energy requirements of elite squash. *Journal of Strength and Conditioning Research* 21 (3), 909-914.

Girard, O., Christian, R.J., Racinais, S., Periard, J.D. (2014). Heat stress does not exacerbate tennis-induced alterations in physical performance. *British Journal of Sports Medicine* 48, i39-i44.

Girard, O., Lattier, G., Maffiuletti, N.A. et al. (2008). Neuromuscular fatigue during a prolonged intermittent exercise: Application to tennis. *Journal of Electromyography and Kinesiology* 18 (6), 1038-1046.

Girard, O., Lattier, G., Micallef, J.P. & Millet, G.P. (2006). Changes in exercise characteristics, maximal voluntary contraction, and explosive strength during prolonged tennis playing. *British Journal of Sports Medicine* 440, 521-526.

Girard, O., Racinais, S., Micallef, J.P. et al. (2007). Changes in motoneuron pool excitability during prolonged tennis playing. *Medicine & Science in Sports & Exercise* 39 (5), S434.

Girard, O., Sciberras, P., Habrad, M., Hot, P., Chevalier, R. & Millet, G.P. (2005). Specific incremental test in elite squash players. *British Journal of Sports Medicine* 39, 921-926.

Green, J.M., Crews, T.R., Bosak, A.M. et al. (2003). A comparison of respiratory compensation thresholds of anaerobic competitors, aerobic competitors and untrained subjects. *European Journal of Applied Physiology* 90, 608-613.

Hornery, D.J., Farrow, D., Mujika, I. & Young, W. (2007a). An integrated physiological and performance profile of professional tennis. *British Journal of Sports Medicine* 41, 531-536.

Hornery, D.J., Farrow, D., Mujika, I. & Young, W. (2007b). Mechanisms of fatigue and effect in tennis. *Sports Medicine* 37 (3), 199-212.

Hughes, M. & Franks, I.M. (1994). Dynamic movement patterns of squash players of different standards in winning and losing rallies. *Ergonomics* 37, 23-29.

International Tennis Federation. (n.d.). www.itftennis.com/about/organisation/history.aspx

Kovacs, M.S. (2006a). Applied physiology of tennis performance. *British Journal of Sports Medicine* 40, 381-386.

Kovacs, M. (2006b). Hydration and temperature in tennis: A practical review. *Journal of Sports Science and Medicine* 55, 1-9.

Martin, C., Thevenet, D., Zouhal, H., Mornet, Y., Deles, R., Crestel, T., Ben Abderrahman, A. & Prioux, J. (2011). Effects of playing surface (hard and clay courts) on heart rate and blood lactate during tennis matches played by high-level players. *Journal of Strength and Conditioning Research* 225, 163-170.

Mendez-Villanueva, A., Fernandez-Fernandez, J., Bishop, D., Fernan-dez-Garcia, B. & Terrados, N. (2007). Activity patterns, blood lactate concentrations and ratings of perceived exertion during a professional singles tennis tournament. *British Journal of Sports Medicine* 41, 296-300.

Morante, S.M. & Brotherhood, J.R. (2008). Autonomic and behavioural thermoregulation in tennis. *British Journal of Sports Medicine* 442, 679-685.

Murray, S. & Hughes, M. (2001). Tactical performance profiling in elite level senior squash. In Hughes, M. & Franks, I.M. (Eds.), pass.com. Cardiff, CPA, UWIC, 185-194. ISBN: 1 901288

Myers, J.B., Guskiewicz, K.M., Schneider, R.A. et al. (1999). Proprioception and neuromuscular control of the shoulder after muscle fatigue. *Journal of Athletic Training* 34, 362-367.

Ojala, T., Hakkinen, K. (2013) Effects of the tennis tournament on player's physical performance, hormonal responses, muscle damage and recovery. *Journal of Sports Science and Medicine* 12, 240-248.

Periard, J.D., Girard, G. & Racinais, S. (2014) Neuromuscular adjustments of the knee extensors and plantar flexors following match-play in the heat. *British Journal of Sports Medicine* 48, i45-i51.

Periard, J.D., Racinais, S., Knez, W.L., Herrara, C.P., Christian, R.J., Girard, G. (2014) Thermal, physiological and perceptual strain mediate alterations in match-play tennis under heat stress. *British Journal of Sports Medicine* 48, i32-i38.

Ranchordas, M.K., Rogerson, D., Ruddock, A., Killer, S.C. & Winter, E.M. (2013). Nutrition for tennis: Practical recommendations. *Journal of Sports Science and Medicine* 12, 211-224.

Reilly, T. & Palmer, J. (1994). Investigation of exercise intensity in male singles lawn tennis. In: Reilly, T., Hughes, M. & Lees, A. (Eds.), *Science and racket sports* (1st ed.). London: E&F Spon, 10-13.

Smekal, G., von Duvillard, S.P., Rihacek, C., Pokan, R., Hofmann, P., Baron, R., Tschan, H. & Bachl, N. (2001). A physiological profile of tennis match play. *Medicine & Science in Sports & Exercise* 333, 999-1005.

Vergauwen, L., Brouns, F. & Hespel, P. (1998). Carbohydrate supplementation improves stroke performance in tennis. *Medicine & Science in Sports & Exercise* 30 (8), 1289-1295.

Vuckovic, G., Pers, J., James, N. & Hughes, M. (2009). Tactical use of the T area in squash by players of differing standard. *Journal of Sports Sciences* 27 (8), 863-871.

Wallbutton, T. (n.d.). World Squash Federation: 140 years of squash. World Squash. Retrieved from www.worldsquash.org/ws/wsf-information/squash-history/140-years-of-squash

Wilkinson, M., Cooke, M., Murray, S., Thompson, K.G., St Clair Gibson, A. & Winter, E.M. (2012). Physiological correlates of multi-sprint ability and performance in international standard squash players. *Journal of Strength and Conditioning Research* 26 (2), 540-547.

Zug, J. (n.d.). The history of squash in 8 1/2 chapters. World Squash. Retrieved from www.worldsquash.org/ws/wsf-information/squash-history/the-history-of-squash-in-8%c2%bd-chapters

Chapter 14

Abdelkrim, N.B., Fazaa, S.E. & Ati, J.E. (2007). Time-motion analysis and physiological data of under-19-year-old basketball players during competition. *British Journal of Sports Medicine* 41, 69-75.

Ainsworth, B.E., Haskell, W.L., Whitt, M.C., Irwin, M.L., Bassett, D.R. Jr., Schmitz, K.H., Empliaincourt, P.O., Jacobs, D.R. Jr. & Leon, A.S. (2000). Compendium of physical activities: An update of activity codes and MET intensities. *Medicine & Science in Sports & Exercise* 32, S498-S504.

Australian Institute of Sport. (n.d.). Basketball. Retrieved from www.ausport.gov.au/ais/nutrition/factsheets/sports/basketball

Crisafulli, A., Melis, F., Tocco, F., Lai, C. & Concu, A. (2002). External mechanical work versus oxidative energy consumption ratio during a basketball field test. *Journal of Sport Medicine and Physical Fitness* 42, 409-417.

Gatorade Sports Science Institute. (n.d.). Nutrition and recovery needs of the basketball athlete: A report from the 2013GSSI taskforce. Retrieved from www.gssiweb.org/docs/default-source/default-document-library/bball-task-force-final.pdf?sfvrsn=2

Gillam, G.M. (1985). Identification of anthropometric and physiological characteristics relative to participation in college basketball. *NSCA Journal* 7 (3), 34-36.

Janeira, M. & Maia, J. (1998). Game intensity in basketball: An inter-actionist view linking time-motion analysis, lactate concentration and heart rate. *Coaching and Sport Science* 2, 26-30.

Lamonte, M.J., McKinney, J.T., Quinn, S.M., Bainbridge, C.N. & Eisenman, P.A. (1999). Comparison of physical and physiological variables for female college basketball players. *Journal of Strength and Conditioning Research* 13(3), 264-270.

McCardle, W.D. (1995). Aerobic capacity, heart rate, and estimated energy cost during women's competitive basketball. *Research Quarterly* 42(2), 178-186.

McInnes, S.E., Carlson, J.S., Jones, C.J. & McKenna, M.J. (1995). The physiological load imposed on basketball players during competition. *Journal of Sports Science* 13, 387-397.

Montgomery, P.G., Pyne, D.B., Hopkins, W.G., Dorman, J.C., Cook, K. & Minahan, C.L. (2008). The effect of recovery strategies on physical performance and cumulative fatigue in competitive basketball. *Journal of Sports Science* 26 (11), 1135-1145.

Montgomery, P.G., Pyne, D.B. & Minahan, C.L. (2010). The physical and physiological demands of basketball training and competition. *International Journal of Sports Physiology and Performance* 5, 75-86.

Narazaki, K., Berg, K. & Shinohara, M. (2006). Bioenergetics and time-motion analysis of competitive basketball. *Medicine & Science in Sports & Exercise* 38, S238-S239.

Nazaraki, K., Berg, K., Stergiou, N. & Chen, B. (2009). Physiological demands of competitive basketball. *Scandinavian Journal of Medicine and Science in Sports* 19, 425-432.

Ostojic, S.M., Mazic, S. & Dikic, N. (2006). Profiling in basketball: Physical and physiological characteristics of elite players. *Journal of Strength and Conditioning Research* 20 (4), 740-744.

Ramsey, J.D., Ayoub, M.M., Dudek, R.A. & Edgar, H.S. (1970). Heart rate recovery during a college basketball game. *Research Quarterly for Exercise and Sport* 41, 528-535.

Rodriguez-Alonso, M., Fernandez-Garcia, B., Perez-Landaluce, J. & Terrados, N. (2003). Blood lactate and heart rate during national and international women's basketball. *Journal of Sports Medicine and Physical Fitness* 43, 432-436.

Smith, H.K. & Thomas, S.G. (1991). Physiological characteristics of elite female basketball players. *Canadian Journal of Sport Science* 16 (4), 289-295.

Note: The italicized *f* and *t* following page numbers refer to figures and tables, respectively.

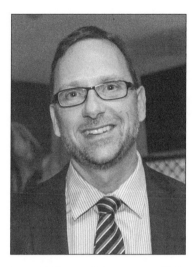

Kevin G. Thompson, PhD, FBASES, FACSM, is director of the Research Institute for Sport and Exercise at the University of Canberra, Australia. He has previously held administrative positions at Canberra and at Northumbria University in the UK. He has held senior positions in elite athlete support, including director of sport sciences and regional director at the English Institute of Sport from 2002 to 2009 and manager of coaching, sport science, and sports medicine at the Welsh Institute of Sport from 1999 to 2002. He is a member of the Australian Institute of Sport High-Performance Sport Research Advisory Panel and former chair of the British Association of Sport and Exercise Sciences (BASES) sport and performance division and special sport science committee. He is a fellow of BASES and a fellow of the American College of Sports Medicine. Thompson is a BASES-accredited high-performance sport physiologist. Since 1994, he has practised as an applied sport scientist supporting professional rugby and soccer players and elite athletes who have competed at Olympic Games and European and World Championships.

Thompson is a section editor of the *European Journal of Sport Sciences* and former associate editor and current advisory board member of the *International Journal of Sport Physiology and Performance*. He has been on the organizing committees of scientific conferences, including the 2005 English Institute of Sport National Conference, the 2010 and 2011 International Sports Science and Sports Medicine Conference in the UK, and the 2013 Sports Medicine Australia-ACT Conference, Science and Medicine in Sport.

Thompson has authored more than 120 articles in peer-reviewed scientific journals and conference proceedings and over 25 articles for sport, professional, and coach education publications. He has written five book chapters and contributed regularly to the *Times* and *Guardian* broadsheet newspapers. Much of his research has been on pacing strategies, physiological monitoring of elite athletes, and fatigue mechanisms.

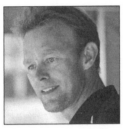

Jos J. de Koning, PhD, FACSM, is Associate Professor at the Faculty of Human Movement Sciences at the VU-University Amsterdam and Adjunct Professor at the Department of Exercise and Sport Science at the University of Wisconsin–La Crosse (USA). His research interests range from biomechanics modeling to high performance exercise physiology. De Koning is internationally recognized for his research on pacing strategies in a range of activities and elite sports performance physiology and biomechanics, particularly in relation to speed skating. He has authored 90 peer-reviewed publications and presented at 70 international conferences with keynote lectures at the ISB, IOC World Congress and ACSM meetings. He is a Fellow of the American College of Sport Medicine and Associate Editor of the International Journal of Sports Physiology and Performance and the European Journal of Sport Science. He was involved in the development and introduction of the innovative Œklapskate in competitive speed skating and was recipient of research grants from the International Olympic Committee to conduct studies at the 1988, 1994 and 2002 Winter Olympic Games.

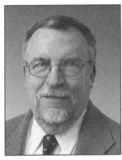

Carl Foster, PhD, FACSM, is a Professor in the Department of Exercise and Sport Science at the University of Wisconsin-La Crosse and a Visiting Professor in the Research Institute MOVE at the VU Amsterdam.

He received his Ph.D. from the University of Texas in 1976 and did post-doctoral work at Ball State University. He is an applied physiologist with wide ranging interests from clinical exercise physiology to elite performance physiology. From 1979-2004 he was a consultant to the U.S. Speedskating Team. He was the President of ACSM in 2005-2006, an Associate Editor for Medicine and Science in Sports and Exercise from 1989-2004, and the Editor of the International Journal of Sports Physiology and Performance from 2009-2013.

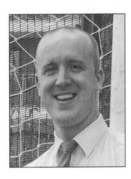

Richard Keegan, PhD, is a Registered Practitioner Psychologist in both the UK (HCPC) and Australia (AHPRA), as well as being a member of both the British Psychological Society and the Australian Psychological Society. He has acted as a sport psychologist across a range of sports, for over 10 years. His research focussed on motivation, and its applications spanning from children's PE to active aging, including the role of motivation in pacing and fatigue. Richard is currently Assistant Professor in Sport and Exercise Psychology and a member of the Research Institute for Sport and Exercise at the University of Canberra, in Australia.

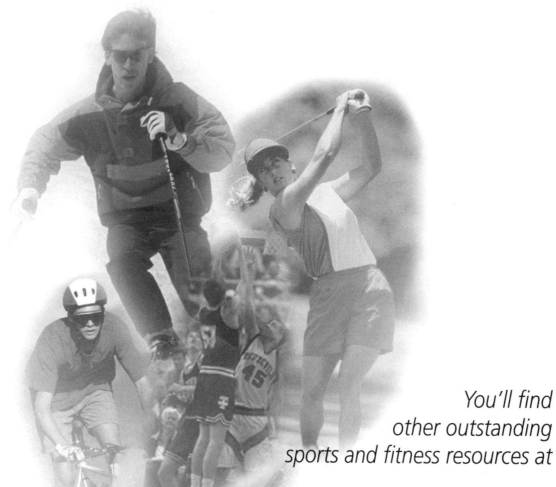

*You'll find
other outstanding
sports and fitness resources at*

www.HumanKinetics.com

In the U.S. call

1-800-747-4457

Australia...08 8372 0999
Canada..1-800-465-7301
Europe...+44 (0) 113 255 5665
New Zealand...0800 222 062

HUMAN KINETICS
The Premier Publisher for Sports & Fitness
P.O. Box 5076 • Champaign, IL 61825-5076 USA